Tarascon Pocket Pharmacopoeia®

2011 Classic Shirt-Pocket Edition

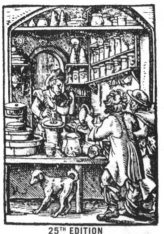

25TH EDITION

"Desire to take medicines ... distinguishes man from animals."
—Sir William Osler

JONES & BARTLETT
LEARNING

World Headquarters

Jones & Bartlett Learning
40 Tall Pine Drive
Sudbury, MA 01776
978-443-5000
info@jblearning.com
www.jblearning.com

Jones & Bartlett Learning
Canada
6339 Ormindale Way
Mississauga, Ontario
L5V 1J2 Canada

Jones & Bartlett Learning
International
Barb House, Barb Mews
London W6 7PA
United Kingdom

Jones & Bartlett Learning books and products are available through most bookstores and online booksellers. To contact Jones & Bartlett Learning directly, call 800-832-0034, fax 978-443-8000, or visit our website www.jblearning.com.

Substantial discounts on bulk quantities of Jones & Bartlett Learning publications are available to corporations, professional associations, and other qualified organizations. For details and specific discount information, contact the special sales department at Jones & Bartlett Learning via the above contact information or send an email to specialsales@jblearning.com.

The information in the *Pocket Pharmacopoeia* is compiled from sources believed to be reliable, and exhaustive efforts have been put forth to make the book as accurate as possible. The *Pocket Pharmacopoeia* is edited by a panel of drug information experts with extensive peer review and input from more than 50 practicing clinicians of multiple specialties. Our goal is to provide health professionals focused, core prescribing information in a convenient, organized, and concise fashion. We include FDA-approved dosing indications and those off-label uses that have a reasonable basis to support their use. *However the accuracy and completeness of this work cannot be guaranteed.* Despite our best efforts this book may contain typographical errors and omissions. The *Pocket Pharmacopoeia* is intended as a quick and convenient reminder of information you have already learned elsewhere. The contents are to be used as a guide only, and healthcare professionals should use sound clinical judgment and individualize therapy to each specific patient care situation. This book is not meant to be a replacement for training, experience, continuing medical education, or studying the latest drug prescribing literature. This book is sold without warranties of any kind, express or implied, and the publisher and editors disclaim any liability, loss, or damage caused by the contents. Although drug companies purchase and distribute our books as promotional items, the Tarascon editorial staff alone determines all book content.

ISSN: 1945-9076

ISBN: 978-0-7637-9305-0

6048

Printed in the United States of America

14 13 12 11 10   10 9 8 7 6 5 4 3 2 1

Production Credits

Chief Executive Officer: Ty Field
President: James Homer
SVP, Chief Operating Officer: Don Jones, Jr.
SVP, Chief Technology Officer: Dean Fossella
SVP, Chief Marketing Officer: Alison M. Pendergast
SVP, Chief Financial Officer: Ruth Siporin
V.P., Design and Production: Anne Spencer
V.P., Manufacturing and Inventory Control: Therese Connell

Executive Publisher: Christopher Davis
Senior Acquisitions Editor: Nancy Anastasi Duffy
Editorial Assistant: Sara Cameron
Production Editor: Daniel Stone
Medicine Marketing Manager: Rebecca Rockel
Composition: Newgen
Text and Cover Design: Anne Spencer
Printing and Binding: Cenveo
Cover Printing: Cenveo

If you obtained your Pocket Pharmacopoeia from a bookstore, please send your address to info@tarascon.com. This allows you to be the first to hear of updates! (We don't sell or distribute our mailing lists, by the way.)

The cover woodcut is The *Apothecary* by Jost Amman, Frankfurt, 1574.

For those of you still trying to solve last year's puzzle, here is the answer:

If the nurses start the IV line and infuse the antibiotic on the first two patients (A and B we'll say) and then do the same for C sequentially, then the entire task will take 20 minutes - A and B will be done in 10 minutes and C has to wait 10 min to start. However, if the nurses start the IV on A and B, then one nurse switches to start the IV on C and the other completes the infusion on B, they can then finally do the infusion on A and C for a total time of 15 minutes. This is an example of how operations research can improve speed and efficiency in medical care, as it does in other industries.

We will send a free copy of next year's edition to the first 25 who can solve the following, algebraic, pharmaceutical puzzle:

Two patients (A & B) are getting an infusion from bags of identical volumes but at different but constant rates. The infusions start at the same time and it takes exactly 5 minutes to change to the 2nd identical bag for each patient. You notice that for the 1st bag, when patient A has 72 mLs left, patient B has received 72 mLs. For the 2nd bag, when patient A has 40 mLs left, patient B has received 40 mLs. How many mLs are in each infusion bag?

CONTENTS

PAGE INDEX FOR TABLES

TARASCON POCKET PHARMACOPOEIA EDITORIAL STAFF*

PREFACE TO THE TARASCON POCKET PHARMACOPOEIA®

The *Tarascon Pocket Pharmacopoeia*® arranges drugs by clinical class with a comprehensive index in the back. Trade names are italicized and capitalized. Drug doses shown in mg/kg are generally intended for children, while fixed doses represent typical adult recommendations. Brackets indicate currently available formulations, although not all pharmacies stock all formulations. The availability of generic, over-the-counter, and scored formulations is mentioned. We have underlined the disease or indication for the pharmaceutical agent. It is meant to function as an aid to find information quickly. Codes are as follows:

▶ **METABOLISM & EXCRETION: L** = primarily liver, **K** = primarily kidney, **LK** = both, but liver > kidney, **KL** = both, but kidney > liver.

♀ **SAFETY IN PREGNANCY: A** = Safety established using human studies, **B** = Presumed safety based on animal studies, **C** = Uncertain safety; no human studies and animal studies show an adverse effect, **D** = Unsafe - evidence of risk that may in certain clinical circumstances be justifiable, **X** = Highly unsafe - risk of use outweighs any possible benefit. For drugs that have not been assigned a category: **+** Generally accepted as safe, **?** Safety unknown or controversial, **–** Generally regarded as unsafe.

▶ **SAFETY IN LACTATION: +** Generally accepted as safe, **?** Safety unknown or controversial, **–** Generally regarded as unsafe. Many of our "+" listings are from the AAP policy "The Transfer of Drugs and Other Chemicals Into Human Milk" (see www.aap.org) and may differ from those recommended by the manufacturer.

© **DEA CONTROLLED SUBSTANCES: I** = High abuse potential, no accepted use (eg, heroin, marijuana), **II** = High abuse potential and severe dependence liability (eg, morphine, codeine, hydromorphone, cocaine, amphetamines, methylphenidate, secobarbital). Some states require triplicates. **III** = Moderate dependence liability (eg, *Tylenol #3, Vicodin*), **IV** = Limited dependence liability (benzodiazepines, propoxyphene, phentermine), **V** = Limited abuse potential (eg, *Lomotil*).

$ **RELATIVE COST:** Cost codes used are "per month" of maintenance therapy (eg, antihypertensives) or "per course" of short-term therapy (eg, antibiotics). Codes are calculated using average wholesale prices (at press time in US dollars) for the most common indication and route of each drug at a typical adult dosage. For maintenance therapy, costs are calculated based upon a 30-day supply or the quantity that might typically be used in a given month. For short-term therapy (ie, 10 days or less), costs are calculated on a single treatment course. When multiple forms are available (eg,

Code	Cost
$	< $25
$$	$25 to $49
$$$	$50 to $99
$$$$	$100 to $199
$$$$$	≥ $200

generics), these codes reflect the least expensive generally available product. When drugs don't neatly fit into the classification scheme above, we have assigned codes based upon the relative cost of other similar drugs. *These codes should be used as a rough guide only,* as (1) they reflect cost, not charges, (2) pricing often varies substantially from location to location and time to time, and (3) HMOs, Medicaid, and buying groups often negotiate quite different pricing. Check with your local pharmacy if you have any questions.

🍁 **CANADIAN TRADE NAMES:** Unique common Canadian trade names not used in the US are listed after a maple leaf symbol. Trade names used in both nations or only in the US are displayed without such notation.

ABBREVIATIONS IN TEXT

AAP – American Academy of Pediatrics
ac – before meals
ADHD – attention deficit hyperactivity disorder
AHA – American Heart Association
Al – aluminum
ANC – absolute neutrophil count
ASA – aspirin
bid – twice per day
BP – blood pressure
BPH – benign prostatic hyperplasia
Ca – calcium
CAD – coronary artery disease
cap – capsule
cm – centimeter
CMV – cytomegalovirus
CNS – central nervous system
COPD – chronic obstructive pulmonary disease
CrCl – creatinine clearance
CVA – stroke
CYP – cytochrome P450
D5W – 5% dextrose
dL – deciliter

DPI – dry powder inhaler
ECG – electrocardiogram
EPS – extrapyramidal symptoms
ET – endotracheal
g – gram
GERD – gastroesophageal reflux disease
gtts – drops
GU – genitourinary
h – hour
HAART – highly active antiretroviral therapy
Hb – hemoglobin
HCTZ – hydrochlorothiazide
HIT – heparin-induced thrombocytopenia
hs – bedtime
HSV – herpes simplex virus
HTN – hypertension
IM – intramuscular
INR – international normalized ratio
IU – international units
IV – intravenous
JRA – juvenile rheumatoid arthritis
kg – kilogram

lbs – pounds
LFT – liver function test
LV – left ventricular
LVEF – left ventricular ejection fraction
m² – square meters
MAOI – monoamine oxidase inhibitor
mcg – microgram
MDI – metered dose inhaler
mEq – milliequivalent
mg – milligram
Mg – magnesium
MI – myocardial infarction
min – minute
mL – milliliter
mm – millimeter
mo – months old
MRSA – methicillin-resistant *Staphylococcus aureus*
ng – nanogram
NHLBI – National Heart, Lung, and Blood Institute
NS – normal saline
N/V – nausea/vomiting
NYHA – New York Heart Association
OA – osteoarthritis
oz – ounces

pc – after meals
PO – by mouth
PR – by rectum
pm – as needed
q – every
qam – every morning
qhs – at bedtime
qid – four times/day
qod – every other day
qpm – every evening
RA – rheumatoid arthritis
RSV – respiratory synctial virus
SC – subcutaneous
sec – second
supp – suppository
susp – suspension
tab – tablet
TB – tuberculosis
TCA – tricyclic antidepressant
tid – three times/day
TNF – tumor necrosis factor
TPN – total parenteral nutrition
UTI – urinary tract infection
wt – weight
y – year
yo – years old

THERAPEUTIC DRUG LEVELS

Drug	Level	Optimal Timing
amikacin peak	20–35 mcg/mL	30 minutes after infusion
amikacin trough	<5 mcg/mL	Just prior to next dose
carbamazepine trough	4–12 mcg/mL	Just prior to next dose
cyclosporine trough	50–300 ng/mL	Just prior to next dose
digoxin	0.8–2.0 ng/mL	Just prior to next dose
ethosuximide trough	40–100 mcg/mL	Just prior to next dose
gentamicin peak	5–10 mcg/mL	30 minutes after infusion
gentamicin trough	<2 mcg/mL	Just prior to next dose
lidocaine	1.5–5 mcg/mL	12–24 hours after start of infusion
lithium trough	0.6–1.2 meq/l	Just prior to first morning dose
NAPA	10–30 mcg/mL	Just prior to next procainamide dose
phenobarbital trough	15–40 mcg/mL	Just prior to next dose
phenytoin trough	10–20 mcg/mL	Just prior to next dose
primidone trough	5–12 mcg/mL	Just prior to next dose
procainamide	4–10 mcg/mL	Just prior to next dose
quinidine	2–5 mcg/mL	Just prior to next dose
theophylline	5–15 mcg/mL	8–12 hours after once daily dose
tobramycin peak	5–10 mcg/mL	30 minutes after infusion
tobramycin trough	<2 mcg/mL	Just prior to next dose
valproate trough (epilepsy)	50–100 mcg/mL	Just prior to next dose
valproate trough (mania)	45–125 mcg/mL	Just prior to next dose
vancomycin trough[1]	10–20 mg/L	Just prior to next dose
zonisamide[2]	10–40 mcg/mL	Just prior to dose

[1] Maintain trough >10 mg/L to avoid resistance; optimal trough for complicated infections is 15–20 mg/L
[2] Ranges not firmly established but supported by clinical trial results

PEDIATRIC DRUGS		*Age*	*2mo*	*4mo*	*6mo*	*9mo*	*12mo*	*15mo*	*2yo*	*3yo*	*5yo*
		Kg	5	6½	8	9	10	11	13	15	19
		Lbs	11	15	17	20	22	24	28	33	42
med	***strength***	***freq***	***teaspoons of liquid per dose*** *(1 tsp = 5 mL)*								
Tylenol (mg)		q4h	80	80	120	120	160	160	200	240	280
Tylenol (tsp)	160/t	q4h	½	½	¾	¾	1	1	1¼	1½	1¾
ibuprofen (mg)		q6h	--	--	75†	75†	100	100	125	150	175
ibuprofen (tsp)	100/t	q6h	--	--	¾†	¾†	1	1	1¼	1½	1¾
amoxicillin or	125/t	bid	1	1¼	1½	1¾	1¾	2	2¼	2¾	3½
Augmentin	200/t	bid	½	¾	1	1	1¼	1¼	1½	1¾	2¼
(not otitis media)	250/t	bid	½	½	¾	¾	1	1	1¼	1¼	1¾
	400/t	bid	¼	½	½	½	¾	¾	¾	1	1
amoxicillin,	200/t	bid	1	1¼	1¾	2	2	2¼	2¾	3	4
(otitis media)‡	250/t	bid	¾	1¼	1½	1½	1¾	1¾	2¼	2½	3¼
	400/t	bid	½	¾	¾	1	1	1¼	1½	1½	2
Augmentin ES‡	600/t	bid	?	½	½	¾	¾	¾	1	1¼	1½
azithromycin*§	100/t	qd	¼†	½†	½	½	½	½	¾	¾	1
(5-day Rx)	200/t	qd	--	¼†	¼	¼	¼	¼	½	½	½
Bactrim/Septra	---	bid	½	¾	1	1	1	1¼	1½	1½	2
cefaclor*	125/t	bid	1	1	1¼	1½	1½	1¾	2	2½	3
"	250/t	bid	½	½	¾	¾	¾	1	1	1¼	1½
cefadroxil	125/t	bid	½	¾	1	1	1¼	1¼	1½	1¾	2¼
"	250/t	bid	¼	½	½	½	¾	¾	¾	1	1
cefdinir	125/t	qd	--	¾†	1	1	1	1¼	1½	1¾	2
cefixime	100/t	qd	½	½	¾	¾	¾	1	1	1¼	1½
cefprozil*	125/t	bid	--	¾†	1	1	1¼	1½	1½	2	2¼
"	250/t	bid	--	½†	½	½	¾	¾	¾	1	1¼
cefuroxime	125/t	bid	--	¾	¾	1	1	1	1½	1¾	2¼
cephalexin	125/t	qid	--	½	¾	¾	1	1	1¼	1½	1¾
"	250/t	qid	--	¼	¼	½	½	½	¾	¾	1
clarithromycin	125/t	bid	½†	½†	½	½	¾	¾	¾	1	1¼
"	250/t	bid	--	--	--	¼	½	½	½	½	¾
dicloxacillin	62½/t	qid	½	¾	1	1	1¼	1¼	1½	1¾	2
nitrofurantoin	25/t	qid	¼	½	½	½	½	¾	¾	¾	1
Pediazole	---	tid	½	½	¾	¾	1	1	1	1¼	1½
penicillin V**	250/t	bid-tid	--	1	1	1	1	1	1	1	1
cetirizine	5/t	qd	--	--	½	½	½	½	½	½	½
Benadryl	12.5/t	q6h	½	½	¾	¾	1	1	1¼	1½	2
prednisolone	15/t	qd	¼	½	½	¾	¾	¾	1	1	1¼
prednisone	5/t	qd	1	1¼	1½	1¾	2	2¼	2½	3	3¾
Robitussin	---	q4h	--	--	¼†	¼†	½	½	¾	¾	1
Tylenol w/ codeine		q4h	--	--	--	--	--	--	--	1	1

* Dose shown is for otitis media only; see dosing in text for alternative indications.

† Dosing at this age/weight not recommended by manufacturer.

‡ AAP now recommends high dose (80-90 mg/kg/d) for all otitis media in children; with Augmentin used as ES only.

§Give a double dose of azithromycin the first day.

**AHA dosing for streptococcal pharyngitis. Treat for 10 days.

tsp = teaspoon; t = teaspoon; q = every; h = hour; kg = kilogram; Lbs = pounds; mL = mililiter; bid = twice per day; qd = every day; qid = four times per day; tid = three times per day

PEDIATRIC VITAL SIGNS AND INTRAVENOUS DRUGS

Age		Pre-matr	New-born	2m	4m	6m	9m	12m	15m	2y	3y	5y
Weight	(Kg)	2	3½	5	6½	8	9	10	11	13	15	19
	(Lbs)	4½	7½	11	15	17	20	22	24	28	33	42
Maint fluids	(mL/h)	8	14	20	26	32	36	40	42	46	50	58
ET tube	(mm)	2½	3/3½	3½	3½	3½	4	4	4½	4½	4½	5
Defib	(Joules)	4	7	10	13	16	18	20	22	26	30	38
Systolic BP	(high)	70	80	85	90	95	100	103	104	106	109	114
	(low)	40	60	70	70	70	70	70	70	75	75	80
Pulse rate	(high)	145	145	180	180	180	160	160	160	150	150	135
	(low)	100	100	110	110	110	100	100	90	90	90	65
Resp rate	(high)	60	60	50	50	50	46	46	30	30	25	25
	(low)	35	30	30	30	24	24	20	20	20	20	20
adenosine	(mg)	0.2	0.3	0.5	0.6	0.8	0.9	1	1.1	1.3	1.5	1.9
atropine	(mg)	0.1	0.1	0.1	0.13	0.16	0.18	0.2	0.22	0.26	0.30	0.38
Benadryl	(mg)	-	-	5	6½	8	9	10	11	13	15	19
bicarbonate	(meq)	2	3½	5	6½	8	9	10	11	13	15	19
dextrose	(g)	1	2	5	6½	8	9	10	11	13	15	19
epinephrine	(mg)	.02	.04	.05	.07	.08	.09	0.1	0.11	0.13	0.15	0.19
lidocaine	(mg)	2	3½	5	6½	8	9	10	11	13	15	19
morphine	(mg)	0.2	0.3	0.5	0.6	0.8	0.9	1	1.1	1.3	1.5	1.9
mannitol	(g)	2	3½	5	6½	8	9	10	11	13	15	19
naloxone	(mg)	.02	.04	.05	.07	.08	.09	0.1	0.11	0.13	0.15	0.19
diazepam	(mg)	0.6	1	1.5	2	2.5	2.7	3	3.3	3.9	4.5	5
fosphenytoin*	(PE)	40	70	100	130	160	180	200	220	260	300	380
lorazepam	(mg)	0.1	0.2	0.35	0.4	0.5	0.5	0.6	0.7	0.8	1.0	
phenobarb	(mg)	30	60	75	100	125	150	175	200	225		275
phenytoin*	(mg)	40	70	100	130	160	180	200	220	260	300	380
ampicillin	(mg)	100	175	250	325	400	450	500	550	650	750	1000
ceftriaxone	(mg)	-	-	250	250	400	450	500	550	650	750	1000
cefotaxime	(mg)	100	175	250	325	400	450	500	550	650	750	1000
gentamicin	(mg)	5	8	12	16	20	22	25	27	32	37	47

*Loading doses; fosphenytoin dosed in "phenytoin equivalents."

CONVERSIONS	Liquid:	Weight:
Temperature:	1 fluid ounce = 30 mL	1 kilogram = 2.2 lbs
F = (1.8) C + 32	1 teaspoon = 5 mL	1 ounce = 30 g
C = (F − 32)/1.8	1 tablespoon = 15 mL	1 grain = 65 mg

FORMULAS

Alveolar-arterial oxygen gradient = A-a = $148 - 1.2(PaCO_2) - PaO_2$
[normal = 10-20 mmHg, breathing room air at sea level]

Calculated osmolality = $2Na + glucose/18 + BUN/2.8 + ethanol/4.6$
[norm 280-295 meq/L. Na in mg/dL, all others in mg/dL]

Pediatric IV maintenance fluids (see table on page xi)
4 mL/kg/hr **or** 100 mL/kg/day for first 10 kg, plus
2 mL/kg/hr **or** 50 mL/kg/day for second 10 kg, plus
1 mL/kg/hr **or** 20 mL/kg/day for all further kg

$$mcg/kg/min = \frac{16.7 \times drug\ conc\ [mg/mL] \times infusion\ rate\ [mL/h]}{weight\ [kg]}$$

$$Infusion\ rate\ [mL/h] = \frac{desired\ mcg/kg/min \times weight\ [kg] \times 60}{drug\ concentration\ [mcg/mL]}$$

Fractional excretion of sodium = $\left[\dfrac{urine\ Na\ /\ plasma\ Na}{urine\ creat\ /\ plasma\ creat}\right] \times 100\%$
[Pre-renal, etc <1%; ATN, etc >1%]

Anion gap = $Na - (Cl + HCO_3)$ [normal = 10-14 meq/L]

Creatinine clearance = $\dfrac{(lean\ kg)(140 - age)(0.85\ if\ female)}{(72)(stable\ creatinine\ [mg/dL])}$
[normal >80]

Glomerular filtration rate using MDRD equation (mL/min/1.73 m²)
= $186 \times (creatinine)^{-1.154} \times (age)^{-0.203} \times (0.742\ if\ ♀) \times (1.210\ if\ African\ American)$

Body surface area (BSA) = square root of: $\left[\dfrac{height\ (cm) \times weight\ (kg)}{3600}\right]$
[in m²]

DRUG THERAPY REFERENCE WEBSITES FORMULAS (selected)

Professional societies or governmental agencies with drug therapy guidelines		
AAP	American Academy of Pediatrics	www.aap.org
ACC	American College of Cardiology	www.acc.org
ACCP	American College of Chest Physicians	www.chestnet.org
ACCP	American College of Clinical Pharmacy	www.accp.com
ADA	American Diabetes Association	www.diabetes.org
AHA	American Heart Association	www.americanheart.org
AHRQ	Agency for Healthcare Research and Quality	www.ahcpr.gov
AMA	American Medical Association	www.ama-assn.org
APA	American Psychiatric Association	www.psych.org
APA	American Psychological Association	www.apa.org
ASHP	Amer. Society Health-Systems Pharmacists	www.ashp.org
ATS	American Thoracic Society	www.thoracic.org
CDC	Centers for Disease Control and Prevention	www.cdc.gov
CDC	CDC bioterrorism and radiation exposures	www.bt.cdc.gov
IDSA	Infectious Diseases Society of America	www.idsociety.org
MHA	Malignant Hyperthermia Association	www.mhaus.org
NHLBI	National Heart, Lung, and Blood Institute	www.nhlbi.nih.gov

Other therapy reference sites	
Cochrane library	www.cochrane.org
Emergency Contraception Website	www.not-2-late.com
Immunization Action Coalition	www.immunize.org
Int'l Registry for Drug-Induced Arrhythmias	www.qtdrugs.org
Managing Contraception	www.managingcontraception.com
Nephrology Pharmacy Associates	www.nephrologypharmacy.com

ANALGESICS

Antirheumatic Agents—Biologic Response Modifiers

NOTE *Death, sepsis, and serious infections (eg, TB and invasive fungal infections) have been reported.*

ADALIMUMAB (*Humira*) RA, psoriatic arthritis, ankylosing spondylitis: 40 mg SC every 2 weeks, alone or in combination with methotrexate or other disease-modifying antirheumatic drugs (DMARDs). May increase frequency to once a week if not on methotrexate. Crohn's disease: 160 mg SC at week 0, 80 mg at week 2, then 40 mg every other week starting with week 4. [Trade only: 40 mg prefilled glass syringes or vials with needles, 2 per pack.] ▶Serum ♀B ▶–$$$$$

ANAKINRA (*Kineret*) RA: 100 mg SC daily. [Trade only: 100 mg prefilled glass syringes with needles, 7 or 28 per box.] ▶K ♀B ▶? $$$$$

ETANERCEPT (*Enbrel*) RA, psoriatic arthritis, ankylosing spondylitis: 50 mg SC once a week. Plaque psoriasis: 50 mg SC 2 times per week for 3 months, then 50 mg SC once a week. JRA age 4 to 17 yo: 0.8 mg/kg SC once a week, to max single dose of 50 mg. Max dose per injection site is 25 mg. [Supplied in a carton containing four dose trays and as single-use prefilled syringes. Each dose tray contains one 25 mg single-use vial of etanercept, one syringe (1 mL sterile bacteriostatic water for injection, containing 0.9% benzyl alcohol), one plunger, and two alcohol swabs. Single-use syringes contain 50 mg/mL.] ▶Serum ♀B ▶–$$$$$

INFLIXIMAB (*Remicade*) RA: 3 mg/kg IV in combination with methotrexate at 0, 2, and 6 weeks. Ankylosing spondylitis: 5 mg/kg IV at 0, 2, and 6 weeks. Plaque psoriasis, psoriatic arthritis, moderately to severely active Crohn's disease, ulcerative colitis, or fistulizing disease: 5 mg/kg IV infusion at 0, 2, and 6 weeks, then q 8 weeks. ▶Serum ♀B ▶? $$$$$

Antirheumatic Agents—Disease Modifying Antirheumatic Drugs (DMARDs)

AZATHIOPRINE (*Azasan, Imuran,* ✦*Immunoprin, Oprisine*) RA: Initial dose 1 mg/kg (50 to 100 mg) PO daily or divided bid. Increase after 6 to 8 weeks. [Generic/Trade: Tabs 50 mg, scored. Trade only (Azasan): 75, 100 mg, scored.] ▶LK ♀D ▶–$$$

HYDROXYCHLOROQUINE (*Plaquenil*) RA: Start 400 to 600 mg PO daily, then taper to 200 to 400 mg daily. SLE: 400 PO daily to bid to start, then taper to 200 to 400 mg daily. [Generic/Trade: Tabs 200 mg, scored.] ▶K ♀C ▶+ $

LEFLUNOMIDE (*Arava*) RA: 100 mg PO daily for 3 days. Maintenance: 10 to 20 mg PO daily. [Generic/Trade: Tabs 10, 20 mg. Trade only: Tab 100 mg.] ▶LK ♀X ▶–$$$$$

METHOTREXATE (*Rheumatrex, Trexall*) RA, psoriasis: Start with 7.5 mg PO single dose once a week or 2.5 mg PO q 12 h for 3 doses given once a week. Max dose 20 mg/week. Supplement with 1 mg/day of folic acid. Chemotherapy doses vary by indication. [Trade only (Trexall): Tabs 5, 7.5, 10, 15 mg. Dose Pak (Rheumatrex) 2.5 mg (# 8, 12, 16, 20, 24). Generic/Trade: Tabs 2.5 mg, scored.] ▶LK ♀X ▶–$$

Muscle Relaxants

BACLOFEN (*Lioresal, Kemstro*)   Spasticity related to MS or spinal cord disease/injury: Start 5 mg PO tid, then increase by 5 mg/dose q 3 day until 20 mg PO tid. Max dose 20 mg qid. [Generic only: Tabs 10, 20 mg. Trade only: (Kemstro) Tabs, orally disintegrating 10, 20 mg.] ▶K ♀C ▶+ $$

CARISOPRODOL (*Soma*)   Acute musculoskeletal pain: 350 mg PO tid to qid. Abuse potential. [Generic/Trade: Tabs 350 mg. Trade only: Tabs 250 mg.] ▶LK ♀? ▶– $

CHLORZOXAZONE (*Parafon Forte DSC*)   Musculoskeletal pain: 500 to 750 mg PO tid to qid to start. Decrease to 250 mg tid to qid. [Generic/Trade: Tabs 250 and 500 mg (Parafon Forte DSC 500 mg tabs, scored).] ▶LK ♀C ▶? $

CYCLOBENZAPRINE (*Amrix, Flexeril, Fexmid*)   Musculoskeletal pain: Start 5 to 10 mg PO tid, max 30 mg/day or 15 to 30 mg (extended-release) PO daily. Not recommended in elderly. [Generic/Trade: Tab 5, 10 mg. Generic only: Tab 7.5 mg. Trade only: (Amrix $$$$$): Extended-release caps 15, 30 mg.] ▶LK ♀B ▶? $

DANTROLENE (*Dantrium*)   Chronic spasticity related to spinal cord injury, CVA, cerebral palsy, MS: 25 mg PO daily to start, up to max of 100 mg bid to qid if necessary. Malignant hyperthermia: 2.5 mg/kg rapid IV push q 5 to 10 min continuing until symptoms subside or to a maximum total dose of 10 mg/kg. [Generic/Trade: Caps 25, 50, 100 mg.] ▶LK ♀C ▶– $$$$$

METAXALONE (*Skelaxin*)   Musculoskeletal pain: 800 mg PO tid to qid. [Generic/Trade: Tabs 800 mg, scored.] ▶LK ♀? ▶? $$$$

METHOCARBAMOL (*Robaxin, Robaxin-750*)   Acute musculoskeletal pain: 1500 mg PO qid or 1000 mg IM/IV tid for 48 to 72 h. Maintenance: 1000 mg PO qid, 750 mg PO q 4 h, or 1500 mg PO tid. Tetanus: Specialized dosing. [Generic/Trade: Tabs 500 and 750 mg. OTC in Canada.] ▶LK ♀C ▶? $$

ORPHENADRINE (*Norflex*)   Musculoskeletal pain: 100 mg PO bid. 60 mg IV/IM bid. [Generic only: 100 mg extended-release. OTC in Canada.] ▶LK ♀C ▶? $$

TIZANIDINE (*Zanaflex*)   Muscle spasticity due to MS or spinal cord injury: 4 to 8 mg PO q 6 to 8 h prn, max 36 mg/day. [Generic/Trade: Tabs 4 mg, scored. Trade only: Caps 2, 4, 6 mg. Generic only: Tabs 2 mg.] ▶LK ♀C ▶? $$$$

Non-Opioid Analgesic Combinations

***ASCRIPTIN* (acetylsalicylic acid + aluminum hydroxide + magnesium hydroxide + calcium carbonate, Aspir-Mox)**   Multiple strengths. 1 to 2 tabs PO q 4 h. [OTC Trade only: Tabs 325 mg aspirin/50 mg Mg hydroxide/50 mg Al hydroxide/50 mg Ca carbonate (Ascriptin and Aspir-Mox). 500 mg aspirin/33 mg Mg hydroxide/33 mg Al hydroxide/ 237 mg Ca carbonate (Ascriptin Maximum Strength).] ▶K ♀D ▶? $

***BUFFERIN* (acetylsalicylic acid + calcium carbonate + magnesium oxide + magnesium carbonate)**   1 to 2 tabs/caplets PO q 4 h. Max 12 in 24 h. [OTC Trade only: Tabs/caplets 325 mg aspirin/158 mg Ca carbonate/63 mg of Mg oxide/34 mg of Mg carbonate. Bufferin ES: 500 mg aspirin/222.3 mg Ca carbonate/88.9 mg of Mg oxide/55.6 mg of Mg carbonate.] ▶K ♀D ▶? $

ESGIC **(acetaminophen + butalbital + caffeine)** 1 to 2 tabs or caps PO q 4 h. Max 6 in 24 h. [Generic only: Tabs/caps, 325 mg acetaminophen/50 mg butalbital/40 mg caffeine. Oral soln 325/50/40 mg per 15 mL. Generic/Trade: Tabs, Esgic Plus is 500/50/40 mg.] ▶LK ♀C ▶? $

EXCEDRIN MIGRAINE **(acetaminophen + acetylsalicylic acid + caffeine)** 2 tabs/caps/geltabs PO q 6 h while symptoms persist. Max 8 in 24 h. [OTC Generic/Trade: Tabs/caplets/geltabs 250 mg acetaminophen/250 mg aspirin/65 mg caffeine.] ▶LK ♀D ▶? $

FIORICET **(acetaminophen + butalbital + caffeine)** 1 to 2 caps PO q 4 h. Max 6 caps in 24 h. [Generic/Trade: Tabs 325 mg acetaminophen/50 mg butalbital/40 mg caffeine.] ▶LK ♀C ▶? $

FIORINAL **(acetylsalicylic acid + butalbital + caffeine)** (*◆Tecnal, Trianal*) 1 to 2 tabs PO q 4 h. Max 6 tabs in 24 h. [Generic/Trade: Caps 325 mg aspirin/50 mg butalbital/40 mg caffeine.] ▶KL ♀D ▶— ©III $

GOODY'S EXTRA STRENGTH HEADACHE POWDER **(acetaminophen + acetylsalicylic acid + caffeine)** 1 powder PO followed with liquid, or stir powder into a glass of water or other liquid. Repeat in 4 to 6 h prn. Max 4 powders in 24 h. [OTC trade only: 260 mg acetaminophen/520 mg aspirin/32.5 mg caffeine per powder paper.] ▶LK ♀D ▶? $

NORGESIC **(orphenadrine + acetaminophen + caffeine)** Multiple strengths; write specific product on Rx. Norgesic: 1 to 2 tabs PO tid to qid. Norgesic Forte, 1 tab PO tid to qid. [Generic/Trade: Tabs Norgesic 25 mg orphenadrine/385 mg aspirin/30 mg caffeine. Norgesic Forte 50/770/60 mg.] ▶KL ♀D ▶? $$

PHRENILIN **(acetaminophen + butalbital)** Tension or muscle contraction headache: 1 to 2 tabs PO q 4 h. Max 6 in 24 h. [Generic/Trade: Tabs, Phrenilin 325 mg acetaminophen/50 mg butalbital. Caps, Phrenilin Forte 650/50 mg.] ▶LK ♀C ▶? $

SEDAPAP **(acetaminophen + butalbital)** 1 to 2 tabs PO q 4 h. Max 6 tabs in 24 h. [Generic only: Tabs 650 mg acetaminophen/50 mg butalbital.] ▶LK ♀C ▶? $

SOMA COMPOUND **(carisoprodol + acetylsalicylic acid)** 1 to 2 tabs PO qid. Abuse potential. [Generic/Trade: Tabs 200 mg carisoprodol/325 mg aspirin.] ▶LK ♀D ▶— $$$

ULTRACET **(tramadol + acetaminophen)** (*◆Tramacet*) Acute pain: 2 tabs PO q 4 to 6 h prn, (up to 8 tabs/day for no more than 5 days). Adjust dose in elderly and renal dysfunction. Avoid in opioid-dependent patients. Seizures may occur if concurrent antidepressants or seizure disorder. [Generic/Trade: Tabs 37.5 mg tramadol/ 325 mg acetaminophen.] ▶KL ♀C ▶— $$

Non-Steroidal Anti-Inflammatories – COX-2 Inhibitors

CELECOXIB (*Celebrex*) OA, ankylosing spondylitis: 200 mg PO daily or 100 mg PO bid. RA: 100 to 200 mg PO bid. Familial adenomatous polyposis: 400 mg PO bid with food. Acute pain, dysmenorrhea: 400 mg single dose, then 200 bid prn. An additional 200 mg dose may be given on day 1 if needed. JRA: Give 50 mg PO bid for age 2 to 17 yo and wt 10 to 25 kg, give 100 mg PO bid for wt greater than 25 kg. Contraindicated in sulfonamide allergy. [Trade only: Caps 50, 100, 200, 400 mg.] ▶L ♀C (D in 3rd trimester) ▶? $$$$$

Non-Steroidal Anti-Inflammatories – Salicylic Acid Derivatives

ACETYLSALICYLIC ACID (*Ecotrin, Empirin, Halfprin, Bayer, Anacin, Zorprin, Aspirin, ✦Asaphen, Entrophen, Novasen*) Analgesia: 325 to 650 mg PO/PR q 4 to 6 h. Platelet aggregation inhibition: 81 to 325 mg PO daily. [Generic/Trade (OTC): Tabs, 325, 500 mg; chewable 81 mg; enteric-coated 81, 162 mg (Halfprin) 81, 325, 500 mg (Ecotrin), 650, 975 mg. Trade only: Tabs, controlled-release 650, 800 mg (ZORprin, Rx). Generic only (OTC): Supps 60, 120, 200, 300, 600 mg.] ▶K ♀D ▶? $

CHOLINE MAGNESIUM TRISALICYLATE (*Trilisate*) RA/OA: 1500 mg PO bid. [Generic only: Tabs 500, 750, 1000 mg. Soln 500 mg/5 mL.] ▶K ♀C (D in 3rd trimester) ▶? $$

DIFLUNISAL (*Dolobid*) Pain: 500 to 1000 mg initially, then 250 to 500 mg PO q 8 to 12 h. RA/OA: 500 mg to 1 g PO divided bid. [Generic/Trade: Tabs 250, 500 mg.] ▶K ♀C (D in 3rd trimester) ▶– $$$

SALSALATE (*Salflex, Disalcid, Amigesic*) RA/OA: 3000 mg/day PO divided q 8 to 12 h. [Generic only: Tabs 500, 750 mg, scored.] ▶K ♀C (D in 3rd trimester) ▶? $$

Non-Steroidal Anti-Inflammatories—Other

ARTHROTEC (diclofenac + misoprostol) OA: One 50/200 tab PO tid. RA: One 50/200 tab PO tid to qid. If intolerant, may use 50/200 or 75/200 PO bid. Misoprostol is an abortifacient. [Trade only: Tabs 50 mg/200 mcg, 75 mg/200 mcg, diclofenac/misoprostol.] ▶LK ♀X ▶– $$$$$

DICLOFENAC (*Voltaren, Voltaren XR, Cataflam, Flector, Zipsor, Cambia, ✦Voltaren Rapide*) Multiple strengths; write specific product on Rx. Immediate- or delayed-release 50 mg PO bid to tid or 75 mg PO bid. Extended-release (Voltaren XR): 100 to 200 mg PO daily. Patch (Flector): apply 1 patch to painful area bid. Gel: 2 to 4 g to affected area qid. Acute migraine with or without aura: 50 mg single dose (Cambia) [Generic/Trade: Tabs, immediate-release (Cataflam) 50 mg, extended-release (Voltaren XR) 100 mg. Generic only: Tabs, delayed-release 25, 50, 75 mg. Trade only: Patch (Flector) 1.3% diclofenac epolamine. Topical gel (Voltaren) 1% 100 g tube. Trade only: Caps, liquid-filled (Zipsor) 25 mg. Trade only: Powder for oral soln (Cambia) 50 mg.] ▶L ♀B (D in 3rd trimester) ▶– $$$

ETODOLAC (*✦Ultradol*) Multiple strengths; write specific product on Rx. Immediate-release 200 to 400 mg PO bid to tid. Extended-release: 400 to 1200 mg PO daily. [Generic only: Caps immediate-release 200, 300 mg, Tabs immediate-release 400, 500 mg, Tabs extended-release 400, 500, 600 mg.] ▶L ♀C (D in 3rd trimester) ▶? $$$

FLURBIPROFEN (*Ansaid, ✦Froben, Froben SR*) 200 to 300 mg/day PO divided bid to qid. [Generic/Trade: Tabs immediate-release 50, 100 mg.] ▶L ♀B (D in 3rd trimester) ▶+ $$$

IBUPROFEN (*Motrin, Advil, Nuprin, Rufen, NeoProfen, Caldolor*) 200 to 800 mg PO tid to qid. Peds older than 6 mo: 5 to 10 mg/kg PO q 6 to 8 h. GI

(cont.)

perforation and necrotizing enterocolitis has been reported with NeoProfen. [OTC Caps/Liqui-Gel Caps 200 mg. Tabs 100, 200 mg. Chewable tabs 50, 100 mg. Susp (infant gtts) 50 mg/1.25 mL (with calibrated dropper), 100 mg/5 mL. Rx Generic/Trade: Tabs 300, 400, 600, 800 mg.] ▶L ♀B (D in 3rd trimester) ▶+ $

INDOMETHACIN (*Indocin, Indocin SR, Indocin IV, ✦Indocid-P.D.A.*) Multiple strengths; write specific product on Rx. Immediate-release preparations 25 to 50 mg cap PO tid. Sustained-release: 75 mg cap PO daily to bid. [Generic/Trade: Caps, sustained-release 75 mg. Generic only: Caps, immediate-release 25, 50 mg. Suppository 50 mg. Trade only: Oral susp 25 mg/5 mL (237 mL)] ▶L ♀B (D in 3rd trimester) ▶+ $

KETOPROFEN (*Orudis, Orudis KT, Actron, Oruvail, ✦Orudis SR*) Immediate-release: 25 to 75 mg PO tid to qid. Extended-release: 100 to 200 mg cap PO daily. [OTC: Tabs, immediate-release 12.5 mg. Rx Generic only: Caps, extended-release 100, 150, 200 mg. Caps, immediate-release 25, 50, 75 mg.] ▶L ♀C (D in 3rd trimester) ▶− $$$

KETOROLAC (*Toradol*) <u>Moderately severe acute pain:</u> 15 to 30 mg IV/IM q 6 h or 10 mg PO q 4 to 6 h prn. Combined duration IV/IM and PO is not to exceed 5 days. [Generic only: Tabs 10 mg.] ▶L ♀C (D in 3rd trimester) ▶+ $

MECLOFENAMATE <u>Mild to moderate pain:</u> 50 mg PO q 4 to 6 h prn. Max dose 400 mg/day. <u>Menorrhagia and primary dysmenorrhea:</u> 100 mg PO tid for up to 6 days. <u>RA/OA:</u> 200 to 400 mg/day PO divided tid to qid. [Generic only: Caps 50, 100 mg.] ▶L ♀B (D in 3rd trimester) ▶− $$$

MEFENAMIC ACID (*Ponstel, ✦Ponstan*) <u>Mild to moderate pain, primary dysmenorrhea:</u> 500 mg PO initially, then 250 mg PO q 6 h prn for no more than 1 week. [Trade only: Caps 250 mg.] ▶L ♀D ▶− $$$$$

MELOXICAM (*Mobic, ✦Mobicox*) <u>RA/OA:</u> 7.5 mg PO daily. <u>JRA</u> age 2 yo or older: 0.125 mg/kg PO daily. [Generic/Trade: Tabs 7.5, 15 mg. Susp 7.5 mg/5 mL (1.5 mg/mL).] ▶L ♀C (D in 3rd trimester) ▶? $

NABUMETONE (*Relafen*) <u>RA/OA:</u> Initial: Two 500 mg tabs (1000 mg) PO daily. May increase to 1500 to 2000 mg PO daily or divided bid. [Generic only: Tabs 500, 750 mg.] ▶L ♀C (D in 3rd trimester) ▶− $$$

NAPROXEN (*Naprosyn, Aleve, Anaprox, EC-Naprosyn, Naprelan, Prevacid, NapraPac*) Immediate-release: 250 to 500 mg PO bid. Delayed-release: 375 to 500 mg PO bid (do not crush or chew). Controlled-release: 750 to 1000 mg PO daily. <u>JRA:</u> give 2.5 mL PO bid for wt 13 kg or less, give 5 mL

(cont.)

NSAIDs − If one class fails, consider another. <u>*Salicylic acid derivatives*</u>: ASA, diflunisal, salsalate, Trilisate. <u>*Propionic acids*</u>: flurbiprofen, ibuprofen, ketoprofen, naproxen, oxaprozin. <u>*Acetic acids*</u>: diclofenac, etodolac, indomethacin, ketorolac, nabumetone, sulindac, tolmetin. <u>*Fenamates*</u>: meclofenamate. <u>*Oxicams*</u>: meloxicam, piroxicam. <u>*COX-2 inhibitors*</u>: celecoxib.

PO bid for 14 to 25 kg, give 7.5 mL PO bid for 26 to 38 kg. 500 mg naproxen equivalent to 550 mg naproxen sodium. [OTC Generic/Trade: (Aleve): Tabs immediate-release 200 mg. OTC Trade only (Aleve): Caps, Gelcaps immediate-release 200 mg. Rx Generic/Trade: Tabs immediate-release (Naprosyn) 250, 375, 500 mg, (Anaprox) 275, 550 mg. Tabs delayed-release enteric coated (EC-Naprosyn) 375, 500 mg. Tabs, controlled-release (Naprelan) 375, 500, 750 mg. Susp (Naprosyn) 125 mg/5 mL. Prevacid NapraPac: 7 lansoprazole 15 mg caps packaged with 14 naproxen tabs 375 mg or 500 mg.] ▶L ♀B (D in 3rd trimester) ▶+ $$$

OXAPROZIN (*Daypro*) 1200 mg PO daily. [Generic/Trade: Tabs 600 mg, trade scored.] ▶L ♀C (D in 3rd trimester) ▶− $$$

PIROXICAM (*Feldene, Fexicam*) 20 mg PO daily. [Generic/Trade: Caps 10, 20 mg.] ▶L ♀B (D in 3rd trimester) ▶+ $$$

SULINDAC (*Clinoril*) 150 to 200 mg PO bid. [Generic/Trade: Tabs 200 mg. Generic only: Tabs 150 mg.] ▶L ♀B (D in 3rd trimester) ▶− $$$

TIAPROFENIC ACID (✦*Surgam, Surgam SR*) Canada only. 600 mg PO daily of sustained-release, or 300 mg PO bid of regular-release. [Generic/Trade: Tabs 300 mg. Trade only: Caps, sustained-release 300 mg. Generic only: Tabs 200 mg.] ▶K ♀C (D in 3rd trimester) ▶− $$

TOLMETIN (*Tolectin*) 200 to 600 mg PO tid. [Generic/Trade: Tabs 200 (trade scored), 600 mg. Caps 400 mg.] ▶L ♀C (D in 3rd trimester) ▶+ $$$$

Opioid Agonist-Antagonists

BUPRENORPHINE (*Buprenex, Subutex*) Analgesia: 0.3 to 0.6 mg IV/IM q 6 h prn. Treatment of opioid dependence: Induction 8 mg SL on day 1, 16 mg SL on day 2. Maintenance: 16 mg SL daily. Can individualize to range of 4 to 24 mg SL daily. [Generic/Trade (Subutex): SL Tabs 2, 8 mg.] ▶L ♀C ▶− ©III $ IV, $$$$$ SL

BUTORPHANOL (*Stadol, Stadol NS*) 0.5 to 2 mg IV or 1 to 4 mg IM q 3 to 4 h prn. Nasal spray (Stadol NS): 1 spray (1 mg) in 1 nostril q 3 to 4 h. Abuse potential. [Generic only: Nasal spray 1 mg/spray, 2.5 mL bottle (14 to 15 doses/bottle).] ▶LK ♀C ▶+ ©IV $$$

NALBUPHINE (*Nubain*) 10 to 20 mg IV/IM/SC q 3 to 6 h prn. [Generic/Trade: 10 mg/mL 10 mL multiple-dose vial, 1 mL ampules (box of 10); 20 mg/mL 10 mL multiple-dose vial, 1 mL ampules (box of 10)] ▶LK ♀? ▶? $

PENTAZOCINE (*Talwin NX*) 30 mg IV/IM q 3 to 4 h prn (Talwin). 1 tab PO q 3 to 4 h. (Talwin NX = 50 mg pentazocine/0.5 mg naloxone). [Generic/Trade: Tabs 50 mg with 0.5 mg naloxone, trade scored.] ▶LK ♀C ▶? ©IV $$$

Opioid Agonists

CODEINE 0.5 to 1 mg/kg up to 15 to 60 mg PO/IM/IV/SC q 4 to 6 h. Do not use IV in children. [Generic only: Tabs 15, 30, 60 mg. Oral soln: 15 mg/5 mL.] ▶LK ♀C ▶− ©II $$

FENTANYL (*Duragesic, Actiq, Fentora, Sublimaze, IONSYS*) Transdermal (Duragesic): 1 patch q 72 h (some with chronic pain may require q 48 h dosing). May wear more than 1 patch to achieve the correct analgesic effect. Transmucosal lozenge (Actiq) for <u>breakthrough cancer pain:</u> 200 to 1600 mcg, goal is 4 lozenges on a stick per day in conjunction with long-acting opioid. Buccal tab (Fentora) for <u>breakthrough cancer pain:</u> 100 to 800 mcg, titrated to pain relief. Buccal soluble film (Onsolis) for <u>breakthrough cancer pain:</u> 200 to 1200 mcg, titrated to pain relief. <u>Adult analgesia/procedural sedation:</u> 50 to 100 mcg slow IV over 1 to 2 min; carefully titrate to effect. <u>Analgesia:</u> 50 to 100 mcg IM q 1 to 2 h prn. [Generic/Trade: Transdermal patches 12.5, 25, 50, 75, 100 mcg/h. Actiq lozenges on a stick, berry flavored 200, 400, 600, 800, 1200, 1600 mcg. Trade only: IONSYS: Iontophoretic transdermal system: 40 mcg fentanyl per activation; max 6 doses/h. Max per system is eighty 40 mcg doses over 24 h. Trade only: (Fentora) buccal tab 100, 200, 300, 400, 600, 800 mcg. Trade only: (Onsolis) buccal soluble film 200, 400, 600, 800, 1200 mcg in child-resistant, protective foil.] ▶L ♀C ▶+ ©II $$$$$

HYDROMORPHONE (*Dilaudid, Dilaudid-5, ✦Hydromorph Contin*) Adults: 2 to 4 mg PO q 4 to 6 h. 0.5 to 2 mg IM/SC or slow IV q 4 to 6 h. 3 mg PR q 6 to 8 h. Titrate dose as high as necessary to relieve cancer pain or other types of nonmalignant pain where chronic opioids are necessary. Peds age younger than or equal to 12 yo: 0.03 to 0.08 mg/kg PO q 4 to 6 h prn or give 0.015 mg/kg/dose IV q 4 to 6 h prn. [Generic/Trade: Tabs 2, 4, 8 mg (8 mg trade scored). Oral soln 5 mg/5 mL. Suppository 3 mg.] ▶L ♀C ▶? ©II $$

LEVORPHANOL (*Levo-Dromoran*) 2 mg PO q 6 to 8 h prn. [Generic only: Tabs 2 mg, scored.] ▶L ♀C ▶? ©II $$$$

MEPERIDINE (*Demerol, pethidine*) 1 to 1.8 mg/kg up to 150 mg IM/SC/PO or slow IV q 3 to 4 h. 75 mg meperidine IV/IM/SC is equivalent to 300 mg meperidine PO. [Generic/Trade: Tabs 50 (trade scored), 100 mg. Syrup 50 mg/5 mL (trade banana flavored).] ▶LK ♀C but ▶ ▶+ ©II $$$

OPIOID EQUIVALENCY*

Opioid	PO	IV/SC/IM	Opioid	PO	IV/SC/IM
buprenorphine	n/a	0.3–0.4 mg	meperidine	300 mg	75 mg
butorphanol	n/a	2 mg	methadone	5–15 mg	2.5–10 mg
codeine	130 mg	75 mg	morphine	30 mg	10 mg
fentanyl	?	0.1 mg	nalbuphine	n/a	10 mg
hydrocodone	20 mg	n/a	oxycodone	20 mg	n/a
hydromorphone	7.5 mg	1.5 mg	oxymorphone	10 mg	1 mg
levorphanol	4 mg	2 mg	pentazocine	50 mg	30 mg

*Approximate equianalgesic doses as adapted from the 2003 American Pain Society (www.ampainsoc.org) guidelines and the 1992 AHCPR guidelines. Not available = "n/a." See drug entries themselves for starting doses. Many recommend initially using lower than equivalent doses when switching between different opioids. IV doses should be titrated slowly with appropriate monitoring. All PO dosing is with immediate-release preparations. Individualize all dosing, especially in the elderly, children, and in those with chronic pain, opioid naïve, or hepatic/renal insufficiency.

METHADONE (*Diskets, Dolophine, Methadose, ✦Metadol*)   Severe pain in opioid-tolerant patients: 2.5 to 10 mg IM/SC/PO q 3 to 4 h prn. Titrate dose as high as necessary to relieve cancer pain or other types of nonmalignant pain where chronic opioids are necessary. Opioid dependence: 20 to 100 mg PO daily. Treatment longer than 3 weeks is maintenance and only permitted in approved treatment programs. [Generic/Trade: Tabs 5, 10 mg. Dispersible tabs 40 mg (for opioid dependence only). Oral concentrate (Intensol): 10 mg/mL. Generic only: Oral soln 5, 10 mg/5 mL.] ▶L ♀C ▶? ⊙II $

MORPHINE (*MS Contin, Kadian, Avinza, Roxanol, Oramorph SR, MSIR, DepoDur, ✦Statex, M.O.S., Doloral*)   Controlled-release tabs (MS Contin, Oramorph SR): Start at 30 mg PO q 8 to 12 h. Controlled-release caps (Kadian): 20 mg PO q 12 to 24 h. Extended-release caps (Avinza): Start at 30 mg PO daily. Do not break, chew, or crush MS Contin or Oramorph SR. Kadian and Avinza caps may be opened and sprinkled in applesauce for easier administration; however, the pellets should not be crushed or chewed: give 0.1 to 0.2 mg/kg up to 15 mg IM/SC or slow IV q 4 h. Titrate dose as high as necessary to relieve cancer pain or other types of nonmalignant pain where chronic opioids are necessary. [Generic/Trade: Tabs, immediate-release 15, 30 mg. Oral soln: 10 mg/5 mL, 20 mg/5 mL, 20 mg/mL (concentrate). Rectal supps 5, 10, 20, 30 mg. Controlled-release tabs (MS Contin) 15, 30, 60, 100, 200 mg. Trade only: Controlled-release caps (Kadian) 10, 20, 30, 50, 60, 80, 100, 200 mg, Controlled-release tabs (Oramorph SR) 15, 30, 60, 100 mg. Extended-release caps (Avinza) 30, 45, 60, 75, 90, 120 mg. Generic only: Tabs, immediate-release 10 mg.] ▶LK ♀C ▶+ ⊙II $$$$

OXYCODONE (*Roxicodone, OxyContin, Percolone, OxyIR, OxyFAST, ✦Endocodone, Supeudol*)   Immediate-release preparations: 5 mg PO q 4 to 6 h prn. Controlled-release (OxyContin): 10 to 40 mg PO q 12 h (no supporting data for shorter dosing intervals for controlled-release tabs). Titrate dose as high as necessary to relieve cancer pain or other types of nonmalignant pain where chronic opioids are necessary. Do not break, chew, or crush controlled-release preparations. [Generic/Trade: Immediate-release: Tabs 5 mg, scored. Caps 5 mg. Tabs 15, 30 mg. Oral soln 5 mg/5 mL. Oral concentrate 20 mg/mL. Generic only: Immediate-release tabs 10, 20 mg. Trade only: Controlled-release tabs: 10, 15, 20, 30, 40, 60, 80 mg.] ▶L ♀B ▶– ⊙II $$$$$

FENTANYL TRANSDERMAL DOSE (Dosing based on ongoing morphine requirement.)

Morphine* (IV/IM)	Morphine* (PO)	Transdermal fentanyl*
10–22 mg/d	60–134 mg/d	25 mcg/h
23–37 mg/d	135–224 mg/d	50 mcg/h
38–52 mg/d	225–314 mg/d	75 mcg/h
53–67 mg/d	315–404 mg/d	100 mcg/h

*For higher morphine doses, see product insert for transdermal fentanyl equivalencies.

OXYMORPHONE (*Opana*) 10 to 20 mg PO q 4 to 6 h (immediate-release) or 5 mg q 12 h (extended-release) in opioid-naive patients, 1 h before or 2 h after meals. 1 to 1.5 mg IM/SC q 4 to 6 h prn. 0.5 mg IV q 4 to 6 h prn, increase dose until pain adequately controlled. [Trade only: Extended-release tabs (Opana ER) 5, 7.5, 10, 15, 20, 30, 40 mg. Immediate-release tabs (Opana IR) 5, 10 mg.] ▶L ♀C ▶? ©II $$$$

PROPOXYPHENE (*Darvon-N, Darvon Pulvules*) 65 to 100 mg PO q 4 h prn. [Generic/Trade: Caps 65 mg. Trade only: Tabs 100 mg (Darvon-N).] ▶L ♀C ▶+ ©IV $$

Opioid Analgesic Combinations

NOTE *Refer to individual components for further information. May cause drowsiness and/or sedation, which may be enhanced by alcohol and other CNS depressants. Opioids, carisoprodol, and butalbital may be habit forming. Avoid exceeding 4 g/day of acetaminophen in combination products. Caution people who drink 3 or more alcoholic drinks/day to limit acetaminophen use to 2.5 g/day due to additive liver toxicity. Opioids commonly cause constipation; concurrent laxatives are recommended. All opioids are pregnancy class D if used for prolonged periods or in high doses at term.*

ANEXSIA (hydrocodone + acetaminophen) Multiple strengths; write specific product on Rx. 1 tab PO q 4 to 6 h prn. [Generic/Trade: Tabs 5/325, 5/500, 7.5/325, 7.5/650, 10/750 mg hydrocodone/mg acetaminophen, scored.] ▶LK ♀C ▶– ©III $$

CAPITAL WITH CODEINE SUSPENSION (acetaminophen + codeine) 15 mL PO q 4 h prn. Give 5 mL q 4 to 6 h prn for age 3 to 6 yo, give 10 mL PO q 4 to 6 h prn pain for age 7 to 12 yo, use adult dose for age older than 12 yo. [Generic equivalent to oral soln. Trade equivalent to susp. Both codeine 12 mg and acetaminophen 120 mg per 5 mL (trade, fruit punch flavor).] ▶LK ♀C ▶? ©V $

COMBUNOX (oxycodone + ibuprofen) 1 tab PO q 6 h prn for no more than 7 days. Max 4 tabs per day. [Generic/Trade: Tabs 5 mg oxycodone/ 400 mg ibuprofen.] ▶L ♀C ▶– ©II $$$

DARVOCET (propoxyphene + acetaminophen) Multiple strengths; write specific product on Rx. 50/325, 2 tabs PO q 4 h prn. 100/500 or 100/650, 1 tab PO q 4 h prn. [Generic/Trade: Tabs 50/325 (Darvocet N-50), 100/650 (Darvocet N-100), 100/500 (Darvocet A500), mg propoxyphene mg acetaminophen.] ▶L ♀C ▶+ ©IV $$

EMPIRIN WITH CODEINE (acetylsalicylic acid + codeine) (✚292 tab) Multiple strengths; write specific product on Rx. 1 to 2 tabs PO q 4 h prn. [Generic only: Tabs 325/30, 325/60 mg aspirin/mg codeine. Empirin brand no longer made.] ▶LK ♀D ▶– ©III $

FIORICET WITH CODEINE (acetaminophen + butalbital + caffeine + codeine) 1 to 2 caps PO q 4 h prn. Max 6 caps per day. [Generic/Trade: Caps 325 mg acetaminophen/50 mg butalbital/40 mg caffeine/30 mg codeine.] ▶LK ♀C ▶– ©III $$$

FIORINAL WITH CODEINE (acetylsalicylic acid + butalbital + caffeine + codeine) (★*Fiorinal C-1/4, Fiorinal C-1/2, Tecnal C-1/4, Tecnal C-1/2*) 1 to 2 caps PO q 4 h prn. Max 6 caps/24 h. [Generic/Trade: Caps 325 mg aspirin/50 mg butalbital/40 mg caffeine/30 mg codeine.] ▶LK ♀D▶– ⊚III $$$

IBUDONE (hydrocodone + ibuprofen) 1 tab PO q 4 to 6 h prn, max dose 5 tabs/day. [Generic/Trade: Tabs 5/200 mg and 10/200 mg hydrocodone/ibuprofen.] ▶LK ♀– ▶? ⊚III $$$

LORCET (hydrocodone + acetaminophen) 1 to 2 caps (5/500) PO q 4 to 6 h prn, max dose 8 caps/day. 1 tab PO q 4 to 6 h prn (7.5/650 and 10/650), max dose 6 tabs/day. [Generic/Trade: Caps 5/500 mg. Tabs 7.5/ 650, 10/650 mg hydrocodone/acetaminophen.] ▶LK ♀C▶– ⊚III $$

LORTAB (hydrocodone + acetaminophen) 1 to 2 tabs (2.5/500 and 5/500) PO q 4 to 6 h prn, max dose 8 tabs/day. 1 tab (7.5/500 and 10/500 PO) q 4 to 6 h prn, max dose 5 tabs/day. Elixir 15 mL PO q 4 to 6 h prn, max 6 doses/day. [Generic/Trade: Lortab 5/500 scored, Lortab 7.5/500 (trade scored), Lortab 10/500 mg hydrocodone/mg acetaminophen. Elixir: 7.5/500 mg hydrocodone/mg acetaminophen/15 mL. Trade only: Tabs 2.5/500 mg.] ▶LK ♀C▶– ⊚III $$

MAXIDONE (hydrocodone + acetaminophen) 1 tab PO q 4 to 6 h prn, max dose 5 tabs/day. [Trade only: Tabs 10/750 mg hydrocodone/acetaminophen.] ▶LK ♀C▶– ⊚III $$$

MERSYNDOL WITH CODEINE (acetaminophen + codeine + doxylamine) Canada only. 1 to 2 tabs PO q 4 to 6 h prn. Max 12 tabs per day. [Canada Trade only: OTC tab 325 mg acetaminophen/8 mg codeine phosphate/5 mg doxylamine.] ▶LK ♀C▶? $

NORCO (hydrocodone + acetaminophen) 1 to 2 tabs PO q 4 to 6 h prn (5/325), max dose 12 tabs/day. 1 tab (7.5/325 and 10/325) PO q 4 to 6 h prn, max dose 8 and 6 tabs/day respectively. [Trade only: Tabs 5/325, 7.5/325, 10/325 mg hydrocodone/acetaminophen, scored.] ▶L ♀C▶? ⊚III $$$

PERCOCET (oxycodone + acetaminophen) (★*Percocet-demi, Oxycocet, Endocet*) Multiple strengths; write specific product on Rx. 1 to 2 tabs PO q 4 to 6 h prn (2.5/325 and 5/325). 1 tab PO q 4 to 6 h prn (7.5/500 and 10/650). [Trade only: Tabs 2.5/325 oxycodone/acetaminophen. Generic/Trade: Tabs 5/325, 7.5/325, 7.5/500, 10/325, 10/650 mg. Generic only: 2.5/300, 5/300, 7.5/300, 10/300, 2.5/400, 5/400, 7.5/400, 10/400, 5/500, 10/500 mg.] ▶L ♀C▶– ⊚III $

PERCODAN (oxycodone + acetylsalicylic acid) (★*Oxycodan, Endodan*) 1 tab PO q 6 h prn. [Generic/Trade: Tabs 4.88/325 mg oxycodone/aspirin (trade scored).] ▶LK ♀D▶– ⊚II $$

ROXICET (oxycodone + acetaminophen) Multiple strengths; write specific product on Rx. 1 tab PO q 6 h prn. Soln: 5 mL PO q 6 h prn. [Generic/Trade: Tabs 5/325 mg. Caps/Caplets 5/500 mg. Soln 5/325 per 5 mL, mg oxycodone/acetaminophen.] ▶L ♀C▶– ⊚II $$

SOMA COMPOUND WITH CODEINE (carisoprodol + acetylsalicylic acid + codeine) <u>Moderate to severe musculoskeletal pain:</u> 1 to 2 tabs PO qid prn. [Generic/Trade: Tabs 200 mg carisoprodol/325 mg aspirin/16 mg codeine.] ▶L ♀D▶– ⊚III $$$

SYNALGOS-DC **(dihydrocodeine + acetylsalicylic acid + caffeine)** 2 caps PO q 4 h prn. [Trade only: Caps 16 mg dihydrocodeine/356.4 mg aspirin/30 mg caffeine. "Painpack" is equivalent to 12 caps.] ▶L ♀C ▶– ⊝III $

TALACEN **(pentazocine + acetaminophen)** 1 tab PO q 4 h prn. [Generic/ Trade: Tabs 25 mg pentazocine/650 mg acetaminophen, trade scored.] ▶L ♀C ▶? ⊝IV $$$

TYLENOL WITH CODEINE **(codeine + acetaminophen)** (✦*Lenoltec, Emtec, Triatec*) Multiple strengths; write specific product on Rx. Give 1 to 2 tabs PO q 4 h prn. Elixir: give 5 mL q 4 to 6 h prn for age 3 to 6 yo; give 10 mL q 4 to 6 h prn for age 7 to 12 yo. [Generic only: Tabs Tylenol #2 (15/300). Tylenol with Codeine Elixir 12/120 per 5 mL, mg codeine/mg acetaminophen. Generic/ Trade: Tabs Tylenol #3 (30/300), Tylenol #4 (60/300). Canadian forms come with (Lenoltec, Tylenol) or without (Empracet, Emtec) caffeine.] ▶LK ♀C ▶? ⊝III (Tabs), V(elixir) $

TYLOX **(oxycodone + acetaminophen)** 1 cap PO q 6 h prn. [Generic/Trade: Caps 5 mg oxycodone/500 mg acetaminophen.] ▶L ♀C ▶– ⊝II $

VICODIN **(hydrocodone + acetaminophen)** 5/500 (max dose 8 tabs/day) and 7.5/750 (max dose of 5 tabs/day): 1 to 2 tabs PO q 4 to 6 h prn. 10/660: 1 tab PO q 4 to 6 h prn (max of 6 tabs/day). [Generic/Trade: Tabs Vicodin (5/500), Vicodin ES (7.5/750), Vicodin HP (10/660), scored, mg hydrocodone/ mg acetaminophen.] ▶LK ♀C ▶? ⊝III $

VICOPROFEN **(hydrocodone + ibuprofen)** 1 tab PO q 4 to 6 h prn, max dose 5 tabs/day. [Generic/Trade: Tabs 7.5/200 mg hydrocodone/ibuprofen. Generic only: Tabs 2.5/200, 5/200, 10/200 mg.] ▶LK ♀– ▶? ⊝III $$$

WYGESIC **(propoxyphene + acetaminophen)** 1 tab PO q 4 h prn. [Generic only: Tabs 65 mg propoxyphene/650 mg acetaminophen.] ▶L ♀C ▶? ⊝IV $

XODOL **(hydrocodone + acetaminophen)** 1 tab PO q 4 to 6 h prn, max 6 doses/day. [Trade only: Tabs 5/300, 7.5/300, 10/300 mg hydrocodone/ acetaminophen.] ▶LK ♀C ▶– ⊝III $$

ZYDONE **(hydrocodone + acetaminophen)** 1 to 2 tabs (5/400) PO q 4 to 6 h prn, max dose 8 tabs/day. 1 tab (7.5/400, 10/400) q 4 to 6 h prn, max dose 6 tabs/day. [Trade only: Tabs 5/400, 7.5/400, 10/400 mg hydrocodone/ mg acetaminophen.] ▶LK ♀C ▶? ⊝III $$

Opioid Antagonists

NALOXONE (***Narcan***) <u>Adult opioid overdose:</u> 0.4 to 2 mg q 2 to 3 min prn. <u>Adult post-op reversal:</u> 0.1 to 0.2 mg q 2 to 3 min prn. <u>Peds opioid overdose:</u> 0.01 mg/kg IV; may give 0.1 mg/kg if inadequate response. <u>Peds post-op reversal:</u> 0.005 to 0.01 mg q 2 to 3 min prn. May use IM/SC/ET if IV not available. ▶LK ♀B ▶? $

Other Analgesics

ACETAMINOPHEN (***Tylenol, Ofirmev, Panadol, Tempra, paracetamol, ✦Abenol, Atasol, Pediatrix***) 325 to 650 mg PO/PR q 4 to 6 h prn. Max dose 4 g/day.

(cont.)

Adults and adolescents wt less than 50 kg, give 15 mg/kg IV q 6 h or 12.5 mg/kg IV q 4 h. Max dose 75 mg/kg/day. Adults and adolescents wt 50 kg or greater, give 1000 mg IV q 6 h or 650 mg IV q 4 h. Max dose 4 g/day. OA: 2 extended-release caplets (ie, 1300 mg) PO q 8 h around the clock. Peds: 10 to 15 mg/kg/dose PO/PR q 4 to 6 h prn. Children age 2 to 12 yo, give 15 mg/kg IV q 6 h or 12.5 mg/kg q 4 h. Max dose 75 mg/kg/day. [OTC: Tabs 325, 500, 650 mg. Chewable Tabs 80 mg. Oral disintegrating tabs 80, 160 mg. Caps/Gelcaps/Caplets 500 mg. Extended-release caplets 650 mg. Liquid 160 mg/5 mL, 500 mg/15 mL. Infant gtts 80 mg/0.8 mL. Supps 80, 120, 325, 650 mg. Trade only (Ofirmev): Injection: 1000 mg/100 mL.] ▶LK ♀C ▶+ $$$$$

TAPENTADOL (*Nucynta*) Moderate to severe acute pain: 50 to 100 mg PO q 4 to 6 h prn, max 600 mg/day. Adjust dose in elderly, renal and hepatic dysfunction. Avoid in opioid-dependent patients. Seizures may occur with concurrent antidepressants or seizure disorder. [Trade only: Tabs 50, 75, 100 mg.] ▶LK ♀C ▶– ©II $$$$

TRAMADOL (*Ultram, Ultram ER, Ryzolt*) Moderate to moderately severe pain: 50 to 100 mg PO q 4 to 6 h prn, max 400 mg/day. Chronic pain, extended-release: 100 to 300 mg PO daily. Adjust dose in elderly, renal and hepatic dysfunction. Avoid in opioid-dependent patients. Seizures may occur with concurrent antidepressants or seizure disorder. [Generic/Trade: Tabs, immediate-release 50 mg. Trade only (Ultram ER, Ryzolt): Extended-release tabs 100, 200, 300 mg.] ▶KL ♀C ▶– $$$

WOMEN'S TYLENOL MENSTRUAL RELIEF (acetaminophen + pamabrom) 2 caplets PO q 4 to 6 h. [OTC: Caplets 500 mg acetaminophen/ 25 mg pamabrom (diuretic).] ▶LK ♀B ▶+ $

ANESTHESIA

Anesthetics & Sedatives

DEXMEDETOMIDINE (*Precedex*) ICU sedation less than 24 h: Load 1 mcg/kg over 10 min followed by infusion 0.2 to 0.7 mcg/kg/h titrated to desired sedation endpoint. Beware of bradycardia and hypotension. ▶LK ♀C ▶? $$$$

ETOMIDATE (*Amidate*) Induction: give 0.3 mg/kg IV. ▶L ♀C ▶? $

FOSPROPOFOL (*Lusedra*) Initial dose 6.5 mg/kg IV (not to exceed 16.5 mL), then give 1.6 mg/kg supplemental dose q 4 min (not to exceed 4 mL). ▶L ♀? ▶? $$$$

KETAMINE (*Ketalar*) 1 to 2 mg/kg IV over 1 to 2 min or 4 mg/kg IM induces 10 to 20 min dissociative state. Concurrent atropine minimizes hypersalivation. ▶L ♀? ▶? ©III $

METHOHEXITAL (*Brevital*) Induction: give 1 to 1.5 mg/kg IV, duration 5 min. ▶L ♀B ▶? ©IV $

MIDAZOLAM (*Versed*) Adult sedation/anxiolysis: 5 mg or 0.07 mg/kg IM; or 1 mg IV slowly q 2 to 3 min up to 5 mg. Peds: 0.25 to 1 mg/kg to max of 20 mg PO, or 0.1 to 0.15 mg/kg IM. IV route (6 mo to 5 yo): initial dose 0.05 to 0.1 mg/kg IV, then titrated to max 0.6 mg/kg. IV route (6 to 12 yo): initial dose 0.025 to 0.05 mg/kg IV, then titrated to max 0.4 mg/kg. Monitor for respiratory depression. [Generic only: Oral liquid 2 mg/mL.] ▶LK ♀D ▶– ©IV $

PENTOBARBITAL (*Nembutal*) Pediatric <u>sedation</u>: 1 to 6 mg/kg IV, adjusted in increments of 1 to 2 mg/kg to desired effect, or 2 to 6 mg/kg IM, max 100 mg. ▶LK ♀D ▶? ©III $$

PROPOFOL (*Diprivan*) <u>Induction dose</u>: 40 mg IV q 10 sec until induction (2 to 2.5 mg/kg). <u>ICU ventilator sedation</u>: Infusion 5 to 50 mcg/kg/min. <u>Deep sedation</u>: 1 mg/kg IV over 20 to 30 seconds. Repeat 0.5 mg/kg IV prn. ▶L ♀B ▶– $$$

THIOPENTAL (*Pentothal*) <u>Induction</u>: 3 to 5 mg/kg IV, duration 5 min. ▶L ♀C ▶? ©III $

Local Anesthetics

ARTICAINE (*Septocaine, Zorcaine*) 4% injection (includes epinephrine). [4% (includes epinephrine 1:100,000).] ▶LK ♀C ▶? $

BUPIVACAINE (*Marcaine, Sensorcaine*) Local and regional anesthesia. [0.25%, 0.5%, 0.75%, all with or without epinephrine.] ▶LK ♀C ▶? $

DUOCAINE (bupivacaine + lidocaine - local anesthetic) <u>Local anesthesia, nerve block for eye surgery.</u> [Vials contain bupivacaine 0.375% + lidocaine 1%.] ▶LK ♀C ▶? $

LIDOCAINE—LOCAL ANESTHETIC (*Xylocaine*) 0.5 to 1% injection with and without epinephrine. [0.5, 1, 1.5, 2%. With epinephrine: 0.5, 1, 1.5, 2%.] ▶LK ♀B ▶? $

MEPIVACAINE (*Carbocaine, Polocaine*) 1 to 2% injection. [1, 1.5, 2, 3%.] ▶LK ♀C ▶? $

Neuromuscular Blockers

CISATRACURIUM (*Nimbex*) <u>Paralysis</u>: 0.15 to 0.2 mg/kg IV. Peds: 0.1 mg/kg. Duration 30 to 60 min. ▶Plasma ♀B ▶? $$

ROCURONIUM (*Zemuron*) <u>Paralysis</u>: 0.6 mg/kg IV. Duration 30 min. ▶L ♀B ▶? $$

SUCCINYLCHOLINE (*Anectine, Quelicin*) <u>Paralysis</u>: 0.6 to 1.1 mg/kg IV. Peds: 2 mg/kg IV. ▶Plasma ♀C ▶? $

VECURONIUM (*Norcuron*) <u>Paralysis</u>: 0.08 to 0.1 mg/kg IV. Duration 15 to 30 min. ▶LK ♀C ▶? $

ANTIMICROBIALS

Aminoglycosides

NOTE *See also dermatology and ophthalmology, Nephrotoxicity, ototoxicity.*

AMIKACIN (*Amikin*) 15 mg/kg/day (up to 1500 mg/day) IM/IV divided q 8 to 12 h. Peak 20 to 35 mcg/mL, trough < 5 mcg/mL. Alternative 15 mg/kg IV q 24 h. ▶K ♀D ▶? $$$

GENTAMICIN (*Garamycin*) Adults: 3 to 5 mg/kg/day IM/IV divided q 8 h. Peak 5 to 10 mcg/mL, trough < 2 mcg/mL. Alternative 5 to 7 mg/kg IV q 24 h. Peds: 2 to 2.5 mg/kg q 8 h. ▶K ♀D ▶+ $

STREPTOMYCIN   Combo therapy for TB: 15 mg/kg (up to 1 g) IM daily. 10 mg/kg (up to 750 mg) for age 60 yo or older. Peds: 20 to 40 mg/kg (up to 1 g) IM daily. ▶K ♀D ▶+ $$$$$

TOBRAMYCIN (*Nebcin, TOBI*)   Adults: 3 to 5 mg/kg/day IM/IV divided q 8 h. Peak 5 to 10 mcg/mL, trough <2 mcg/mL. Alternative 5 to 7 mg/kg IV q 24 h. Peds: 2 to 2.5 mg/kg q 8 h. Cystic fibrosis (TOBI): 300 mg neb bid 28 days on, then 28 days off. [Trade only: TOBI 300 mg ampules for nebulizer.]   ▶K ♀D ? $$

Antifungal Agents—Azoles

CLOTRIMAZOLE (*Mycelex*)   Oral troches 5 times per day for 14 days. [Generic/Trade: Oral troches 10 mg.]   ▶L ♀C ▶? $$$$

FLUCONAZOLE (*Diflucan*)   Vaginal candidiasis: 150 mg PO single dose ($). All other dosing regimens IV/PO. Oropharyngeal candidiasis: 100 to 200 mg daily for 7 to 14 days. Esophageal candidiasis: 200 to 400 mg daily for 14 to 21 days. Candidemia: 800 mg on first day, then 400 mg daily. Cryptococcal meningitis in AIDS: 400 mg daily for 8 weeks, then 200 mg daily until immune reconstitution. Peds: Oropharyngeal candidiasis: 6 mg/kg on first day, then 3 mg/kg daily for 7 to 14 days. Esophageal candidiasis: 12 mg/kg on first day, then 6 mg/kg daily for 14 to 21 days. Systemic candidiasis: Cryptococcal meningitis in AIDS: 12 mg/kg on first day, then 6 to 12 mg/kg daily. [Generic/Trade: Tabs 50, 100, 150, 200 mg. 150 mg tab in single-dose blister pack. Susp 10, 40 mg/mL (35 mL).]   ▶K ♀C ▶+ $$$$

ITRACONAZOLE (*Hyphanox, Sporanox*)   Oral caps for onychomycosis "pulse dosing": 200 mg PO bid for first week of month for 2 months (fingernails) or 3 to 4 months (toenails). Standard regimen, toenail onychomycosis: 200 mg PO daily with full meal for 12 weeks. Fluconazole-refractory oropharyngeal or esophageal candidiasis: Oral soln 200 mg PO daily for 14 to 21 days. Contraindicated with dofetilide, ergot alkaloids, lovastatin, PO midazolam, pimozide, quinidine, simvastatin, triazolam. Negative inotrope; do not use for onychomycosis if ventricular dysfunction. [Trade: Tabs 200 mg. Oral soln 10 mg/mL (150 mL). Generic/Trade: Caps 100 mg. Oral soln 10 mg/mL (150 mL).]   ▶L ♀C ▶− $$$$$

KETOCONAZOLE (*Nizoral*)   200 to 400 mg PO daily. Hepatotoxicity. Contraindicated with midazolam, pimozide, triazolam. H2 blockers, proton pump inhibitors, antacids impair absorption. [Generic/Trade: Tabs 200 mg.]   ▶L ♀C ▶? $$$

MICONAZOLE-BUCCAL (*Oravig*)   Oropharyngeal candidiasis: Apply 50 mg buccal tab to gums once daily for 14 days. Increased INR with warfarin. [Trade: Buccal tabs, 50 mg.]   ▶L - ♀C ▶?

POSACONAZOLE (*Noxafil*)   Prevention of invasive Aspergillus or Candida infection, age 13 yo or older: 200 mg (5 mL) PO tid. Oropharyngeal candidiasis, age 13 yo or older: 100 mg (2.5 mL) PO bid on day 1, then 100 mg PO once daily for 13 days. Oropharyngeal candidiasis resistant to itraconazole/fluconazole, age 13 yo or older: 400 mg (10 mL) PO bid. Take with full meal or liquid nutritional supplement. CYP3A4 inhibitor. [Trade only: Oral susp 40 mg/mL, 105 mL bottle.]   ▶Glucuronidation ♀C ▶− $$$$$

VORICONAZOLE (*Vfend*) <u>Aspergillosis, systemic Candida infections:</u> 6 mg/kg IV q 12 h for 2 doses, then 3 to 4 mg/kg IV q 12 h (use 4 mg/kg for aspergillosis). <u>Esophageal candidiasis or maintenance therapy of aspergillosis/candidiasis:</u> 200 mg PO bid. For wt less than 40 kg, reduce to 100 mg PO bid. Dosage adjustment for efavirenz: Voriconazole 400 mg PO bid with efavirenz 300 mg PO once daily (use caps). Peds less than 12 yo: 7 mg/kg IV q 12 h. Infuse IV over 2 h. Take tabs and/or susp 1 h before or after meals. CYP3A4 inhibitor. Many drug interactions. [Trade only: Tabs 50, 200 mg (contains lactose). Susp 40 mg/mL (75 mL).] ▶L ♀D ▶? $$$$$

Antifungal Agents—Echinocandins

ANIDULAFUNGIN (*Eraxis*) <u>Candidemia:</u> 200 mg IV load on day 1, then 100 mg IV once daily. <u>Esophageal candidiasis:</u> 100 mg IV load on day 1, then 50 mg IV once daily. Max infusion rate of 1.1 mg/min to prevent histamine reactions. ▶Degraded chemically ♀C ▶? $$$$$
CASPOFUNGIN (*Cancidas*) Infuse over 1 h, give 70 mg IV loading dose on day 1, then 50 mg once daily. Peds: 70 mg/m^2 IV loading dose on day 1, then 50 mg/m^2 once daily (max of 70 mg/day). ▶KL ♀C ▶? $$$$$
MICAFUNGIN (*Mycamine*) Infuse IV over 1 h. <u>Esophageal candidiasis:</u> 150 mg once daily. <u>Prevention of candidal infections in bone marrow transplant patients:</u> 50 mg once daily. <u>Candidemia, acute disseminated candidiasis, Candida peritonitis/abscess:</u> 100 mg once daily. ▶L, feces ♀C ▶? $$$$$

Antifungal Agents—Polyenes

NOTE See www.idsociety.org for guidelines on the management of fungal infections. See www.aidsinfo.nih.gov for management of fungal infections in HIV-infected patients.

AMPHOTERICIN B DEOXYCHOLATE (*Fungizone*) Test dose 0.1 mg/kg up to 1 mg slow IV. Wait 2 to 4 h, and if tolerated then begin 0.25 mg/kg IV daily and advance to 0.5 to 1.5 mg/kg/day depending on fungal type. Maximum dose 1.5 mg/kg/day. ▶Tissues ♀B ▶? $$$$
AMPHOTERICIN B LIPID FORMULATIONS (*Amphotec, Abelcet, AmBisome*) Abelcet: 5 mg/kg/day IV at 2.5 mg/kg/h. AmBisome: 3 to 5 mg/kg/day IV over 2 h. Amphotec: Test dose of 10 mL over 15 to 30 min, observe for 30 min, then 3 to 4 mg/kg/day IV at 1 mg/kg/h. ▶? ♀B ▶? $$$$$

Antifungal Agents—Other

FLUCYTOSINE (*Ancobon*) 50 to 150 mg/kg/day PO divided qid. Myelosuppression. [Trade only: Caps 250, 500 mg.] ▶K ♀C ▶− $$$$$
GRISEOFULVIN (*Grifulvin V, ◆Fulvicin*) <u>Tinea capitis:</u> 500 mg PO daily in adults; 15 to 20 mg/kg (up to 1 g) PO daily in peds. Treat for 4 to 6 weeks, continuing for 2 weeks past symptom resolution. [Generic/Trade: Susp 125 mg/5 mL (120 mL). Trade only: Tabs 250, 500 mg.] ▶Skin ♀C ▶? $$$$

NYSTATIN (*Mycostatin, ✦Nilstat, Candistatin*) Thrush: 4 to 6 mL PO swish and swallow qid. Infants: 2 mL/dose with 1 mL in each cheek qid. [Generic only: Susp 100,000 units/mL (60, 480 mL).] ▶Not absorbed ♀B ▶? $$

TERBINAFINE (*Lamisil*) Onychomycosis: 250 mg PO daily for 6 weeks to treat fingernails, for 12 weeks to treat toenails. Tinea capitis, age 4 yo or older: Give granules PO once daily with food for 6 weeks: 125 mg for wt less than 25 kg, 187.5 mg for wt 25 to 35 kg, 250 mg for wt more than 35 kg. [Generic/ Trade: Tabs 250 mg. Trade only: Oral granules 125, 187.5 mg/packet.] ▶LK ♀B ▶– $

Antimalarials

NOTE For help treating malaria or getting antimalarials, see www.cdc.gov/ malaria or call the CDC "malaria hotline" (770) 488–7788 Monday-Friday 9 am to 5 pm EST; after hours/weekend (770) 488–7100. Pediatric doses of antima-larials should never exceed adult doses.

CHLOROQUINE (*Aralen*) Malaria prophylaxis, chloroquine-sensitive areas: 8 mg/kg up to 500 mg PO q week starting 1 to 2 weeks before exposure to 4 weeks after exposure. Chloroquine resistance is widespread. Can prolong QT interval and cause torsades. [Generic only: Tabs 250 mg. Generic/Trade: Tabs 500 mg (500 mg phosphate equivalent to 300 mg base).] ▶KL ♀C but ▶+ $

COARTEM (artemether + lumefantrine) (*coartemether*) Uncomplicated malaria: Take PO with food bid for 3 days. On day 1, give 2nd dose 8 h after first dose. Dose based on wt: 1 tab for 5 to 14 kg; 2 tabs for 15 to 24 kg; 3 tabs for 25 to 34 kg; 4 tabs for 35 kg or greater. Repeat dose if vomiting occurs within 1 to 2 h. Can prolong QT interval. [Trade only: Tabs, artemether 20 mg + lumefantrine 120 mg.] ▶L ♀C ▶? $$$

MALARONE (atovaquone + proguanil) Prevention of malaria: Give the following dose PO once daily from 1 to 2 days before exposure until 7 days after. Dose based on wt: ½ ped tab for wt 5 to 8 kg; ¾ ped tab for wt 9 to 10 kg; 1 ped tab for wt 11 to 20 kg; 2 ped tabs for 21 to 30 kg; 3 ped tabs for 31 to 40 kg; 1 adult tab for all patients wt greater than 40 kg. Treatment of malaria: Give the following dose PO once daily for 3 days. Dose based on wt: 2 ped tabs for 5 to 8 kg; 3 ped tabs for 9 to 10 kg; 1 adult tab for 11 to 20 kg; 2 adult tabs for 21 to 30 kg; 3 adult tabs for 31 to 40 kg; 4 adult tabs for all patients wt greater than 40 kg. Take with food or milky drink. [Trade only: Adult tabs atovaquone 250 mg + proguanil 100 mg; pediatric tabs 62.5 mg + 25 mg.] ▶feces; LK ♀C ▶? $$$$$

MEFLOQUINE (*Lariam*) Malaria prophylaxis for chloroquine-resistant areas: 250 mg PO once a week from 1 week before exposure to 4 weeks after. Treatment: 1250 mg PO single dose. Peds Malaria prophylaxis: Give the following dose PO once a week starting 1 week before exposure to 4 weeks after: Dose based on wt: 5 mg/kg (prepared by pharmacist) for wt 9 kg or less; ¼ tab for wt greater than 9 kg to 19 kg; give ½ tab for wt greater than 19 kg to 30 kg; give ¾ tab for wt greater than 30 to 45 kg; give 1 tab for wt 45 kg or greater. Peds Treatment: 20 to 25 mg/kg PO single dose or divided into 2 doses given 6 to 8 h apart. Take on full stomach. [Generic only: Tabs 250 mg.] ▶L ♀C ▶? $$

PRIMAQUINE   Prevention of relapse, P vivax/ovale malaria: 0.5 mg/kg (up to 30 mg) base PO daily for 14 days. Do not use unless normal G6PD level. [Generic only: Tabs 26.3 mg (equiv to 15 mg base).]   ▶L ♀– ▶– $$

QUININE (*Qualaquin*)   Malaria: 648 mg PO tid. Peds: 25 to 30 mg/kg/day (up to 2 g/day) PO divided q 8 h. Treat for 3 days (Africa/South America) or 7 days (Southeast Asia). Also give 7-day course of doxycycline, tetracycline, or clindamycin. Nocturnal leg cramps: 325 mg PO at bedtime. FDA warns that risks exceed potential benefit for this indication. Can cause life-threatening adverse effects: Cinchonism with overdose; hemolysis with G6PD deficiency; hypersensitivity; thrombocytopenia; HUS/TTP; QT interval prolongation; many drug interactions. [Trade only: Caps 324 mg.]   ▶L ♀C ▶+? $$$$

Antimycobacterial Agents

NOTE *Treat active mycobacterial infection with at least 2 drugs. See guidelines at www.thoracic.org/statements/index.php and www.aidsinfo.nih.gov.*

DAPSONE (*Aczone*)   Pneumocystis prophylaxis, leprosy: 100 mg PO daily. Pneumocystis treatment: 100 mg PO daily with trimethoprim 5 mg/kg PO tid for 21 days. Acne (Aczone): Apply bid. [Generic only: Tabs 25, 100 mg. Trade only (Aczone): Topical gel 5% 30 g.]   ▶LK ♀C ▶– $

ETHAMBUTOL (*Myambutol*, ◆*Etibi*)   15 to 20 mg/kg PO daily. Dose with whole tabs: Give 800 mg PO daily for wt 40 to 55 kg, 1200 mg for wt 56 to 75 kg, 1600 mg for wt 76 to 90 kg. Base dose on estimated lean body wt. Peds: 15 to 20 mg/kg (up to 1 g) PO daily. [Generic/Trade: Tabs 100, 400 mg.]   ▶LK ♀C but + ▶+ $$$$

ISONIAZID (*INH*, ◆*Isotamine*)   Adults: 5 mg/kg (up to 300 mg) PO daily. Peds: 10 to 15 mg/kg (up to 300 mg) PO daily. Hepatotoxicity. Consider supplemental pyridoxine up to 50 mg per day to prevent neuropathy. [Generic only: Tabs 100, 300 mg. Syrup 50 mg/5 mL.]   ▶LK ♀C but + ▶+ $

PYRAZINAMIDE (*PZA*, ◆*Tebrazid*)   20 to 25 mg/kg (up to 2000 mg) PO daily. Dose with whole tabs: Give 1000 mg PO daily for wt 40 to 55 kg, 1500 mg for wt 56 to 75 kg, 2000 mg for wt 76 to 90 kg. Base dose on estimated lean body wt. Peds: 15 to 30 mg/kg (up to 2000 mg) PO daily. Hepatotoxicity. [Generic only: Tabs 500 mg.]   ▶LK ♀C ▶? $$$$

RIFABUTIN (*Mycobutin*)   300 mg PO daily or 150 mg PO bid. Dosage reduction required with protease inhibitors. [Trade only: Caps 150 mg.]   ▶L ♀B ▶? $$$$$

RIFAMATE (isoniazid + rifampin)   2 caps PO daily on empty stomach. [Generic/Trade: Caps isoniazid 150 mg + rifampin 300 mg.]   ▶LK ♀C but + ▶+ $$$$

RIFAMPIN (*Rimactane*, *Rifadin*, ◆*Rofact*)   TB: 10 mg/kg (up to 600 mg) PO/IV daily. Peds: 10 to 20 mg/kg (up to 600 mg) PO/IV daily. Neisseria meningitidis carriers: 600 mg PO bid for 2 days. Peds: Age 1 mo or older: 10 mg/kg (up to 600 mg) PO bid for 2 days. Age younger than 1 mo: 5 mg/kg PO bid for 2 days. IV and PO doses are the same. Take oral doses on empty stomach. [Generic/Trade: Caps 150, 300 mg. Pharmacists can make oral susp.]   ▶L ♀C but + ▶+ $$$

RIFAPENTINE (*Priftin*) <u>TB:</u> 600 mg PO twice a week for 2 months, then once a week for 4 months. Use for continuation therapy only in selected HIV-negative patients. [Trade only: Tabs 150 mg.] ▶Esterases, fecal ♀C ▶? $$$$

RIFATER (isoniazid + rifampin + pyrazinamide) <u>TB:</u> 4 tabs daily for wt less than 45 kg, 5 tabs daily for wt 45 to 54 kg, 6 tabs daily for wt 55 kg or greater. [Trade only: Tabs Isoniazid 50 mg + rifampin 120 mg + pyrazinamide 300 mg.] ▶LK ♀C ▶? $$$$$

Antiparasitics

ALBENDAZOLE (*Albenza*) <u>Hydatid disease, neurocysticercosis:</u> 15 mg/kg/day (up to 800 mg/day) for wt less than 60 kg, 400 mg PO bid for wt 60 kg or greater. [Trade only: Tabs 200 mg.] ▶L ♀C ▶? $$$$

ATOVAQUONE (*Mepron*) <u>Pneumocystis treatment:</u> 750 mg PO bid for 21 days. <u>Pneumocystis prevention:</u> 1500 mg PO daily. Take with meals. [Trade only: Susp 750 mg/5 mL (210 mL), foil pouch 750 mg/5 mL (5, 10 mL).] ▶Fecal ♀C ▶? $$$$$

IVERMECTIN (*Stromectol*) Single PO dose of 200 mcg/kg for <u>strongyloidiasis,</u> 200 mcg/kg for <u>scabies</u> (may need to repeat dose in 10 to 14 days), 150 mcg/kg for <u>onchocerciasis.</u> Peds head lice: 200 to 400 mcg/kg PO single dose; repeat in 7 days. Not for children less than 15 kg. Take on empty stomach with water. [Trade only: Tabs 3 mg.] ▶L ♀C ▶? $$

MEBENDAZOLE (*Vermox*) <u>Pinworm:</u> 100 mg PO once; repeat in 2 weeks. <u>Roundworm, whipworm, hookworm:</u> 100 mg PO bid for 3 days. [Generic only: Chewable tabs 100 mg.] ▶L ♀C ▶? $$

NITAZOXANIDE (*Alinia*) <u>Cryptosporidial or Giardial diarrhea:</u> 100 mg bid for age 1 to 3 yo, 200 mg bid for 4 to 11 yo, 500 mg bid for adults and children 12 yo or older. Give PO with food for 3 days. Use susp if less than 12 yo. [Trade only: Oral susp 100 mg/5 mL, 60 mL bottle. Tabs 500 mg.] ▶L ♀B ▶? $$$$

PAROMOMYCIN 25 to 35 mg/kg/day PO divided tid with or after meals. [Generic only: Caps 250 mg.] ▶Not absorbed ♀C ▶? $$$$

PENTAMIDINE (*Pentam, NebuPent*) <u>Pneumocystis treatment:</u> 4 mg/kg IM/IV daily for 21 days. <u>Pneumocystis prevention:</u> 300 mg nebulized q 4 weeks. [Trade only: Aerosol 300 mg.] ▶K ♀C ▶– $$$$

PRAZIQUANTEL (*Biltricide*) <u>Schistosomiasis:</u> 20 mg/kg PO q 4 to 6 h for 3 doses. [Trade only: Tabs 600 mg.] ▶LK ♀B ▶– $$$

PYRANTEL (*Antiminth, Pin-X, Pinworm, ✦Combantrin*) <u>Pinworm, roundworm:</u> 11 mg/kg (up to 1 g) PO single dose. Repeat in 2 weeks for pinworm. [OTC Trade only (Pin-X): Susp 144 mg/mL (equivalent to 50 mg/mL of pyrantel base) 30, 60 mL. Tabs 720.5 mg (equivalent to 250 mg of pyrantel base). OTC Generic only: Caps 180 mg (equivalent to 62.5 mg of pyrantel base).] ▶Not absorbed ♀– ▶? $$

PYRIMETHAMINE (*Daraprim*) <u>CNS toxoplasmosis in AIDS. Acute therapy:</u> First dose 200 mg PO, then 50 mg PO daily for wt less than 60 kg; use 75 mg PO once daily for 60 kg or greater. Treat for at least 6 weeks with pyrimethamine + sulfadiazine + leucovorin 10 to 25 mg PO once daily (can increase leucovorin to 50 mg/day). Secondary prevention: Pyrimethamine 25

(cont.)

to 50 mg PO once daily + sulfadiazine + leucovorin 10 to 25 mg PO once daily. [Trade only: Tabs 25 mg.] ▶L ♀C ▶+ $$

TINIDAZOLE (*Tindamax*) Adults: 2 g PO daily for 1 day for <u>trichomoniasis or giardiasis</u>, for 3 days for <u>amebiasis</u>. <u>Bacterial vaginosis</u>: 2 g PO once daily for 2 days or 1 g PO once daily for 5 days. Peds, age older than 3 yo: 50 mg/kg (up to 2 g) PO daily for 1 day for <u>giardiasis</u>, for 3 days for <u>amebiasis</u>. Take with food. [Trade only: Tabs 250, 500 mg. Pharmacists can compound oral susp.] ▶KL ♀C ▶?- $

Antiviral Agents—Anti-CMV

CIDOFOVIR (*Vistide*) <u>CMV retinitis in AIDS</u>: 5 mg/kg IV once a week for 2 weeks, then 5 mg/kg every 2 weeks. Severe nephrotoxicity. ▶K ♀C ▶– $$$$$

FOSCARNET (*Foscavir*) <u>CMV retinitis</u>: 60 mg/kg IV (over 1 h) q 8 h or 90 mg/kg IV (over 1.5 to 2 h) q 12 h for 2 to 3 weeks, then 90 to 120 mg/kg IV daily over 2 h. <u>HSV infection</u>: 40 mg/kg (over 1 h) q 8 to 12 h. Nephrotoxicity, seizures. ▶K ♀C ▶? $$$$$

GANCICLOVIR (*Cytovene*) <u>CMV retinitis</u>: Induction 5 mg/kg IV q 12 h for 14 to 21 days. Maintenance 6 mg/kg IV daily for 5 days per week. Myelosuppression. Potential carcinogen, teratogen. May impair fertility. [Generic only: Caps 250, 500 mg.] ▶K ♀C ▶– $$$$$

VALGANCICLOVIR (*Valcyte*) <u>CMV retinitis</u>: 900 mg PO bid for 21 days, then 900 mg PO daily. Prevention of CMV disease in high-risk transplant patients: 900 mg PO daily given within 10 days post-transplant until 100 days post-transplant for heart or kidney-pancreas or 200 days for kidney transplant. See package insert for peds dose. Greater bioavailability than oral ganciclovir. Give with food. Impaired fertility, myelosuppression, potential carcinogen and teratogen. [Trade only: Tabs 450 mg. Oral soln 50 mg/mL.] ▶K ♀C ▶– $$$$$

Antiviral Agents—Anti-Herpetic

ACYCLOVIR (*Zovirax*) <u>Genital herpes</u>: 400 mg PO tid for 7 to 10 days for first episode, or for 5 days for recurrent episodes. <u>Chronic suppression of genital herpes</u>: 400 mg PO bid; in HIV infection use 400 to 800 mg PO bid to tid. <u>Zoster</u>: 800 mg PO 5 times a day for 7 to 10 days. <u>Chickenpox</u>: 20 mg/kg (up to 800 mg) PO qid for 5 days. <u>Adult IV</u>: 5 to 10 mg/kg IV q 8 h, each dose over 1 h. <u>Herpes encephalitis</u>: 20 mg/kg IV q 8 h for 10 days for age 3 mo to 12 yo; 10 mg/kg IV q 8 h for 10 days for age 12 yo or older. <u>Neonatal herpes</u>: 20 mg/kg IV q 8 h for 21 days for disseminated/CNS disease, for 14 days for skin/mucous membrane infections. [Generic/Trade: Caps 200 mg. Tabs 400, 800 mg. Susp 200 mg/5 mL.] ▶K ♀B ▶+ $

FAMCICLOVIR (*Famvir*) <u>First episode genital herpes</u>: 250 mg PO tid for 7 to 10 days. <u>Recurrent genital herpes</u>: 1000 mg PO bid for 2 doses; give 500 mg bid for 7 days if HIV infected. <u>Chronic suppression of genital herpes</u>: 250 mg PO bid; 500 mg PO bid if HIV infected. <u>Recurrent herpes labialis</u>: 1500 mg PO single dose; 500 mg bid for 7 days if HIV-infected. <u>Zoster</u>: 500 mg PO tid for 7 days. [Generic/Trade: Tabs 125, 250, 500 mg.] ▶K ♀B ▶? $$

VALACYCLOVIR (*Valtrex*) First episode genital herpes: 1 g PO bid for 10 days. Recurrent genital herpes: 500 mg PO bid for 3 days; if HIV infected give 1 g PO bid for 5 to 10 days. Chronic suppression of genital herpes: 500 to 1000 mg PO daily; if HIV infected give 500 mg PO bid. Reduction of genital herpes transmission in immunocompetent patients with no more than 9 recurrences per year: 500 mg PO daily for source partner, in conjunction with safer sex practices. Herpes labialis: age 12 yo or older: 2 g PO q 12 h for 2 doses. Zoster: 1000 mg PO tid for 7 days. Chicken pox, age 2 to 18 yo: 20 mg/kg (max of 1 g) PO tid for 5 days. [Generic/Trade: Tabs 500, 1000 mg.] ▶K ♀B ▶+ $$$$$

NOTE *Many serious drug interactions: Always check before prescribing. See www.aidsinfo.nih.gov for AIDS treatment guidelines and the use of rifamycins with NNRTIs. Consider monitoring LFTs in patients receiving HAART.*

Antiviral Agents—Anti-HIV—CCR5 Antagonists

MARAVIROC (*Selzentry, MVC*) 150 mg PO bid with strong CYP3A4 inhibitors (most protease inhibitors, ketoconazole, itraconazole, clarithromycin); 300 mg PO bid with drugs that are not strong CYP3A4 inducers/inhibitors (NRTIs, tipranavir-ritonavir, nevirapine, raltegravir; rifabutin without a strong CYP3A4 inhibitor or inducer); 600 mg PO bid with strong CYP3A4 inducers (efavirenz, etravirine, rifampin, carbamazepine, phenobarbital, phenytoin). Tropism test before treatment; not for dual/mixed or CXCR4-tropic HIV infection. Hepatotoxicity with allergic features. [Trade only: Tabs 150, 300 mg.] ▶LK ♀B ▶– $$$$$

Antiviral Agents—Anti-HIV—Combinations

ATRIPLA (efavirenz + emtricitabine + tenofovir) 1 tab PO once daily on empty stomach, preferably at bedtime. [Trade only: Tabs efavirenz 600 mg + emtricitabine 200 mg + tenofovir 300 mg.] ▶KL ♀D ▶– $$$$$
COMBIVIR (lamivudine + zidovudine) 1 tab PO bid for wt 30 kg or greater. [Trade only: Tabs lamivudine 150 mg + zidovudine 300 mg.] ▶LK ♀C ▶– $$$$$
EPZICOM (abacavir + lamivudine) 1 tab PO daily. [Trade only: Tabs abacavir 600 mg + lamivudine 300 mg.] ▶LK ♀C ▶– $$$$$
TRIZIVIR (abacavir + lamivudine + zidovudine) 1 tab PO bid. [Trade only: Tabs abacavir 300 mg + lamivudine 150 mg + zidovudine 300 mg.] ▶LK ♀C ▶– $$$$$
TRUVADA (emtricitabine + tenofovir) 1 tab PO daily. [Trade only: Tabs emtricitabine 200 mg + tenofovir 300 mg.] ▶K ♀B ▶– $$$$$

Antiviral Agents—Anti-HIV—Integrase Strand Transfer Inhibitor

RALTEGRAVIR (*Isentress, RAL*) 400 mg PO bid. Increase to 800 mg PO bid if given with rifampin. [Trade only: Tabs 400 mg.] ▶Glucuronidation ♀C ▶– $$$$$

*Antiviral Agents—Anti-HIV—Non-Nucleoside Reverse
Transcriptase Inhibitors*

EFAVIRENZ (*Sustiva, EFV*)   Adults and children wt 40 kg or greater: 600 mg PO at bedtime. With voriconazole: Use voriconazole 400 mg PO bid and efavirenz 300 mg PO once daily. Peds, age 3 yo or older: Give PO at bedtime 200 mg for wt 10 kg to less than 15 kg, 250 mg for wt 15 kg to less than 20 kg, 300 mg for wt 20 kg to less than 25 kg, 350 mg for wt 25 kg to less than 32.5 kg, 400 mg for wt 32.5 kg to less than 40 kg. Do not give with high-fat meal. [Trade only: Caps 50, 100, 200 mg. Tabs 600 mg.]   ▶L ♀C ▶– $$$$$

ETRAVIRINE (*Intelence, ETR*)   Combination therapy for treatment-resistant HIV infection: 200 mg PO bid after meals. [Trade only: Tabs 100 mg.]   ▶L ♀B ▶– $$$$$

NEVIRAPINE (*Viramune, NVP*)   200 mg PO daily for 14 days initially. If tolerated, increase to 200 mg PO bid. Peds, age 15 days or older: 150 mg/m2 PO once daily for 14 days, then 150 mg/m2 bid (max dose 200 mg bid). Severe skin reactions and hepatotoxicity. [Trade only: Tabs 200 mg, susp 50 mg/5 mL (240 mL).]   ▶LK ♀C ▶– $$$$$

*Antiviral Agents—Anti-HIV—Nucleoside/Nucleotide Reverse
Transcriptase Inhibitors*

ABACAVIR (*Ziagen, ABC*)   Adult: 300 mg PO bid or 600 mg PO daily. Peds. Oral soln, age 3 mo or older: 8 mg/kg (up to 300 mg) PO bid. Peds, tabs: 150 mg PO bid for wt 14 to 21 kg, 150 mg PO q am and 300 mg PO q pm for wt 22 to 29 kg, 300 mg PO bid for wt 30 kg or greater. Potentially fatal hypersensitivity. HLA-B*5701 predisposes to hypersensitivity; screen before starting and avoid if positive test. Never rechallenge with abacavir after suspected reaction. [Trade only: Tabs 300 mg scored. Oral soln 20 mg/mL (240 mL).]   ▶L ♀C ▶– $$$$$

DIDANOSINE (*Videx, Videx EC, ddI*)   Videx EC. Give 200 mg PO once daily for wt 20 to 24 kg, 250 mg PO once daily for wt 25 to 59 kg, 400 mg PO once daily for wt 60 kg or greater. Dosage reduction of Videx EC with tenofovir in adults: 200 mg for wt less than 60 kg, 250 mg for wt 60 kg or greater. Dosage reduction unclear with tenofovir if CrCl <60 mL/min. Buffered powder, peds: 100 mg/m2 PO bid for age 2 weeks to 8 mo; 120 mg/m2 PO bid for age older than 8 mo. All formulations usually taken on empty stomach. [Generic/Trade: Pediatric powder for oral soln 10 mg/mL (buffered with antacid). Delayed-release caps (Videx EC): 125, 200, 250, 400 mg.]   ▶LK ♀B ▶– $$$$$

EMTRICITABINE (*Emtriva, FTC*)   200 mg cap or 240 mg oral soln PO once daily. Peds, oral soln: 3 mg/kg PO once daily for age 3 mo or younger; 6 mg/kg PO once daily (up to 240 mg) for age older than 3 mo. Can give 200 mg cap PO once daily if wt greater than 33 kg. [Trade only: Caps 200 mg. Oral soln 10 mg/mL (170 mL).]   ▶K ♀B ▶– $$$$$

LAMIVUDINE (*Epivir, Epivir-HBV, 3TC, ◆Heptovir*)   Epivir for HIV infection. Adults and teens older than 16 yo: 150 mg PO bid or 300 mg PO daily. Peds: 4 mg/kg (up to 150 mg) PO bid. Use tabs if wt 14 kg or greater. Epivir-HBV

(cont.)

for hepatitis B: Adults: 100 mg PO daily. Peds: 3 mg/kg (up to 100 mg) PO daily. [Trade only: Epivir, 3TC: Tabs 150 (scored), 300 mg, oral soln 10 mg/mL. Epivir-HBV, Heptovir: Tabs 100 mg, oral soln 5 mg/mL.] ▸K ♀C ▶– $$$$$

TENOFOVIR (Viread, TDF) Adults and adolescents: 300 mg PO daily. [Trade only: Tabs 300 mg.] ▸K ♀B ▶– $$$$$

ZIDOVUDINE (Retrovir, AZT, ZDV) 600 mg/day PO divided bid or tid for wt 30 kg or greater. Peds dose based on wt: give 24 mg/kg/day PO divided bid or tid for wt 4 to 8 kg, 18 mg/kg/day PO divided bid or tid for wt 9 to 29 kg. [Generic/Trade: Caps 100 mg. Tabs 300 mg. Syrup 50 mg/5 mL (240 mL).] ▸LK ♀C ▶– $$$$$

Antiviral Agents—Anti-HIV—Protease Inhibitors

ATAZANAVIR (Reyataz, ATV) Adults, therapy-naive: 400 mg PO once daily (without ritonavir) OR 300 mg + ritonavir 100 mg PO both once daily. With tenofovir, therapy-naive: 300 mg + ritonavir 100 mg PO both once daily. With efavirenz, therapy-naive: 400 mg + ritonavir 100 mg PO both once daily. Do not give atazanavir with efavirenz in therapy-experienced patients. Therapy-experienced: 300 mg + ritonavir 100 mg PO both once daily. Peds, therapy-naive, age 6 yo or older: Give following dose PO once daily based on wt: atazanavir 8.5 mg/kg for wt 15 to 19 kg; 7 mg/kg (up to 300 mg) for wt 20 kg or greater. Give with ritonavir 4 mg/kg (up to 100 mg) PO once daily. Peds, therapy-experienced, age 6 yo or older and wt 25 kg or greater: atazanavir 7 mg/kg (up to 300 mg) with ritonavir 4 mg/kg (up to 100 mg) PO once daily. Therapy-naive, ritonavir-intolerant, age 13 yo or older and wt 39 kg or greater: 400 mg PO once daily. Give caps with food. Give atazanavir 2 h before or 1 h after buffered didanosine. [Trade only: Caps 100, 150, 200, 300 mg.] ▸L ♀B ▶– $$$$$

DARUNAVIR (Prezista, DRV) Therapy-experienced, adult: 800 mg + ritonavir 100 mg PO both once daily. Therapy-experienced, adult: 600 mg + ritonavir 100 mg PO both bid. Peds, age 6 yo or older: 375 mg + ritonavir 50 mg PO both bid for wt 20 to 29 kg; 450 mg + ritonavir 60 mg PO both bid for wt 30 kg to 39 kg; 600 mg + ritonavir 100 mg PO both bid for wt 40 kg or greater. Take with food. Do not use without ritonavir. [Trade only: Tabs 75, 150, 300, 400, 600 mg.] ▸L ♀B ▶– $$$$$

FOSAMPRENAVIR (Lexiva, FPV, ✦Telzir) Therapy-naive adults: 1400 mg PO bid (without ritonavir) OR 1400 mg + ritonavir 100/200 mg PO both once daily OR 700 mg + ritonavir 100 mg PO both bid. Protease inhibitor-experienced adults: 700 mg + ritonavir 100 mg PO both bid. Peds, therapy-naive, 2 to 5 yo: Susp 30 mg/kg PO bid. Therapy-naive, 6 yo or older: Susp 30 mg/kg PO bid OR susp 18 mg/kg + ritonavir 3 mg/kg PO both bid. Therapy-experienced, 6 yo or older: Susp 18 mg/kg + ritonavir 3 mg/kg PO both bid. Do not exceed adult dose in children. For unboosted fosamprenavir, can use tabs for peds patients with wt 47 kg or greater. For ritonavir-boosted fosamprenavir, can use tabs for peds patients with wt 39 kg or greater. Take tabs without regard to meals. Adults should take susp without food; children should take with food. [Trade only: Tabs 700 mg. Susp 50 mg/mL.] ▸L ♀C ▶– $$$$$

INDINAVIR (Crixivan, IDV) 800 mg PO q 8 h between meals with water (at least 48 ounces/day to prevent kidney stones). [Trade only: Caps 100, 200, 400 mg.] ▸LK ♀C ▶– $$$$$

LOPINAVIR-RITONAVIR (*Kaletra, LPV/r*)   Adults: 400/100 mg PO bid (tabs or oral soln). Can use 800/200 mg PO once daily in patients with less than 3 lopinavir resistance-associated substitutions. Coadministration with efavirenz, nevirapine, fosamprenavir, or nelfinavir: 500/125 mg tabs (use two 200/50 mg + one 100/25 mg tab) or 533/133 mg oral soln (6.5 mL) PO bid. Infants, age 14 days to 6 mo: Lopinavir 16 mg/kg PO bid. Peds, age 6 mo to 12 yo: Lopinavir 12 mg/kg PO bid for wt less than 15 kg, use 10 mg/kg PO bid for wt 15 to 40 kg. Coadministration with efavirenz, nevirapine, fosamprenavir, or nelfinavir: Lopinavir 13 mg/kg PO bid for wt less than 15 kg, 11 mg/kg PO bid for wt 15 to 45 kg. Do not exceed adult dose in children. No once daily dosing for pediatric or pregnant patients; coadministration with carbamazepine, phenobarbital, phenytoin, efavirenz, nevirapine, fosamprenavir, or nelfinavir; or in patients with 3 or more lopinavir resistance-associated substitutions. Give tabs without regard to meals; give oral soln with food. [Trade only: Tabs 200/50 mg, 100/25 mg. Oral soln 80/20 mg/mL (160 mL).]   ▶L ♀C ▶– $$$$$

NELFINAVIR (*Viracept, NFV*)   750 mg PO tid or 1250 mg PO bid. Peds: 45 to 55 mg/kg PO bid (up to 2500 mg/day). Take with meals. [Trade only: Tabs 250, 625 mg. Oral powder 50 mg/g (114 g).]   ▶L ♀B ▶– $$$$$

RITONAVIR (*Norvir, RTV*)   Adult doses of 100 mg PO bid to 400 mg PO bid used to boost levels of other protease inhibitors. Full-dose regimen (600 mg PO bid) is poorly tolerated. Peds, full-dose regimen: Start with 250 mg/m2 bid and increase every 2 to 3 days by 50 mg/m2 bid to achieve usual dose of 350 to 400 mg/m2 (up to 600 mg) PO bid for age older than 1 mo. If 400 mg/m2 twice daily not tolerated, consider other alternatives. See specific protease inhibitor entries (atazanavir, darunavir, fosamprenavir, tipranavir) for pediatric boosting doses of ritonavir. [Trade only: Caps 100 mg, tabs 100 mg. Oral soln 80 mg/mL (240 mL).]   ▶L ♀B ▶– $$$$$

SAQUINAVIR (*Invirase, SQV*)   Regimens must contain ritonavir. Saquinavir 1000 mg + ritonavir 100 mg both PO bid within 2 h after meals. Saquinavir 1000 mg + Kaletra 400/100 mg PO both bid. [Trade only: Invirase (hard gel) Caps 200 mg. Tabs 500 mg.]   ▶L ♀B ▶– $$$$$

TIPRANAVIR (*Aptivus, TPV*)   500 mg boosted by ritonavir 200 mg PO bid with food. Peds: 14 mg/kg with 6 mg/kg ritonavir PO bid; do not exceed adult dose. Hepatotoxicity. [Trade only: Caps 250 mg. Oral soln 100 mg/mL (95 mL in unit-of-use amber glass bottle).]   ▶Feces ♀C ▶– $$$$$

Antiviral Agents—Anti-Influenza

AMANTADINE (*Symmetrel, ♦Endantadine*)   Parkinsonism: 100 mg PO bid. Max 300 to 400 mg/day divided tid to qid. Prevention/treatment of influenza A: 5 mg/kg/day up to 150 mg/day PO divided bid for age 1 to 9 yo and any child wt less than 40 kg. Give 100 mg PO bid for adults and children age 10 yo or older; reduce to 100 mg PO daily if age 65 yo or older. The CDC generally recommends against amantadine/rimantadine for treatment/prevention of influenza A in the United States due to high levels of resistance. [Generic only: Caps 100 mg. Tabs 100 mg. Syrup 50 mg/5 mL (480 mL).]   ▶K ♀C ▶? $$

OVERVIEW OF BACTERIAL PATHOGENS (Selected)

Gram Positive Aerobic Cocci: *Staph epidermidis* (coagulase negative), *Staph aureus* (coagulase positive), *Streptococci: S pneumoniae* (pneumococcus), *S pyogenes* (Group A), *S agalactiae* (Group B), enterococcus

Gram Positive Aerobic/Facultatively Anaerobic Bacilli: *Bacillus*, *Corynebacterium diphtheriae*, *Erysipelothrix rhusiopathiae*, *Listeria monocytogenes*, *Nocardia*

Gram Negative Aerobic Diplococci: *Moraxella catarrhalis*, *Neisseria gonorrhoeae*, *Neisseria meningitidis*

Gram Negative Aerobic Coccobacilli: *Haemophilus ducreyi*, *Haemoph. Influenzae*

Gram Negative Aerobic Bacilli: *Acinetobacter*, *Bartonella* species, *Bordetella pertussis*, *Brucella*, *Burkholderia cepacia*, *Campylobacter*, *Francisella tularensis*, *Helicobacter pylori*, *Legionella pneumophila*, *Pseudomonas aeruginosa*, *Stenotrophomonas maltophilia*, *Vibrio cholerae*, *Yersinia*

Gram Negative Facultatively Anaerobic Bacilli: *Aeromonas hydrophila*, *Eikenella corrodens*, *Pasteurella multocida*, Enterobacteriaceae: *E coli*, *Citrobacter*, *Shigella*, *Salmonella*, *Klebsiella*, *Enterobacter*, *Hafnia*, *Serratia*, *Proteus*, *Providencia*

Anaerobes: *Actinomyces*, *Bacteroides fragilis*, *Clostridium botulinum*, *Clostridium difficile*, *Clostridium perfringens*, *Clostridium tetani*, *Fusobacterium*, *Lactobacillus*, *Peptostreptococcus*

Defective Cell Wall Bacteria: *Chlamydia pneumoniae*, *Chlamydia psittaci*, *Chlamydia trachomatis*, *Coxiella burnetii*, *Mycoplasma pneumoniae*, *Rickettsia prowazekii*, *Rickettsia rickettsii*, *Rickettsia typhi*, *Ureaplasma urealyticum*

Spirochetes: *Borrelia burgdorferi*, *Leptospira*, *Treponema pallidum*

Mycobacteria: *M avium complex*, *M kansasii*, *M leprae*, *M TB*

OSELTAMIVIR (*Tamiflu*) <u>Influenza A/B:</u> For treatment, give each dose bid for 5 days starting within 2 days of symptom onset. For prevention, give each dose once daily for 10 days starting within 2 days of exposure. For adults each dose is 75 mg. For peds, age 1 yo or older, each dose is 30 mg for wt 15 kg or less; 45 mg for wt 16 to 23 kg; 60 mg for wt 24 to 40 kg; and 75 mg for wt greater than 40 kg or age 13 yo or older. <u>Influenza treatment in infants younger than 1 yo:</u> 3 mg/kg/dose PO bid for 5 days. <u>Influenza prophylaxis in infants 3 to 11 months old:</u> 3 mg/kg/dose PO once daily. Due to limited data, prophylaxis is not recommended for infants younger than 3 mo unless the situation is critical. Can take with food to improve tolerability. [Trade only: Caps 30, 45, 75 mg. Susp 12 mg/mL (25 mL). Pharmacist can compound suspension (15 mg/mL).] ▶LK ♀C ▶? $$$

RIMANTADINE (*Flumadine*) <u>Treatment or prevention of influenza A in adults:</u> 100 mg PO bid. Reduce dose to 100 mg PO once daily for age older than 65 yo. <u>Peds influenza A prophylaxis:</u> 5 mg/kg (up to 150 mg/day) PO once daily for age 1 to 9 yo. Use adult dose for age 10 yo or older. Start treatment within 2 days of symptom onset and continue for 7 days. The CDC generally recommends against amantadine/rimantadine for treatment/prevention of influenza A in the United States due to high levels of resistance. [Generic/Trade: Tabs 100 mg. Pharmacist can compound suspension.] ▶LK ♀C ▶– $$$

ZANAMIVIR (*Relenza*) <u>Influenza A/B treatment:</u> 2 puffs bid for 5 days for adults and children 7 yo or older. <u>Influenza A/B prevention:</u> 2 puffs once daily for 10 days for adults and children 5 yo or older starting within 2 days of exposure. Do not use if chronic airway disease. [Trade only: Rotadisk inhaler 5 mg/puff (20 puffs).] ▶K ♀C ▶? $$$

Antiviral Agents—Other

ADEFOVIR (*Hepsera*) <u>Chronic hepatitis B:</u> 10 mg PO daily. Nephrotoxic; lactic acidosis and hepatic steatosis; discontinuation may exacerbate hepatitis B; may result in HIV resistance in untreated HIV infection. [Trade only: Tabs 10 mg.] ▶K ♀C ▶– $$$$$

ENTECAVIR (*Baraclude*) <u>Chronic hepatitis B:</u> 0.5 mg PO once daily if treatment-naive; give 1 mg if lamivudine-resistant, history of viremia despite lamivudine treatment, or HIV coinfected. Give on empty stomach. [Trade only: Tabs 0.5, 1 mg.] ▶K ♀C ▶– $$$$$

INTERFERON ALFA-2B (*Intron A*) <u>Chronic hepatitis B:</u> 5 million units/day or 10 million units 3 times per week SC/IM for 16 weeks if HBeAg+, for 48 weeks if HBeAg-. [Trade only: Powder/soln for injection 18, 50 million units/vial. Soln for injection 18, 25 million units/multidose vial. Multidose injection pens 3, 5, 10 million units/0.2 mL (1.5 mL), 6 doses/pen.] ▶K ♀C ▶?+ $$$$$

PALIVIZUMAB (*Synagis*) <u>Prevention of respiratory syncytial virus pulmonary disease in high-risk infants:</u> 15 mg/kg IM once monthly during RSV season. ▶L ♀C ▶? $$$$$

PEGINTERFERON ALFA-2A (*Pegasys*) <u>Chronic hepatitis C:</u> 180 mcg SC in abdomen or thigh once a week for 48 weeks with or without PO ribavirin. <u>Hepatitis B:</u> 180 mcg SC in abdomen or thigh once a week for 48 weeks. May cause or worsen severe autoimmune, neuropsychiatric, ischemic, and infectious diseases. Frequent clinical and lab monitoring. [Trade only: 180 mcg/1 mL soln in single-use vial, 180 mcg/0.5 mL prefilled syringe.] ▶LK ♀C ▶– $$$$$

PEGINTERFERON ALFA-2B (*PEG-Intron*) <u>Chronic hepatitis C:</u> Give SC once a week on same day each week. Monotherapy 1 mcg/kg/week. In combo with oral ribavirin: 1.5 mcg/kg/week with ribavirin 800 to 1400 mg/day PO divided bid. Peds, age older than 3 yo: 60 mcg/m2 SC once a week with ribavirin 15 mg/kg/day PO divided bid. May cause or worsen severe autoimmune, neuropsychiatric, ischemic, and infectious diseases. Frequent clinical and lab monitoring. [Trade only: 50, 80, 120, 150 mcg/ 0.5 mL single-use vials with diluent, 2 syringes, and alcohol swabs. Disposable single-dose Redipen 50, 80, 120, 150 mcg.] ▶K? ♀C ▶– $$$$$

RIBAVIRIN—INHALED (*Virazole*) <u>Severe respiratory syncytial virus infection in children:</u> Aerosol 12 to 18 h/day for 3 to 7 days. Beware of sudden pulmonary deterioration; drug precipitation can cause ventilator dysfunction. ▶Lung ♀X ▶– $$$$$

RIBAVIRIN—ORAL (*Rebetol, Copegus, Ribasphere*) In combination with ribavirin for chronic hepatitis C, peginterferon is preferred over interferon alfa because of substantially higher response rate. Regimen and duration of treatment is based on genotype. Divide daily dose of ribavirin bid and give with food. <u>Chronic hepatitis C, genotypes 1 and 4:</u> Treat for 48 weeks, evaluating response after 12 weeks. Ribavirin in combo with peginterferon alfa-2b (PegIntron): 800 mg/day PO for wt 65 kg or less, 1000 mg/day for wt 66 kg to 85 kg, 1200 mg/day for wt 86 kg to 105 kg, 1400 mg/day

(cont.)

for wt greater than 105 kg. Ribavirin in combo with peginterferon alfa-2a (Pegasys): 1000 mg/day PO for wt less than 75 kg, 1200 mg/day for wt 75 kg or greater. <u>Chronic hepatitis C, genotypes 2 and 3:</u> Treat for 24 weeks with ribavirin 800 mg/day in combo with peginterferon. <u>Chronic hepatitis C, children age 2 yo and older:</u> Treat for 48 weeks with peginterferon alfa-2b in combo with ribavirin 15 mg/kg/day PO divided bid. Can cause hemolytic anemia; dosage adjustments required based on Hb. [Generic/Trade: Caps 200 mg, Tabs 200, 500 mg. Generic only: Tabs 400, 600 mg. Trade only (Rebetol): Oral soln 40 mg/mL (100 mL).] ▶Cellular, K ♀X ▶− $$$$$

TELBIVUDINE (*Tyzeka*)   <u>Chronic hepatitis B:</u> 600 mg PO once daily. [Trade only: Tabs 600 mg. Oral soln 100 mg/5 mL (300 mL).] ▶K ♀B ▶− $$$$$

Carbapenems

DORIPENEM (*Doribax*)   500 mg IV q 8 h. ▶K ♀B ▶? $$$$$
ERTAPENEM (*Invanz*)   1 g IV/IM q 24 h. <u>Prophylaxis, colorectal surgery:</u> 1 g IV 1 h before incision. Peds, younger than 13 yo: 15 mg/kg IV/IM q 12 h (up to 1 g/day). Infuse IV over 30 min. ▶K ♀B ▶? $$$$$
IMIPENEM-CILASTATIN (*Primaxin*)   250 to 1000 mg IV q 6 to 8 h. Peds, age older than 3 mo: 15 to 25 mg/kg IV q 6 h. Seizures (especially if given with ganciclovir, elderly with renal dysfunction, or cerebrovascular or seizure disorder). ▶K ♀C ▶? $$$$$
MEROPENEM (*Merrem IV*)   <u>Complicated skin infections:</u> 10 mg/kg up to 500 mg IV q 8 h. <u>Intra-abdominal infections:</u> 20 mg/kg up to 1 g IV q 8 h. <u>Peds meningitis:</u> 40 mg/kg IV q 8 h for age 3 mo or older; 2 g IV q 8 h for wt greater than 50 kg. ▶K ♀B ▶? $$$$$

Cephalosporins—1st Generation

CEFADROXIL (*Duricef*)   1 to 2 g/day PO once daily or divided bid. Peds: 30 mg/kg/day divided bid. [Generic/Trade: Tabs 1 g. Caps 500 mg. Susp 125, 250, 500 mg/5 mL.] ▶K ♀B ▶+ $$$
CEFAZOLIN (*Ancef*)   0.5 to 1.5 g IM/IV q 6 to 8 h. Peds: 25 to 50 mg/kg/day divided q 6 to 8 h (up to 100 mg/kg for severe infections). ▶K ♀B ▶+ $$
CEPHALEXIN (*Keflex, Panixine DisperDose*)   250 to 500 mg PO qid. Peds: 25 to 50 mg/kg/day. Not for otitis media, sinusitis. [Generic/Trade: Caps 250, 500 mg. Generic only: Tabs 250, 500 mg. Susp 125, 250 mg/5 mL. Panixine DisperDose 125, 250 mg scored tabs for oral susp. Trade only: Caps 333, 750 mg.] ▶K ♀B ▶? $$$

Cephalosporins—2nd Generation

CEFACLOR (*Ceclor, Raniclor*)   250 to 500 mg PO tid. Peds: 20 to 40 mg/kg/day PO divided tid. <u>Otitis media:</u> 40 mg/kg/day PO divided bid. <u>Group A streptococcal</u>

(cont.)

pharyngitis: 20 mg/kg/day PO divided bid. Serum sickness-like reactions with repeated use. [Generic only: Caps 250, 500 mg, Susp, Chewable tabs 125, 187, 250, 375 mg per 5 mL or tab.] ▶K ♀B ▶? $$$$

CEFOXITIN (*Mefoxin*) 1 to 2 g IM/IV q 6 to 8 h. Peds: 80 to 160 mg/kg/day IV divided q 4 to 8 h. ▶K ♀B ▶+ $$$$$

CEFPROZIL (*Cefzil*) 250 to 500 mg PO bid. Peds otitis media: 15 mg/kg/dose PO bid. Peds group A streptococcal pharyngitis (2nd line to penicillin): 7.5 mg/kg/dose PO bid for 10 days. [Generic/Trade: Tabs 250, 500 mg. Susp 125, 250 mg/5 mL.] ▶K ♀B ▶+ $$$$

CEFUROXIME (*Zinacef, Ceftin*) Adult: 750 to 1500 mg IM/IV q 8 h. 250 to 500 mg PO bid. Peds: 50 to 100 mg/kg/day IV divided q 6 to 8 h; not for meningitis; 20 to 30 mg/kg/day susp PO divided bid. [Generic/Trade: Tabs 125, 250, 500 mg. Susp 125, 250 mg/5 mL.] ▶K ♀B ▶? $$$

Cephalosporins—3rd Generation

CEFDINIR (*Omnicef*) 14 mg/kg/day up to 600 mg/day PO once daily or divided bid. [Generic/Trade: Caps 300 mg. Susp 125, 250 mg/5 mL.] ▶K ♀B ▶? $$$$

CEFDITOREN (*Spectracef*) 200 to 400 mg PO bid with food. [Trade only: Tabs 200, 400 mg.] ▶K ♀B ▶? $$$$$

CEFIXIME (*Suprax*) 400 mg PO once daily. Gonorrhea: 400 mg PO single dose. Peds: 8 mg/kg/day once daily or divided bid. [Trade only: Susp 100, 200 mg/5 mL. Tabs 400 mg.] ▶K/Bile ♀B ▶? $$

CEFOTAXIME (*Claforan*) Usual dose: 1 to 2 g IM/IV q 6 to 8 h. Peds: 50 to 180 mg/kg/day IM/IV divided q 4 to 6 h. AAP dose for pneumococcal meningitis: 225 to 300 mg/kg/day IV divided q 6 to 8 h. ▶KL ♀B ▶+ $$$$$

CEFPODOXIME (*Vantin*) 100 to 400 mg PO bid. Peds: 10 mg/kg/day divided bid. [Generic/Trade: Tabs 100, 200 mg. Susp 50, 100 mg/5 mL.] ▶K ♀B ▶? $$$$

CEFTAZIDIME (*Ceptaz, Fortaz, Tazicef*) 1 g IM/IV or 2 g IV q 8 to 12 h. Peds: 30 to 50 mg/kg IV q 8 h. ▶K ♀B ▶+ $$$$$

CEFTIBUTEN (*Cedax*) 400 mg PO once daily. Peds: 9 mg/kg (up to 400 mg) PO once daily. [Trade only: Caps 400 mg. Susp 90 mg/5 mL.] ▶K ♀B ▶? $$$$$

CEPHALOSPORINS – GENERAL ANTIMICROBIAL SPECTRUM

1st generation: gram positive (including Staph aureus); basic gram neg. coverage

2nd generation: diminished Staph aureus, improved gram negative coverage compared to 1st generation; some with anaerobic coverage

3rd generation: further diminished Staph aureus, further improved gram negative coverage compared to 1st & 2nd generation; some with Pseudomonal coverage & diminished gram positive coverage

4th generation: same as 3rd generation plus coverage against Pseudomonas

CEFTIZOXIME (*Cefizox*) 1 to 2 g IV q 8 to 12 h. Peds: 50 mg/kg/dose IV q 6 to 8 h. ▶K ♀B ▶? $$$$$

CEFTRIAXONE (*Rocephin*) 1 to 2 g IM/IV q 24 h. <u>Meningitis:</u> 2 g IV q 12 h. <u>Gonorrhea:</u> Single dose 125 mg IM (250 mg if PID). Peds: 50 to 75 mg/kg/day (up to 2 g/day) divided q 12 to 24 h. <u>Peds meningitis:</u> 100 mg/kg/day (up to 4 g/day) IV divided q 12 to 24 h. <u>Otitis media:</u> 50 mg/kg up to 1 g IM single dose. May dilute in 1% lidocaine for IM. Contraindicated in neonates who require (or are expected to require) IV calcium (including calcium in TPN); fatal lung/kidney precipitation of calcium ceftriaxone has been reported in neonates. In other patients, do not give ceftriaxone and calcium-containing solns simultaneously, but sequential administration is acceptable if lines are flushed with a compatible fluid between infusions. ▶K/Bile ♀B ▶+ $$$

Cephalosporins—4th Generation

CEFEPIME (*Maxipime*) 0.5 to 2 g IM/IV q 12 h. Peds: 50 mg/kg IV q 8 to 12 h. ▶K ♀B ▶? $$$$$

Macrolides

AZITHROMYCIN (*Zithromax, Zmax*) 500 mg IV daily. 10 mg/kg (up to 500 mg) PO on day 1, then 5 mg/kg (up to 250 mg) daily for 4 days. <u>Otitis media:</u> 30 mg/kg PO single dose or 10 mg/kg PO daily for 3 days. <u>Peds sinusitis:</u> 10 mg/kg PO daily for 3 days. <u>Group A streptococcal pharyngitis</u> (second-line to penicillin): 12 mg/kg (up to 500 mg) PO daily for 5 days. <u>Adult acute sinusitis or exacerbation of chronic bronchitis:</u> 500 mg PO daily for 3 days. Zmax for <u>community-acquired pneumonia, acute sinusitis:</u> 60 mg/kg (up to 2 g) PO single dose on empty stomach; give adult dose of 2 g for wt 34 kg or greater. <u>Chlamydia (including pregnancy), chancroid:</u> 1 g PO single dose. <u>Prevention of disseminated Mycobacterium avium complex disease:</u> 1200 mg PO once a week. <u>Pertussis treatment/post-exposure prophylaxis:</u> 10 mg/kg PO once daily for 5 days for infants age younger than 6 mo; 10 mg/kg (max 500 mg) PO on day 1, then 5 mg/kg (max 250 mg) PO once daily for 4 days for children 6 mo of age and older; 500 mg PO on day 1, then 250 mg PO daily for 4 days for adolescents and adults. [Generic/Trade: Tabs 250, 500, 600 mg. Susp 100, 200 mg/5 mL. Trade only: Packet 1000 mg. Z-Pak: #6, 250 mg tab. Tri-Pak: #3, 500 mg tab. Zmax extended-release oral susp: 2 g in 60 mL single-dose bottle.] ▶L ♀B ▶? $$

CLARITHROMYCIN (*Biaxin, Biaxin XL*) 250 to 500 mg PO bid. Peds: 7.5 mg/kg PO bid. <u>H pylori:</u> See table in GI section. See table for prophylaxis of <u>bacterial endocarditis. Mycobacterium avium complex disease prevention:</u> 7.5 mg/kg up to 500 mg PO bid. Biaxin XL: 1000 mg PO daily with food. [Generic/Trade: Tabs 250, 500 mg. Extended-release tab 500 mg. Susp 125, 250 mg/ 5 mL. Trade only: Biaxin XL-Pak: #14, 500 mg tabs. Generic only: Extended-release tab 1000 mg.] ▶KL ♀C ▶? $$$

ERYTHROMYCIN BASE (*Eryc, E-mycin, Ery-Tab, ✦Erybid, Erythromid, P.C.E.*) Adult: 250 to 500 mg PO qid, 333 mg PO tid, or 500 mg PO bid. Peds: 30 to 50 mg/kg/day PO divided qid. [Generic/Trade: Tabs 250, 333, 500 mg, delayed-release cap 250.] ▶L ♀B ▶+ $

SEXUALLY TRANSMITTED DISEASES & VAGINITIS*

Bacterial vaginosis: (1) metronidazole 5 g of 0.75% gel intravaginally daily for 5 days OR 500 mg PO bid for 7 days. (2) clindamycin 5 g of 2% cream intravaginally at bedtime for 7 days. In pregnancy: (1) metronidazole 500 mg PO bid for 7 days OR 250 mg PO tid for 7 days. (2) clindamycin 300 mg PO bid for 7 days.
Candidal vaginitis: (1) intravaginal clotrimazole, miconazole, terconazole, nystatin, tioconazole, or butoconazole. (2) fluconazole 150 mg PO single dose.
Chancroid: Single dose of: (1) azithromycin 1 g PO or (2) ceftriaxone 250 mg IM.
Chlamydia: First line either azithromycin 1 g PO single dose or doxycycline 100 mg PO bid for 7 days. Second line fluoroquinolones or erythromycin. In pregnancy: (1) azithromycin 1 g PO single dose. (2) amoxicillin 500 mg PO tid for 7 days. Repeat NAAT[‡] 3 weeks after treatment.
Epididymitis: (1) ceftriaxone 250 mg IM single dose + doxycycline 100 mg PO bid for 10 days. (2) ofloxacin 300 mg PO bid or levofloxacin 500 mg PO daily for 10 days if enteric organisms suspected, or negative gonococcal culture or NAAT.[‡]
Gonorrhea: Single dose of (1) ceftriaxone 125 mg IM (2) cefixime 400 mg PO (not for pharyngeal).[§,†] Treat chlamydia empirically.
Gonorrhea, disseminated: Initially treat with ceftriaxone 1 g IM/IV q 24 h until 24 to 48 h after improvement. Second-line alternatives: (1) cefotaxime 1 g IV q 8 h. (2) ceftizoxime 1 g IV q 8 h.[§] Complete 1 week of treatment with: (1) cefixime tabs 400 mg PO bid. (2) cefixime susp 500 mg PO bid. (3) cefpodoxime 400 mg PO bid.[†]
Gonorrhea, meningitis: ceftriaxone 1 to 2 g IV q 12 h for 10 to 14 days.[†]
Gonorrhea, endocarditis: ceftriaxone 1 to 2 g IV q 12 h for at least 4 weeks.[§]
Granuloma inguinale: doxycycline 100 mg PO bid for at least 3 weeks and until lesions completely healed. Alternative azithromycin 1 g PO once weekly for 3 weeks.
Herpes simplex (genital, first episode): (1) acyclovir 400 mg PO tid for 7 to 10 days. (2) famciclovir 250 mg PO tid for 7 to 10 days. (3) valacyclovir 1 g PO bid for 7 to 10 days.
Herpes simplex (genital, recurrent): (1) acyclovir 400 mg PO tid for 5 days. (2) acyclovir 800 mg PO tid for 2 days or bid for 5 days. (3) famciclovir 125 mg PO bid for 5 days. (4) famciclovir 1 g PO bid for 1 day. (5) valacyclovir 500 mg PO bid for 3 days. (6) valacyclovir 1 g PO daily for 5 days.
Herpes simplex (suppressive therapy): (1) acyclovir 400 mg PO bid. (2) famciclovir 250 mg PO bid. (3) valacyclovir 500 to 1000 mg PO daily.
Herpes simplex (genital, recurrent in HIV infection): (1) Acyclovir 400 mg PO tid for 5 to 10 days. (2) famciclovir 500 mg PO bid for 5 to 10 days. (3) Valacyclovir 1 g PO bid for 5 to 10 days.
Herpes simplex (suppressive therapy in HIV infection): (1) Acyclovir 400 to 800 mg PO bid to tid. (2) Famciclovir 500 mg PO bid. (3) Valacyclovir 500 mg PO bid.
Herpes simplex (prevention of transmission in immunocompetent patients with not more than 9 recurrences/year): Valacyclovir 500 mg PO daily by source partner, in conjunction with safer sex practices.
Lymphogranuloma venereum: (1) doxycycline 100 mg PO bid for 21 days. Alternative: erythromycin base 500 mg PO qid for 21 days.
Pelvic inflammatory disease (PID), inpatient regimens: (1) cefoxitin 2 g IV q6h + doxycycline 100 mg PO/IV q 12 h. (2) clindamycin 900 mg IV q 8 h + gentamicin 2 mg/kg IM/IV loading dose, then 1.5 mg/kg IM/IV q 8 h (See gentamicin entry for alternative daily dosing). Can switch to PO therapy within 24 h of improvement.
Pelvic inflammatory disease (PID), outpatient treatment: (1) ceftriaxone 250 mg IM single dose + doxycycline 100 mg PO bid +/− metronidazole 500 mg PO bid for 14 days.

(cont.)

SEXUALLY TRANSMITTED DISEASES & VAGINITIS* (continued)

Proctitis, proctocolitis, enteritis: ceftriaxone 125 mg IM single dose + doxycycline 100 mg PO bid for 7 days.

Sexual assault prophylaxis: ceftriaxone 125 mg IM single dose + metronidazole 2 g PO single dose + azithromycin 1 g PO single dose/doxycycline 100 mg PO bid for 7 days. Consider giving antiemetic.

Syphilis (primary and secondary): (1) benzathine penicillin 2.4 million units IM single dose. (2) doxycycline 100 mg PO bid for 2 weeks if penicillin-allergic.

Syphilis (early latent, i.e. duration less than 1 year): (1) benzathine penicillin 2.4 million units IM single dose. (2) doxycycline 100 mg PO bid for 2 weeks if penicillin-allergic.

Syphilis (late latent or unknown duration): (1) benzathine penicillin 2.4 million units IM q week for 3 doses. (2) doxycycline 100 mg PO bid for 4 weeks if penicillin-allergic.

Syphilis (tertiary): (1) benzathine penicillin 2.4 million units IM q week for 3 doses. (2) doxycycline 100 mg PO bid for 4 weeks if penicillin-allergic.

Syphilis (neuro): (1) penicillin G 18 to 24 million units/day continuous IV infusion or 3 to 4 million units IV q 4 h for 10 to 14 days. (2) procaine penicillin 2.4 million units IM daily + probenecid 500 mg PO qid, both for 10 to 14 days.

Syphilis in pregnancy: Treat only with penicillin regimen for stage of syphilis as noted above. Use penicillin desensitization protocol if penicillin-allergic.

Trichomoniasis: metronidazole (can use in pregnancy) or tinidazole, each 2 g PO single dose.

Urethritis, Cervicitis: Test for Chlamydia and gonorrhea with NAAT.[‡] Treat based on test results or treat presumptively if high-risk of infection (Chlamydia: age 25 yo or younger, new/multiple sex partners, or unprotected sex. Gonorrhea: population prevalence greater than 5%), esp. if NAAT[‡] unavailable or patient unlikely to return for follow-up.

Urethritis (persistent/recurrent): metronidazole/ tinidazole 2 g PO single dose + azithromycin 2 g PO single dose (if not used in first episode).

---

* MMWR 2006;55:RR-11 or http://www.cdc.gov/STD/treatment/. Treat sexual partners for all except herpes, candida, and bacterial vaginosis.

[†] As of April 2007, the CDC no longer recommends fluoroquinolones for gonorrhea because of high resistance rates. Do not consider fluoroquinolone unless antimicrobial susceptibility can be documented by cultures. If parenteral cephalosporin not feasible for PID (and NAAT is negative or culture documents fluoroquinolone susceptibility), can consider levofloxacin 500 mg PO once daily or ofloxacin 400 mg PO bid +/− metronidazole 500 mg PO bid for 14 days.

[‡] NAAT = nucleic acid amplification test.

§Cephalosporin desensitization advised for cephalosporin-allergic patients (e.g. pregnant women).

ERYTHROMYCIN ETHYL SUCCINATE (_EES, Eryped_)   400 mg PO qid. Peds: 30 to 50 mg/kg/day PO divided qid. [Generic/Trade: Tabs 400. Susp 200, 400 mg/5 mL. Trade only (EryPed): Susp 100 mg/2.5 mL (50 mL).]   ▶L ♀B ▶+ $

ERYTHROMYCIN LACTOBIONATE (✦_Erythrocin IV_)   15 to 20 mg/kg/day (max 4 g) IV divided q 6 h. Peds: 15 to 50 mg/kg/day IV divided q 6 h.   ▶L ♀B ▶+ $$$$$

PEDIAZOLE (erythromycin ethyl succinate + sulfisoxazole) 50 mg/kg/day (based on EES dose) PO divided tid to qid. [Generic/Trade: Susp, erythromycin ethyl succinate 200 mg + sulfisoxazole 600 mg/5 mL.] ▶KL ♀C ▶– $$

Penicillins—1st generation—Natural

BENZATHINE PENICILLIN (*Bicillin L-A*, *✦Megacillin*) Adults and peds wt greater than 27 kg: 1.2 million units IM. Peds wt 27 kg or less: 600,000 units IM. Doses last 2 to 4 weeks. Give IM q month for secondary prevention of rheumatic fever (q 3 weeks for high-risk patients). [Trade only: For IM use, 600,000 units/mL; 1, 2, 4 mL syringes.] ▶K ♀B ▶? $$

BICILLIN C-R (procaine penicillin + benzathine penicillin) For IM use. Not for treatment of syphilis. [Trade only: For IM use 300/300 thousand units/mL procaine/benzathine penicillin; 1, 2, 4 mL syringes.] ▶K ♀B ▶? $$$

PENICILLIN G Pneumococcal pneumonia and severe infections: 250,000 to 400,000 units/kg/day (8 to 12 million units/day in adult) IV divided q 4 to 6 h. Pneumococcal meningitis: 250,000 to 400,000 units/kg/day (24 million units/day in adult) in 4 to 6 divided doses. ▶K ♀B ▶? $$$$

PENICILLIN V (*Veetids*, *✦PVF-K, Nadopen-V*) Adults: 250 to 500 mg PO qid. Peds: 25 to 50 mg/kg/day divided bid to qid. AHA doses for pharyngitis: 250 mg (peds 27 kg or less) or 500 mg (adults and peds greater than 27 kg) PO bid to tid for 10 days. [Generic/Trade: Tabs 250, 500 mg, oral soln 125, 250 mg/5 mL.] ▶K ♀B ▶? $

PROCAINE PENICILLIN (*Wycillin*) 0.6 to 1 million units IM daily (peak 4 h, lasts 24 h). [Generic: For IM use, 600,000 units/mL; 1, 2 mL syringes.] ▶K ♀B ▶? $$$$$

Penicillins—2nd generation—Penicillinase-Resistant

DICLOXACILLIN (*Dynapen*) 250 to 500 mg PO qid. Peds: 12.5 to 25 mg/kg/day PO divided qid. [Generic only: Caps 250, 500 mg.] ▶KL ♀B ▶? $$

NAFCILLIN 1 to 2 g IM/IV q 4 h. Peds: 50 to 200 mg/kg/day IM/IV divided q 4 to 6 h. ▶L ♀B ▶? $$$$$

OXACILLIN (*Bactocill*) 1 to 2 g IM/IV q 4 to 6 h. Peds 150 to 200 mg/kg/day IM/IV divided q 4 to 6 h. ▶KL ♀B ▶? $$$$$

Penicillins—3rd generation—Aminopenicillins

AMOXICILLIN (*Amoxil, DisperMox, Moxatag, Trimox*, *✦Novamoxin*) 250 to 500 mg PO tid, or 500 to 875 mg PO bid. High-dose for community-acquired pneumonia, acute sinusitis: 1 g PO tid. Lyme disease: 500 mg PO tid for 14 days for early disease, for 28 days for Lyme arthritis. Chlamydia in pregnancy: 500 mg PO tid for 7 days. AHA dosing for group A streptococcal pharyngitis: 50 mg/kg (max 1 g) PO once daily for 10 days. Group A streptococcal pharyngitis/ tonsillitis: 775 mg ER tab (Moxatag) PO for 10 days for age 12 yo or older. Peds AAP otitis media: 90 mg/kg/day divided bid. AAP recommends 5 to 7 days of therapy for age 6 yo or older with non-severe otitis media, and 10 days for younger children and those with severe disease. Peds infections other

(cont.)

<u>than otitis media</u>: 40 mg/kg/day PO divided tid or 45 mg/kg/day divided bid. [Generic/Trade: Caps 250, 500 mg, Tabs 500, 875 mg, Chewable tabs 125, 200, 250, 400 mg. Susp 125, 250 mg/5 mL. Susp 200, 400 mg/5 mL. Trade only: Infant gtts 50 mg/mL (Amoxil). DisperMox 200, 400, 600 mg tabs for oral susp, Moxatag 775 mg extended-release tab.] ▶K ♀B ▶+ $

AMOXICILLIN-CLAVULANATE (*Augmentin, Augmentin ES-600, Augmentin XR, ✦Clavulin*) 500 to 875 mg PO bid or 250 to 500 mg tid. Augmentin XR: 2 tabs PO q 12 h with meals. Peds AAP otitis media: Augmentin ES 90 mg/kg/day divided bid. AAP recommends 5 to 7 days of therapy for age 6 yo or older non-severe otitis media, and 10 days for younger children and those with severe disease. Peds: 45 mg/kg/day PO divided tid or 40 mg/kg/day divided tid for <u>sinusitis, pneumonia, otitis media</u>; 25 mg/kg/day divided bid or 20 mg/kg/day divided tid for less severe infections. [Generic/Trade: (amoxicillin/clavulanate) Tabs 250/125, 500/125, 875/125 mg, Chewables, Susp 200/28.5, 400/57 per tab or 5 mL, 250/62.5 mg per 5 mL, (ES) Susp 600/42.9 mg per 5 mL. Trade only: Chewables, Susp 125/31.25 per tab or 5 mL, 250/62.5 mg per tab. Extended-release tabs (Augmentin XR) 1000/62.5 mg.] ▶K ♀B ▶? $$$$

AMPICILLIN (*Principen, ✦Penbritin*) Usual dose: 1 to 2 g IV q 4 to 6 h. <u>Sepsis, meningitis</u>: 150 to 200 mg/kg/day IV divided q 3 to 4 h. Peds: 10 to 400 mg/kg/day IM/IV divided q 4 to 6 h. [Generic/Trade: Caps 250, 500 mg. Susp 125, 250 mg/5 mL.] ▶K ♀B ▶? $ PO $$$$$ IV

AMPICILLIN-SULBACTAM (*Unasyn*) 1.5 to 3 g IM/IV q 6 h. Peds: 100 to 400 mg/kg/day of ampicillin divided q 6 h. ▶K ♀B ▶? $$$$$

Penicillins—4th generation—Extended Spectrum

PIPERACILLIN Usual dose: 3 to 4 g IM/IV q 4 to 6 h. ▶K/Bile ♀B ▶? $$$$$
PIPERACILLIN-TAZOBACTAM (*Zosyn, ✦Tazocin*) 3.375 to 4.5 g IV q 6 h. Peds appendicitis or peritonitis: 80 mg/kg IV q 8 h for age 2 to 9 mo, 100 mg/kg piperacillin IV q 8 h for age older than 9 mo, use adult dose for wt greater than 40 kg. ▶K ♀B ▶? $$$$$

PROPHYLAXIS FOR BACTERIAL ENDOCARDITIS*

Limited to dental or respiratory tract procedures in patients at highest risk. All regimens are single doses administered 30-60 minutes prior to procedure.	
Standard regimen	amoxicillin 2 g PO
Unable to take oral meds	ampicillin 2 g IM/IV; or cefazolin† or ceftriaxone† 1 g IM/IV
Allergic to penicillin	clindamycin 600 mg PO; or cephalexin† 2 g PO; or azithromycin or clarithromycin 500 mg PO
Allergic to penicillin and unable to take oral meds	clindamycin 600 mg IM/IV; or cefazolin† or ceftriaxone† 1 g IM/IV
Pediatric drug doses	Pediatric dose should not exceed adult dose. Amoxicillin 50 mg/kg, ampicillin 50 mg/kg, azithromycin 15 mg/kg, cephalexin† 50 mg/kg, cefazolin† 50 mg/kg, ceftriaxone† 50 mg/kg, clarithromycin 15 mg/kg, clindamycin 20 mg/kg.

*For additional details of the 2007 AHA guidelines, see http://www.americanheart.org.
†Avoid cephalosporins if prior penicillin-associated anaphylaxis, angioedema, or urticaria.

PENICILLINS — GENERAL ANTIMICROBIAL SPECTRUM

1st generation: Most streptococci; oral anaerobic coverage
2nd generation: Most streptococci; *Staph aureus* (but not MRSA)
3rd generation: Most streptococci; basic gram negative coverage
4th generation: *Pseudomonas*

TICARCILLIN-CLAVULANATE (*Timentin*) 3.1 g IV q 4 to 6 h. Peds: 50 mg/kg up to 3.1 g IV q 4 to 6 h. ▶K ♀B ▶? $$$$$

Quinolones—2nd Generation

CIPROFLOXACIN (*Cipro, Cipro XR, ProQuin XR*) 200 to 400 mg IV q 8 to 12 h. 250 to 750 mg PO bid. <u>Simple UTI:</u> 250 mg bid for 3 days or Cipro XR/ ProQuin XR 500 mg PO daily for 3 days. Give ProQuin XR with main meal of day. Cipro XR for <u>pyelonephritis or complicated UTI:</u> 1000 mg PO daily for 7 to 14 days. [Generic/Trade: Tabs 100, 250, 500, 750 mg. Extended-release tabs 500, 1000 mg. Trade only (ProQuin XR): Extended-release tabs 500 mg, blister pack 500 mg (#3 tabs).] ▶LK ♀C but teratogenicity unlikely ▶?+ $
NORFLOXACIN (*Noroxin*) <u>Simple UTI:</u> 400 mg PO bid for 3 days. [Trade only: Tabs 400 mg.] ▶LK ♀C ▶? $
OFLOXACIN (*Floxin*) 200 to 400 mg PO bid. [Generic/Trade: Tabs 200, 300, 400 mg.] ▶LK ♀C ▶?+ $$$

Quinolones—3rd Generation

LEVOFLOXACIN (*Levaquin*) 250 to 750 mg PO/IV daily. [Trade only: Tabs 250, 500, 750 mg, Oral soln 25 mg/mL. Leva-Pak: #5, 750 mg tabs.] ▶KL ♀C ▶? $$$$

Quinolones—4th Generation

GEMIFLOXACIN (*Factive*) 320 mg PO daily for 5 to 7 days. [Trade only: Tabs 320 mg.] ▶Feces, K ♀C ▶− $$$$
MOXIFLOXACIN (*Avelox*) 400 mg PO/IV daily for 5 days (<u>chronic bronchitis exacerbation</u>), 5 to 14 days (<u>complicated intra-abdominal infection</u>), 7 days (<u>uncomplicated skin infections</u>), 10 days (<u>acute sinusitis</u>), 7 to 14 days (<u>community-acquired pneumonia</u>), 7 to 21 days (<u>complicated skin infections</u>). [Trade only: Tabs 400 mg.] ▶LK ♀C ▶− $$$

QUINOLONES—GENERAL ANTIMICROBIAL SPECTRUM

1st generation: gram negative (excluding *Pseudomonas*), urinary tract only, no atypicals
2nd generation: gram negative (including *Pseudomonas*); *Staph aureus* (but not MRSA or *pneumococcus*); some atypicals
3rd generation: gram negative (including *Pseudomonas*); gram positive, including *pneumococcus* and *Staph aureus* (but not MRSA); expanded atypical coverage
4th generation: same as 3rd generation plus enhanced coverage of *pneumococcus*, decreased activity vs. *Pseudomonas*

Sulfonamides

SULFADIAZINE CNS toxoplasmosis in AIDS. Acute treatment: 1000 mg PO qid for wt less than 60 kg to 1500 mg PO qid for wt 60 kg or greater. Secondary prevention: 2000 to 4000 mg/day PO divided bid to qid. Give with pyrimethamine + leucovorin. [Generic only: Tabs 500 mg.] ▶K ♀C ▶+ $$$$

TRIMETHOPRIM-SULFAMETHOXAZOLE (*Bactrim, Septra, Sulfatrim, cotrimoxazole*) 1 tab PO bid, double-strength (DS, 160 mg/800 mg) or single-strength (SS, 80 mg/400 mg). Pneumocystis treatment: 15 to 20 mg/kg/day (based on TMP) IV divided q 6 to 8 h or PO divided tid for 21 days total. Pneumocystis prophylaxis: 1 DS tab PO daily. Peds usual dose: 1 mL/kg/day susp PO divided bid (up to 20 mL PO bid). Community-acquired MRSA skin infections. Adults: 1 to 2 DS tabs PO bid for 7 to 10 days. Peds: 8 to 12 mg/kg/day (based on TMP) PO divided bid. [Generic/Trade: Tabs 80 mg TMP/400 mg SMX (single strength), 160 mg TMP/800 mg SMX (double strength; DS). Susp 40 mg TMP/200 mg SMX per 5 mL. 20 mL susp is equivalent to 2 SS tabs or equivalent to 1 DS tab.] ▶K ♀C ▶+ $

Tetracyclines

DEMECLOCYCLINE (*Declomycin*) Usual dose: 150 mg PO qid or 300 mg PO bid on empty stomach. SIADH: 600 to 1200 mg/day PO given in 3 to 4 divided doses. [Generic/Trade: Tabs 150, 300 mg.] ▶K, feces ♀D ▶?+ $$$$

DOXYCYCLINE (*Adoxa, Doryx, Monodox, Oracea, Periostat, Vibramycin, Vibra-Tabs, ✦Doxycin*) 100 mg PO bid on first day, then 50 mg bid or 100 mg daily. Severe infections: 100 mg PO/IV bid. Community-acquired MRSA skin infections: 100 mg PO bid. Lyme disease: 100 mg PO bid for 14 days for early disease, for 28 days for Lyme arthritis. Acne: Up to 100 mg PO bid. Periostat ($$$$$) for periodontitis: 20 mg PO bid. Oracea ($$$$$) for inflammatory rosacea: 40 mg PO once every morning on empty stomach. Malaria prophylaxis: 2 mg/kg/day up to 100 mg PO daily starting 1 to 2 days before exposure until 4 weeks after. Avoid in children age younger than 8 yo due to teeth staining. [Generic/Trade: Tabs 75, 100 mg, Caps 20, 50, 100 mg. Susp 25 mg/5 mL (60 mL). Trade only: (Vibramycin) Syrup 50 mg/5 mL (480 mL). Delayed-release: Tabs 75, 100 mg (Doryx $$$$$), Caps 40 mg (Oracea $$$$$). Generic only: Caps 75, 150 mg tabs 50, 150 mg.] ▶LK ♀D ▶?+ $

MINOCYCLINE (*Minocin, Dynacin, Solodyn, ✦Enca*) 200 mg IV/PO initially, then 100 mg q 12 h. Community-acquired MRSA skin infections: 100 mg PO bid. Acne (traditional dosing, not Solodyn): 50 mg PO bid. Solodyn ($$$$$) for inflammatory acne in adults and children 12 yo and older: Give PO once daily at dose of 45 mg for wt 45 to 54 kg, 65 mg for wt 55 to 77 kg, 90 mg for wt 78 to 102 kg, 115 mg for wt 103 to 125 kg, 135 mg for wt 126 to 136 kg. [Generic/Trade: Caps, Tabs 50, 75, 100 mg. Tabs, extended-release (Solodyn) 45, 90, 135 mg. Trade only: Tabs, extended-release (Solodyn) 65, 115 mg.] ▶LK ♀D ▶?+ $$

TETRACYCLINE (*Sumycin*) 250 to 500 mg PO qid. [Generic only: Caps 250, 500 mg.] ▶LK ♀D ▶?+ $

Other Antimicrobials

AZTREONAM (*Azactam*)   0.5 to 2 g IM/IV q 6 to 12 h. Peds: 30 mg/kg IV q 6 to 8 h. ▶K ♀B ▶+ $$$$$

CHLORAMPHENICOL (*Chloromycetin*)   50 to 100 mg/kg/day IV divided q 6 h. Aplastic anemia. ▶LK ♀C ▶− $$$$$

CLINDAMYCIN (*Cleocin*, ◆*Dalacin C*)   150 to 450 mg PO qid. 600 to 900 mg IV q 8 h. <u>Community-acquired MRSA skin infections:</u> 300 mg PO tid for adults; 30 mg/kg/day PO divided tid for peds. Peds: 20 to 40 mg/kg/day IV divided q 6 to 8 h or give 8 to 25 mg/kg/day susp PO divided q 6 to 8 h. [Generic/Trade: Caps 75, 150, 300 mg. Oral soln 75 mg/5 mL (100 mL).] ▶L ♀B ▶+ $$$

DAPTOMYCIN (*Cubicin, Cidecin*)   <u>Complicated skin infections (including MRSA):</u> 4 mg/kg IV daily for 7 to 14 days. <u>S. aureus bacteremia (including MRSA):</u> 6 mg/kg IV daily for at least 2 to 6 weeks. Infuse over 30 min. Not for pneumonia (inactived by surfactant). Not approved in children. ▶K ♀B ▶? $$$$$

DROTRECOGIN (*Xigris*)   To reduce mortality in <u>sepsis:</u> 24 mcg/kg/h IV for 96 h. ▶Plasma ♀C ▶? $$$$$

FOSFOMYCIN (*Monurol*)   <u>Simple UTI:</u> One 3 g packet PO single dose. [Trade only: 3 g packet of granules.] ▶K ♀B ▶? $$

LINEZOLID (*Zyvox*, ◆*Zyvoxam*)   <u>Pneumonia, complicated skin infections (including MRSA), vancomycin-resistant E faecium infections:</u> 10 mg/kg (up to 600 mg) IV/PO q 8 h for age younger than 12 yo, 600 mg IV/PO q 12 h for adults and age 12 yo or older. Myelosuppression, drug interactions due to MAO inhibition. Limit tyramine foods to less than 100 mg/meal. [Trade only: Tabs 600 mg. Susp 100 mg/ 5 mL.] ▶Oxidation/K ♀C ▶? $$$$$

METRONIDAZOLE (*Flagyl, Flagyl ER*, ◆*Florazole ER, Trikacide, Nidazol*)   <u>Bacterial vaginosis:</u> 500 mg PO bid or Flagyl ER 750 mg PO daily for 7 days. <u>H pylori:</u> See table in GI section. <u>Anaerobic bacterial infections:</u> Load 1 g or 15 mg/kg IV, then 500 mg or 7.5 mg/kg (up to 4 g/day) IV/PO q 6 to 8 h, each IV dose over 1 h. Peds: 7.5 mg/kg IV q 6 h. <u>C. difficile-associated diarrhea:</u> Adults: 500 mg PO tid for 10 to 14 days. Peds: 30 mg/kg/day PO divided qid for 10 to 14 days. See table for management of C. difficile infection. <u>Trichomoniasis:</u> 2 g PO single dose for patient and sex partners (may be used in pregnancy per CDC). <u>Giardia:</u> 250 mg (5 mg/kg/dose for peds) PO tid for 5 to 7 days. [Generic/Trade: Tabs 250, 500 mg, Caps 375 mg. Trade only: Tabs, extended-release 750 mg.] ▶KL ♀B ▶?- $

NITROFURANTOIN (*Furadantin, Macrodantin, Macrobid*)   50 to 100 mg PO qid. Peds: 5 to 7 mg/kg/day divided qid. Macrobid: 100 mg PO bid. [Generic/Trade (Macrodantin): Caps 25, 50, 100 mg, Generic/Trade (Macrobid): Caps 100 mg. Trade only (Furadantin): Susp 25 mg/5 mL.] ▶KL ♀B ▶+? $

RIFAXIMIN (*Xifaxan*)   <u>Traveler's diarrhea:</u> 200 mg PO tid for 3 days. <u>Prevention of recurrent hepatic encephalopathy ($$$$$):</u> 550 mg PO bid. [Trade only: Tabs 200, 550 mg.] ▶Feces, no GI absorption ♀C ▶? $$$

SYNERCID (quinupristin + dalfopristin)   7.5 mg/kg IV q 8 to 12 h, each dose over 1 h. Not active against E faecalis. ▶Bile ♀B ▶? $$$$$

C DIFFICILE INFECTION IN ADULTS: IDSA/SHEA TREATMENT RECOMMENDATIONS

Severity	Clinical signs	Treatment
Initial episode		
Mild to moderate	Leukocytosis with WBC count 15,000 or lower AND Serum creatinine less than 1.5 times premorbid level	Metronidazole 500 mg PO q8h for 10 to 14 days
Severe	Leukocytosis with WBC count 15,000 or higher OR Serum creatinine at least 1.5 times greater than premorbid level	Vancomycin 125 mg PO q6h for 10 to 14 days
Severe complicated	Hypotension or shock, ileus, megacolon	Vancomycin 500 mg PO/NG q6h plus metronidazole 500 mg IV q8h. Consider vancomycin 500 mg/100 mL normal saline retention enema q6h if complete ileus.
Recurrent episodes		
First recurrence	--	Same as initial episode, stratified by severity. Use vancomycin if WBC count 15,000 or higher, or serum creatinine is increasing.
Second recurrence	--	Vancomycin taper* and/or pulsed regimen

Adapted from Infect Control Hosp Epidemiol 2010; 31(5):000-000. Available online at: http://www.idsociety.org.
* Example: Vancomycin 125 mg PO QID for 10 to 14 days, then 125 mg BID for 7 days, then 125 mg every 2 or 3 days for 2 to 8 weeks

TELAVANCIN (*Vibativ*) Complicated skin infections including MRSA: 10 mg/kg IV once daily for 7 to 14 days. Infuse over 1 h. Teratogenic; get serum pregnancy test before use in women of childbearing potential. Nephrotoxicity. Not approved in children. ▶K ♀C ▶? $$$$$

TELITHROMYCIN (*Ketek*) 800 mg PO daily for 7 to 10 days for community-acquired pneumonia. No longer indicated for acute sinusitis or acute exacerbation of chronic bronchitis (risks exceed potential benefit). Contraindicated in myasthenia gravis. [Trade only: Tabs 300, 400 mg. Ketek Pak: #10, 400 mg tabs.] ▶LK ♀C ▶? $$$

TIGECYCLINE (*Tygacil*) Complicated skin infections, complicated intra-abdominal infections, community-acquired pneumonia: 100 mg IV first dose, then 50 mg IV q 12 h. Infuse over 30 to 60 min. Consider other antibiotics for severe infection because mortality is higher with tigecycline, especially in ventilator-associated pneumonia. ▶Bile, K ♀D ▶?+ $$$$$

TRIMETHOPRIM (*Primsol*, ✦*Proloprim*)   100 mg PO bid or 200 mg PO daily. [Generic only: Tabs 100 mg. Trade only (Primsol): Oral soln 50 mg/5 mL.] ▶K ♀C ▶– $

VANCOMYCIN (*Vancocin*)   Usual dose: 15 to 20 mg/kg IV q 8 to 12 h; consider loading dose of 25 to 30 mg/kg for severe infection. Infuse over 1 h; infuse over 1.5 to 2 h if dose greater than 1 g. Peds: 10 to 15 mg/kg IV q 6 h. C difficile diarrhea: 40 to 50 mg/kg/day PO up to 500 mg/day divided qid for 10 to 14 days. IV administration ineffective for this indication. Dose depends on severity and complications, see table for management of C. difficile infection. [Trade only: Caps 125, 250 mg.] ▶K ♀C ▶? $$$$$

CARDIOVASCULAR

ACE Inhibitors

NOTE *See also antihypertensive combinations. Hyperkalemia possible, especially if used concomitantly with other drugs that increase K+ (including K+ containing salt substitutes) and in patients with heart failure, diabetes mellitus, or renal impairment. Monitor closely for hypoglycemia, especially during first month of treatment when combined with insulin or oral antidiabetic agents. ACE inhibitors are contraindicated during pregnancy. Contraindicated with a history of angioedema. Renoprotection and decreased cardiovascular morbidity/mortality seen with some ACE inhibitors are most likely a class effect.*

BENAZEPRIL (*Lotensin*)   HTN: Start 10 mg PO daily, usual maintenance dose 20 to 40 mg PO daily or divided bid, max 80 mg/day. [Generic/Trade: Tabs unscored 5, 10, 20, 40 mg.] ▶LK ♀– ▶? $$

ACE INHIBITOR DOSING	HTN		Heart Failure	
	Initial	Max/day	Initial	Max
benazepril (*Lotensin*)	10 mg daily*	80 mg	-	-
captopril (*Capoten*)	25 mg bid/tid	450 mg	6.25 mg tid	50 mg tid
enalapril (*Vasotec*)	5 mg daily*	40 mg	2.5 mg bid	10–20 mg bid
fosinopril (*Monopril*)	10 mg daily*	80 mg	5–10 mg daily	40 mg daily
lisinopril (*Zestril/ Prinivil*)	10 mg daily	80 mg	2.5–5 mg daily	20–40 mg daily
moexipril (*Univasc*)	7.5 mg daily*	30 mg	-	-
perindopril (*Aceon*)	4 mg daily*	16 mg	2 mg daily	8–16 mg daily
quinapril (*Accupril*)	10–20 mg daily*	80 mg	5 mg bid	20 mg bid
ramipril (*Altace*)	2.5 mg daily*	20 mg	1.25–2.5 mg bid	10 mg daily
trandolapril (*Mavik*)	1–2 mg daily*	8 mg	1 mg daily	4 mg daily

Data taken from prescribing information and *Circulation* 2009;119:e391–e479.
*May require bid dosing for 24-h BP control.

CAPTOPRIL (*Capoten*) HTN: Start 25 mg PO bid to tid, usual maintenance dose 25 to 150 mg bid to tid, max 450 mg/day. <u>Heart failure:</u> Start 6.25 to 12.5 mg PO tid, usual dose 50 to 100 mg PO tid, max 450 mg/day. <u>Diabetic nephropathy:</u> 25 mg PO tid. [Generic/Trade: Tabs scored 12.5, 25, 50, 100 mg.] ▶LK ♀– ▶+ $

CILAZAPRIL (*✦Inhibace*) Canada only. <u>HTN:</u> 1.25 to 10 mg PO daily. [Generic/Trade: Tabs scored 1, 2.5, 5 mg.] ▶LK ♀– ▶? $

ENALAPRIL (*enalaprilat, Vasotec*) <u>HTN:</u> Start 5 mg PO daily, usual maintenance dose 10 to 40 mg PO daily or divided bid, max 40 mg/day. If oral therapy not possible, can use enalaprilat 1.25 mg IV q 6 h over 5 min, and increase up to 5 mg IV q 6 h if needed. Renal impairment or concomitant diuretic therapy: Start 2.5 mg PO daily. <u>Heart failure:</u> Start 2.5 mg PO bid, usual 10 to 20 mg PO daily, max 40 mg/day. [Generic/Trade: Tabs scored 2.5, 5 mg; unscored 10, 20 mg.] ▶LK ♀– ▶+ $$

FOSINOPRIL (*Monopril*) <u>HTN:</u> Start 10 mg PO daily, usual maintenance dose 20 to 40 mg PO daily or divided bid, max 80 mg/day. <u>Heart failure:</u> Start 5-10 mg PO daily, usual dose 20 to 40 mg PO daily, max 40 mg/day. [Generic/Trade: Tabs scored 10, unscored 20, 40 mg.] ▶LK ♀– ▶? $

LISINOPRIL (*Prinivil, Zestril*) <u>HTN:</u> Start 10 mg PO daily, usual maintenance dose 20 to 40 mg PO daily, max 80 mg/day. <u>Heart failure, acute MI:</u> Start 2.5 to 5 mg PO daily, usual dose 5 to 20 mg PO daily, max dose 40 mg. [Generic/Trade: Tabs unscored (Zestril) 2.5, 5, 10, 20, 30, 40 mg. Tabs scored (Prinivil) 10, 20, 40 mg.] ▶K ♀– ▶? $

MOEXIPRIL (*Univasc*) <u>HTN:</u> Start 7.5 mg PO daily, usual maintenance dose 7.5 to 30 mg PO daily or divided bid, max 30 mg/day. [Generic/Trade: Tabs scored 7.5, 15 mg.] ▶LK ♀– ▶? $$

PERINDOPRIL (*Aceon, ✦Coversyl*) <u>HTN:</u> Start 4 mg PO daily, usual maintenance dose 4 to 8 mg PO daily or divided bid, max 16 mg/day. <u>Reduction of cardiovascular events in stable CAD:</u> Start 4 mg PO daily for 2 weeks, max 8 mg/day. Elderly (age older than 70 yo): 2 mg PO daily for 1 week, 4 mg PO daily for 1 week, then 8 mg/day. [Generic/Trade: Tabs scored 2, 4, 8 mg.] ▶K ♀– ▶? $$

QUINAPRIL (*Accupril*) <u>HTN:</u> Start 10 to 20 mg PO daily (start 10 mg/day if elderly), usual maintenance dose 20 to 80 mg PO daily or divided bid, max 80 mg/day. <u>Heart failure:</u> Start 5 mg PO bid, usual maintenance dose 10 to 20 mg bid. [Generic/Trade: Tabs scored 5, unscored 10, 20, 40 mg.] ▶LK ♀– ▶? $$

RAMIPRIL (*Altace*) <u>HTN:</u> 2.5 mg PO daily, usual maintenance dose 2.5 to 20 mg PO daily or divided bid, max 20 mg/day. <u>Heart failure post MI:</u> Start 2.5 mg PO bid, usual maintenance dose 5 mg PO bid. <u>Reduce risk of MI, CVA, death from cardiovascular causes:</u> 2.5 mg PO daily for 1 week, then 5 mg daily for 3 weeks, increase as tolerated to max 10 mg/day. [Generic/Trade: Caps 1.25, 2.5, 5, 10 mg.] ▶LK ♀– ▶? $$$

TRANDOLAPRIL (*Mavik*) <u>HTN:</u> Start 1 mg PO daily, usual maintenance dose 2 to 4 mg PO daily or divided bid, max 8 mg/day. <u>Heart failure/post MI:</u> Start 0.5 to 1 mg PO daily, usual maintenance dose 4 mg PO daily. [Generic/Trade: Tabs scored 1, unscored 2,4 mg.] ▶LK ♀– ▶? $$

Aldosterone Antagonists

EPLERENONE (*Inspra*) HTN: Start 50 mg PO daily; max 50 mg bid. Improve survival of stable patients with LV systolic dysfunction (LVEF 40% or less) and heart failure post MI: Start 25 mg PO daily; titrate to target dose 50 mg daily within 4 weeks, if tolerated. [Trade only: Tabs unscored 25, 50 mg.] ▶L ♀B ▶? $$$$

SPIRONOLACTONE (*Aldactone*) HTN: 50 to 100 mg PO daily or divided bid. Edema: 25 to 200 mg/day. Hypokalemia: 25 to 100 mg PO daily. Primary hyperaldosteronism, maintenance: 100 to 400 mg/day PO. Cirrhotic ascites: Start 100 mg once daily or in divided doses. Maintenance 25 to 200 mg/day. [Generic/Trade: Tabs unscored 25 mg scored 50, 100 mg.] ▶LK ♀D ▶+ $

Angiotensin Receptor Blockers (ARBs)

NOTE *See also antihypertensive combinations.*

CANDESARTAN (*Atacand*) HTN: Start 16 mg PO daily, maximum 32 mg/day. Heart failure (NYHA II-IV and LVEF 40% or less): Start 4 mg PO daily, maximum 32 mg/day; has added effect when used with ACE inhibitor. [Trade only: Tabs unscored 4, 8, 16, 32 mg.] ▶K ♀− ▶? $$$

EPROSARTAN (*Teveten*) HTN: Start 600 mg PO daily, maximum 800 mg/day given daily or divided bid. [Trade only: Tabs unscored 400, 600 mg.] ▶Fecal excretion ♀− ▶? $$$

IRBESARTAN (*Avapro*) HTN: Start 150 mg PO daily, maximum 300 mg/day. Type 2 diabetic nephropathy: Start 150 mg PO daily, target dose 300 mg daily. [Trade only: Tabs unscored 75, 150, 300 mg.] ▶L ♀− ▶? $$$

HTN THERAPY[1]

Area of Concern	BP Target	Preferred Therapy[2]	Comments
General CAD prevention	<140/90 mm Hg	ACEI, ARB, CCB, thiazide, or combination	Start 2 drugs if systolic BP ≥ 160 or diastolic BP ≥ 100
High CAD risk[3]	<130/80 mm Hg		
Stable angina, un-stable angina, MI	<130/80 mm Hg	Beta-blocker[4] + (ACEI or ARB)[5]	May add dihydropyridine CCB or thiazide
Left heart failure[6,7]	<120/80 mm Hg	Beta-blocker + (ACEI or ARB) + diuretic[8] + aldosterone antagonist[9]	

1. ACEI = angiotensin converting enzyme inhibitor; ARB = angiotensin-receptor blocker; CCB = calcium-channel blocker; MI = myocardial infarction. Adapted from *Circulation* 2007;115:2761–2788. **2.** All patients should attempt lifestyle modifications: optimize wt, healthy diet, sodium restriction, exercise, smoking cessation, alcohol moderation. **3.** Diabetes mellitus, chronic kidney disease, known CAD or risk equivalent (eg, peripheral artery disease, abdominal aortic aneurysm, carotid artery disease, and prior ischemic CVA/TIA), 10-year Framingham risk score ≥ 10%. **4.** Use only if hemodynamically stable. If beta-blocker contraindications or intolerable side effects (and no bradycardia or heart failure), may substitute verapamil or diltiazem. **5.** Preferred if anterior wall MI, persistent HTN, heart failure, or diabetes mellitus. **6.** Avoid verapamil, diltiazem, clonidine, beta-blockers. **7.** For blacks with NYHA class III or IV HF, consider adding hydralazine/isosorbide dinitrate. **8.** Loop or thiazide. **9.** Use if NYHA class III or IV, or if clinical heart failure + LVEF < 40%.

LOSARTAN (*Cozaar*)   HTN: Start 50 mg PO daily, max 100 mg/day given daily or divided bid. Volume-depleted patients or history of hepatic impairment: Start 25 mg PO daily. CVA risk reduction in patients with HTN and LV hypertrophy (may not be effective in black patients): Start 50 mg PO daily. If need more BP reduction add HCTZ 12.5 mg PO daily, then increase losartan to 100 mg/day, then increase HCTZ to 25 mg/day. Type 2 diabetic nephropathy: Start 50 mg PO daily, target dose 100 mg daily. [Generic/Trade: Tabs unscored 25, 50, 100 mg.]   ▶L ♀− ▶? $$$

OLMESARTAN (*Benicar*)   HTN: Start 20 mg PO daily, max 40 mg/day. [Trade only: Tabs unscored 5, 20, 40 mg.]   ▶K ♀− ▶? $$$

TELMISARTAN (*Micardis*)   HTN: Start 40 mg PO daily, max 80 mg/day. Cardiovascular risk reduction: Start 80 mg PO daily, max 80 mg/day. [Trade only: Tabs unscored 20, 40, 80 mg.]   ▶L ♀− ▶? $$$

VALSARTAN (*Diovan*)   HTN: Start 80 to 160 mg PO daily, max 320 mg/day. Heart failure: Start 40 mg PO bid, target dose 160 mg bid; there is no evidence of added benefit when used with adequate dose of ACE inhibitor. Reduce mortality/morbidity post MI with LV systolic dysfunction/failure: Start 20 mg PO bid, target dose 160 mg bid. [Trade only: Tabs scored 40 mg, unscored 80, 160, 320 mg.]   ▶L ♀− ▶? $$$

Antiadrenergic Agents

CLONIDINE (*Catapres, Catapres-TTS, ✦Dixarit*)   HTN: Start 0.1 mg PO bid, usual maintenance dose 0.2 to 1.2 mg/day divided bid to tid, max 2.4 mg/day. Rebound HTN with abrupt discontinuation, especially at doses that exceed 0.7 mg/day. Transdermal (Catapres-TTS): Start 0.1 mg/24 h patch once a week, titrate to desired effect, max effective dose 0.6 mg/24 h (two 0.3 mg/24 h patches). Transdermal Therapeutic System (TTS) is designed for 7 days use so that a TTS-1 delivers 0.1 mg/day for 7 days. May supplement first dose of TTS with oral for 2 to 3 days while therapeutic level is achieved. ADHD (unapproved peds): Start 0.05 mg PO at bedtime, titrate based on response over 8 weeks to max 0.2 mg/day (for wt less than 45 kg) or to max 0.4 mg/day (for wt 45 kg or greater) in 2 to 4 divided doses. Tourette's syndrome (unapproved peds and adult): 3 to 5 mcg/kg/day PO divided bid to qid. Opioid withdrawal, adjunct: 0.1 to 0.3 mg PO tid to qid or 0.1 to 0.2 mg PO q 4 h for 3 days tapering off over 4 to 10 days. Alcohol withdrawal, adjunct: 0.1 to 0.2 mg PO q 4 h prn. Smoking cessation: Start 0.1 mg PO bid, increase 0.1 mg/day at weekly intervals to 0.75 mg/day as tolerated; transdermal (Catapres TTS): 0.1 to 0.2 mg/24 h patch once a week for 2 to 3 weeks after cessation. Menopausal flushing: 0.1 to 0.4 mg/day PO divided bid to tid. Transdermal system applied weekly: 0.1 mg/day. [Generic/Trade: Tabs unscored 0.1, 0.2, 0.3 mg. Transdermal weekly patch 0.1 mg/day (TTS-1), 0.2 mg/day (TTS-2), 0.3 mg/day (TTS-3). Generic only: Oral Susp, Extended-release, 0.09 mg/mL (118 mL). Tabs Extended-release 0.17, 0.26 mg.]   ▶LK ♀C ▶? $$

DOXAZOSIN (*Cardura, Cardura XL*)   BPH: Immediate-release: Start 1 mg PO at bedtime, max 8 mg/day. Extended-release (not approved for HTN): 4 mg

(cont.)

PO qam with breakfast, max 8 mg/day. <u>HTN:</u> Start 1 mg PO at bedtime, max 16 mg/day. Take first dose at bedtime to minimize orthostatic hypotension. [Generic/Trade: Tabs scored 1, 2, 4, 8 mg. Trade only (Cardura XL): Tabs extended-release 4, 8 mg.] ▶L ♀C ▶? $$

GUANFACINE (Tenex) <u>HTN:</u> Start 1 mg PO at bedtime, increase to 2 to 3 mg at bedtime if needed after 3 to 4 weeks, max 3 mg/day. <u>ADHD in children:</u> Start 0.5 mg PO daily, titrate by 0.5 mg q 3 to 4 days as tolerated to 0.5 mg PO tid. [Generic/Trade: Tabs unscored 1, 2 mg.] ▶K ♀B ▶? $

METHYLDOPA (Aldomet) <u>HTN:</u> Start 250 mg PO bid to tid, maximum 3000 mg/day. May cause hemolytic anemia. [Generic only: Tabs unscored 125, 250, 500 mg.] ▶LK ♀B ▶+ $

PRAZOSIN (Minipress) <u>HTN:</u> Start 1 mg PO bid to tid, max 40 mg/day. Take first dose at bedtime to minimize orthostatic hypotension. [Generic/Trade: Caps 1, 2, 5 mg.] ▶L ♀C ▶? $$

TERAZOSIN (Hytrin) <u>HTN:</u> Start 1 mg PO at bedtime, usual effective dose 1 to 5 mg PO daily or divided bid, max 20 mg/day. Take first dose at bedtime to minimize orthostatic hypotension. <u>BPH:</u> Start 10 mg/day at bedtime, usual effective dose 10 mg/day, max 20 mg/day. [Generic/Trade: Tabs Caps 1, 2, 5, 10 mg.] ▶LK ♀C ▶? $$

Anti-Dysrhythmics/Cardiac Arrest

ADENOSINE (Adenocard) <u>PSVT conversion (not A-fib):</u> Adult and peds wt 50 kg or greater: 6 mg rapid IV and flush, preferably through a central line. If no response after 1 to 2 min, then 12 mg. A 3rd dose of 12 mg may be given prn. Peds wt less than 50 kg: Initial dose 50 to 100 mcg/kg, subsequent doses 100 to 200 mcg/kg q 1 to 2 min prn up to a max single dose of 300 mcg/kg or 12 mg, whichever is less. Half-life is less than 10 sec. Give doses by rapid IV push followed by NS flush. Need higher dose if on theophylline or caffeine, lower dose if on dipyridamole or carbamazepine ▶Plasma ♀C ▶? $$$

AMIODARONE (Cordarone, Pacerone) <u>Life-threatening ventricular arrhythmia without cardiac arrest:</u> Load 150 mg IV over 10 min, then 1 mg/min for 6 h, then 0.5 mg/min for 18 h. Mix in D5W. Oral loading dose 800 to 1600 mg PO daily for 1 to 3 weeks, reduce to 400 to 800 mg PO daily for 1 month when arrhythmia is controlled, reduce to lowest effective dose thereafter, usually 200 to 400 mg PO daily. Photosensitivity with oral therapy. Pulmonary and hepatic toxicity. Hypo or hyperthyroidism possible. Coadministration of fluoroquinolones, macrolides, or azoles may prolong QTc. May increase digoxin levels; discontinue digoxin or decrease dose by 50%. May increase INR with warfarin by up to 100%; decrease warfarin dose by 33 to 50%. Do not use with grapefruit juice. Do not use with simvastatin dose greater than 20 mg/day, lovastatin dose greater than 40 mg/day; caution with atorvastatin; increases risk of myopathy and rhabdomyolysis. Caution with beta-blockers and calcium channel blockers. IV therapy may cause hypotension. Contraindicated with marked sinus bradycardia and 2nd or 3rd degree heart block in the absence of a functioning pacemaker. [Trade only (Pacerone): tabs unscored 100 mg. Generic/Trade: Tabs scored 200, 400 mg.] ▶L ♀D ▶– $$$$

ATROPINE (*AtroPen*) Bradyarrhythmia/CPR: 0.5 to 1 mg IV q 3 to 5 min to max 0.04 mg/kg (3 mg). Peds: 0.02 mg/kg/dose; minimum single dose, 0.1 mg; max cumulative dose, 1 mg. AtroPen: Injector pens for insecticide or nerve agent poisoning. [Trade only: Prefilled auto-injector pens: 0.25 mg (yellow), 0.5 mg (blue), 1 mg (dark red), 2 mg (green).] ▶K ♀C ▶– $

BICARBONATE Severe acidosis: 1 mEq/kg IV up to 50 to 100 mEq/dose. ▶K ♀C ▶? $

DIGOXIN (*Lanoxin, Lanoxicaps, Digitek*) Systolic heart failure/rate control of chronic A-fib: 0.125 to 0.25 mg PO daily; impaired renal function: 0.0625 to 0.125 mg PO daily. Rapid A-fib: Load 0.5 mg IV, then 0.25 mg IV q 6 h for 2 doses, maintenance 0.125 to 0.375 mg IV/PO daily. [Generic/Trade: Tabs scored (Lanoxin, Digitek) 0.125, 0.25 mg; elixir 0.05 mg/mL. Trade only: Caps (Lanoxicaps), 0.1, 0.2 mg.] ▶KL ♀C ▶+ $

DIGOXIN IMMUNE FAB (*Digibind, Digifab*) Digoxin toxicity: Dose varies. Acute ingestion of known amount: 1 vial binds approximately 0.5 mg digoxin. Acute ingestion of unknown amount: 10 vials IV, may repeat once. Toxicity during chronic therapy: 6 vials usually adequate; one formula is: Number vials is equivalent to (serum dig level in ng/mL) × (kg)/100. ▶K ♀C ▶? $$$$$

DISOPYRAMIDE (*Norpace, Norpace CR, ✦Rythmodan, Rythmodan-LA*) Rarely indicated, consult cardiologist. Ventricular arrhythmia: 400 to 800 mg PO daily in divided doses (immediate-release is divided q 6 h: extended-release is divided q 12 h). Proarrhythmic. [Generic/Trade: Caps immediate-release 100, 150 mg; extended-release 150 mg. Trade only: Caps, extended-release 100 mg.] ▶KL ♀C ▶+ $$$$

DRONEDARONE (*Multaq*) Reduce risk of CV hospitalization with paroxysmal or persistent atrial fib/flutter, with recent episode of atrial fib/flutter and CV risk factors (ie, age older than 70 yo, HTN, diabetes, prior CVA, left atrial diameter 50 mm or greater, or LVEF less than 40%), who are in sinus rhythm or will be converted: 400 mg PO BID with morning and evening meals. Do not use with any of the following: 2nd or 3rd degree AV block or sick sinus syndrome without functioning pacemaker; bradycardia < 50 bpm; QTc Bazett interval > 500 ms; or severe hepatic impairment. Do not use with grapefruit juice; other antiarrhythmic agents; potent inhibitors of CYP 3A4 enzyme system (clarithromycin, erythromycin, itraconazole, ketoconazole, nefazodone, ritonavir, voriconazole); or inducers of CYP 3A4 enzyme system (carbamazepine, phenytoin, phenobarbital, rifampin, St. John's Wort). May increase digoxin levels; discontinue digoxin or decrease dose by 50%. Caution with beta-blockers and calcium channel blockers. May increase levels of sirolimus, tacrolimus, and CYP3A4 substrates with narrow therapeutic index. [Trade: Tabs unscored 400 mg.] ▶L ♀X ▶– $$$$

FLECAINIDE (*Tambocor*) Proarrhythmic. Prevention of paroxysmal atrial fib/flutter or PSVT, with symptoms and no structural heart disease: Start 50 mg PO q 12 h, may increase by 50 mg bid q 4 days, max 300 mg/day. Use with AV nodal slowing agent (beta-blocker, verapamil, diltiazem) to minimize risk of 1:1 atrial flutter. Life-threatening ventricular arrhythmias without structural heart disease: Start 100 mg PO q 12 h, may increase by 50 mg bid q 4 days, max 400 mg/day. With severe renal impairment (CrCl < 35 mL/min): Start 50 mg PO bid. [Generic/Trade: Tabs unscored 50, scored 100, 150 mg.] ▶K ♀C ▶– $$$$

SELECTED DRUGS THAT MAY PROLONG THE QT INTERVAL

alfuzosin	erythromycin*†	nicardipine	sertraline
amiodarone*†	felbamate	octreotide	sotalol*†
apomorphine	flecainide*	ofloxacin	sunitinib
arsenic trioxide*	foscarnet	ondansetron	tacrolimus
azithromycin*	fosphenytoin	pentamidine*†	tamoxifen
chloroquine*	gemifloxacin	phenothiazines‡	telithromycin*
chlorpromazine	granisetron	pimozide*†	thioridazine
cisapride*†	haloperidol*‡	polyethylene	tizanidine
clarithromycin*	ibutilide*†	glycol (PEG-salt	tolterodine
clozapine	indapamide*	soln)§	vardenafil
cocaine*	isradipine	procainamide*	venlafaxine
dasatinib	levofloxacin*	quetiapine‡	visicol§
disopyramide*†	lithium	quinidine*†	voriconazole*
dofetilide*	mefloquine	quinine	vorinostat
dolasetron	methadone*†	ranolazine	ziprasidone‡
droperidol*	moexipril/HCTZ	risperidone‡	
epirubicin	moxifloxacin	salmeterol	

Note. This table may not include all drugs that prolong the QT interval or cause torsades. Risk of drug-induced QT prolongation may be increased in women, elderly, hypokalemia, hypomagnesemia, bradycardia, starvation, CHF, & CNS injuries. Hepatorenal dysfunction & drug interactions can increase the concentration of QT interval-prolonging drugs. Coadministration of QT interval-prolonging drugs can have additive effects. Avoid these (and other) drugs in congenital prolonged QT syndrome (www.qtdrugs.org). *Torsades reported in product labeling/case reports. †Increased risk in women. ‡QT prolongation: thioridazine > ziprasidone > risperidone, quetiapine, haloperidol. §May be due to electrolyte imbalance.

IBUTILIDE (Corvert) Recent onset A-fib/flutter: 0.01 mg/kg up to 1 mg IV over 10 min, may repeat once if no response after 10 additional min. Keep on cardiac monitor at least 4 h. ▶K ♀C ▶? $$$$$

ISOPROTERENOL (Isuprel) Refractory bradycardia or 3rd degree AV block: bolus method: 0.02 to 0.06 mg IV: infusion method, dilute 2 mg in 250 mL D5W (8 mcg/mL), a rate of 37.5 mL/h delivers 5 mcg/min. Peds infusion method: 0.05 to 2 mcg/kg/min. Using the same concentration as adult for a 10 kg child, a rate of 8 mL/h delivers 0.1 mcg/kg/min. ▶LK ♀C ▶? $$$

LIDOCAINE (Xylocaine, Xylocard) Ventricular arrhythmia: Load 1 mg/kg IV, then 0.5 mg/kg q 8 to 10 min as needed to max 3 mg/kg. IV infusion: 4 g in 500 mL D5W (8 mg/mL) run at rate of 7.5 to 30 mL/h to deliver 1 to 4 mg/min. Peds: 20 to 50 mcg/kg/min. ▶LK ♀B ▶? $

MEXILETINE (Mexitil) Proarrhythmic. Rarely indicated, consult cardiologist. Ventricular arrhythmia: Start 200 mg PO q 8 h with food or antacid, max dose 1200 mg/day. [Generic only: Caps 150, 200, 250 mg.] ▶L ♀C ▶- $$$

PROCAINAMIDE (Pronestyl) Ventricular arrhythmia: Loading dose: 100 mg IV q 10 min or 20 mg/min (150 mL) until QRS widens more than 50%, dysrhythmia suppressed, hypotension, or total of 17 mg/kg or 1000 mg delivered. Infusion: dilute 2 g in 250 mL D5W (8 mg/mL) rate of 15 to 45 mL/h to deliver 2 to 6 mg/min. Proarrhythmic. ▶LK ♀C ▶? $

PROPAFENONE (*Rythmol, Rythmol SR*) Proarrhythmic. <u>Prevention of paroxysmal atrial fib/flutter or PSVT, with symptoms and no structural heart disease;</u> or <u>life-threatening ventricular arrhythmias:</u> Start (immediate-release) 150 mg PO q 8 h; may increase after 3 to 4 days to 225 mg PO q 8 h; max 900 mg/day. <u>Prolong time to recurrence of symptomatic atrial fib without structural heart disease:</u> 225 mg SR PO q 12 h, may increase after 5 days to 325 mg SR PO q 12 h, max 425 mg SR PO q 12 h. Consider using with AV nodal blocking agent (beta-blocker, verapamil, diltiazem) to minimize risk of 1:1 atrial flutter. [Generic/Trade: Tabs immediate-release scored 150, 225, 300 mg. Trade only: SR, Caps 225, 325, 425 mg.] ▶L ♀C ▶? $$$$

QUINIDINE (✦*Biquin durules*) <u>Arrhythmia:</u> Gluconate, extended-release: 324 to 648 mg PO q 8 to 12 h; sulfate, immediate-release: 200 to 400 mg PO q 6 to 8 h; sulfate, extended-release: 300 to 600 mg PO q 8 to 12 h. Proarrhythmic. [Generic gluconate: Tabs extended-release unscored 324 mg. Generic sulfate: Tabs scored immediate-release 200, 300 mg; Tabs extended-release 300 mg.] ▶LK ♀C ▶+ $$$- gluconate, $-sulfate

SOTALOL (*Betapace, Betapace AF, ✦Rylosol*) <u>Ventricular arrhythmia</u> (Betapace), <u>A-fib/A-flutter</u> (Betapace AF): Start 80 mg PO bid, max 640 mg/day. Proarrhythmic. [Generic/Trade: Tabs scored 80, 120, 160, 240 mg; Tabs scored (Betapace AF) 80, 120, 160 mg.] ▶K ♀B ▶– $$$$

Anti-Hyperlipidemic Agents—Bile Acid Sequestrants

CHOLESTYRAMINE (*Questran, Questran Light, Prevalite, LoCHOLEST, LoCHOLEST Light*) <u>Elevated LDL-C:</u> Powder: Start 4 g PO daily to bid before meals, increase up to max 24 g/day. [Generic/Trade: Powder for oral susp, 4 g cholestyramine resin/9 g powder (Questran, LoCHOLEST), 4 g cholestyramine resin/5 g powder (Questran Light), 4 g cholestyramine resin/5.5 g powder (Prevalite, LoCHOLEST Light). Each available in bulk powder and single-dose packets.] ▶Not absorbed ♀C ▶+ $$$

COLESEVELAM (*Welchol*) <u>Glycemic control of type 2 diabetes or LDL-C reduction:</u> 6 tabs once daily or 3 tabs PO bid, max dose 6 tabs/day; or 3.75 g powder once daily or 1.875 g powder bid, max dose 3.75 g/day. Give with meal. Give tabs with liquid. Mix powder in 4 to 8 ounces water. [Trade only: Tabs unscored 625 mg. Powder single-dose packets 1.875, 3.75 g.] ▶Not absorbed ♀B ▶+ $$$$$

COLESTIPOL (*Colestid, Colestid Flavored*) <u>Elevated LDL-C:</u> Tabs: Start 2 g PO daily to bid, max 16 g/day. Granules: Start 5 g PO daily to bid, max 30 g/day. [Generic/Trade: Tabs 1 g. Granules for oral susp, 5 g/7.5 g powder.] ▶Not absorbed ♀B ▶+ $$$$

Anti-Hyperlipidemic Agents—HMG-CoA Reductase Inhibitors ("Statins") and Combinations

NOTE *Hepatotoxicity: Monitor LFTs initially, approximately 12 weeks after starting/titrating therapy, then annually or more frequently if indicated. Evaluate muscle symptoms before starting therapy, 6 to 12 weeks after starting/increasing therapy, and at each follow-up visit. Obtain creatine kinase when patient*

(cont.)

complains of muscle soreness, tenderness, weakness, or pain. These factors increase the risk for myopathy: Advanced age (especially age older than 80 yo, women > men); multisystem disease (eg, chronic renal insufficiency, especially due to diabetes); multiple medications; perioperative periods; alcohol abuse; grapefruit juice (more than 1 quart/day); specific concomitant medications: fibrates (especially gemfibrozil), nicotinic acid (rare), cyclosporine, erythromycin, clarithromycin, itraconazole, ketoconazole, protease inhibitors, nefazodone, verapamil, amiodarone. Weigh potential risk of combination therapy against potential benefit.

ADVICOR (lovastatin + niacin) <u>Hyperlipidemia:</u> 1 tab PO at bedtime with a low-fat snack. Establish dose using extended-release niacin first, or if already on lovastatin, substitute combo product with lowest niacin dose. Aspirin or ibuprofen 30 min prior may decrease niacin flushing reaction. [Trade only: Tabs unscored extended- release lovastatin/niacin 20/500, 20/750, 20/1000, 40/1000.] ▶LK ♀X ▶– $$$$

ATORVASTATIN (*Lipitor*) <u>Hyperlipidemia/prevention of cardiovascular events, including type 2 DM:</u> Start 10 to 40 mg PO daily, max 80 mg/day. See package insert for dosing restrictions when used with clarithromycin, cyclosporine, itraconazole, or protease inhibitor combinations that include ritonavir. [Trade only: Tabs unscored 10, 20, 40, 80 mg.] ▶L ♀X ▶– $$$$

CADUET (amlodipine + atorvastatin) <u>Simultaneous treatment of HTN and hypercholesterolemia:</u> Establish dose using component drugs first. Dosing interval: Daily [Trade only: Tabs 2.5/10, 2.5/20, 2.5/40, 5/10, 5/20, 5/40, 5/80, 10/10, 10/20, 10/40, 10/80 mg.] ▶L ♀X ▶– $$$$

FLUVASTATIN (*Lescol, Lescol XL*) <u>Hyperlipidemia:</u> Start 20 to 80 mg PO at bedtime, max 80 mg daily (XL) or divided bid. <u>Post percutaneous coronary intervention:</u> 80 mg of extended-release PO daily, max 80 mg daily. [Trade only: Caps 20, 40 mg. Tabs extended-release unscored 80 mg.] ▶L ♀X ▶– $$$

LIPID REDUCTION BY CLASS/AGENT[1]

Drug class/agent	LDL	HDL	TG
Bile acid sequestrants[2]	↓ 15–30%	↑ 3–5%	No change or ↑
Cholesterol absorption inhibitor[3]	↓ 18%	↑ 1%	↓ 8%
Fibrates[4]	↓ 5–20%	↑ 10–20%	↓ 20–50%
Lovastatin+ext'd release niacin[5]*	↓ 30–42%	↑ 20–30%	↓ 32–44%
Niacin[6]*	↓ 5–25%	↑ 15–35%	↓ 20–50%
Omega 3 fatty acids[7]	No change or ↑	↑ 9%	↓ 45%
Statins[8]	↓18–63%	↑ 5–15%	↓ 7–35%
Simvastatin+ezetimibe[9]	↓ 45–60%	↑ 6–10%	↓ 23–31%

1. LDL = low density lipoprotein. HDL = high density lipoprotein. TG = triglycerides. Adapted from NCEP: *JAMA* 2001; 285:2486 and prescribing information. 2. Cholestyramine (4–16 g), colestipol (5–20 g), colesevelam (2.6–3.8 g). 3. Ezetimibe (10 mg). When added to statin therapy, will ↓ LDL 25%, ↑ HDL 3%, ↓ TG 14% in addition to statin effects. 4. Fenofibrate (145–200 mg), gemfibrozil (600 mg BID). 5. Advicor® (20/1000–40/2000 mg). 6. Extended release nicotinic acid (Niaspan® 1–2 g), immediate release (crystalline) nicotinic acid (1.5–3 g), sustained release nicotinic acid (Slo-Niacin® 1–2 g). 7. Lovaza (4 g) 8. Atorvastatin (10–80 mg), fluvastatin (20–80 mg), lovastatin (20–80 mg), pravastatin (20–80 mg), rosuvastatin (5–40 mg), simvastatin (20–80 mg). 9. Vytorin® (10/10–10/80 mg). *Lowers lipoprotein a.

LOVASTATIN (*Mevacor, Altoprev*) <u>Hyperlipidemia/prevention of cardiovascular events:</u> Start 20 mg PO q pm, max 80 mg/day daily or divided bid. See package insert for dosing restrictions when used with amiodarone, cyclosporine, danazol, fibrates, niacin, or verapamil. [Generic/Trade: Tabs unscored 20, 40 mg. Trade only: Tabs extended-release (Altoprev) 20, 40, 60 mg.] ▶L ♀X ▶– $

PITAVASTATIN (*Livalo*) <u>Hyperlipidemia:</u> Start 2 mg PO at bedtime, max 4 mg daily. Renal impairment (GFR 30-60 mL/min) or end stage renal disease receiving hemodialysis: Max start 1 mg PO daily, max 2 mg daily. See package insert for dosing restrictions when used for patients taking erythromycin or rifampin. Do not use with cyclosporine, protease inhibitor combination lopinavir/ritonavir, or with severe renal impairment (GFR < 30 mL/min) not on hemodialysis. [Trade only: Tabs 1, 2, 4 mg.] ▶L – ♀X ▶– $$$$

PRAVASTATIN (*Pravachol*) <u>Hyperlipidemia/prevention of cardiovascular events:</u> Start 40 mg PO daily, max 80 mg/day. [Generic/Trade: Tabs unscored 10, 20, 40, 80 mg. Generic only: Tabs 30 mg.] ▶L ♀X ▶– $$$

ROSUVASTATIN (*Crestor*) <u>Hyperlipidemia/slow progression of atherosclerosis/ primary prevention of cardiovascular disease:</u> Start 10 to 20 mg daily, max 40 mg/day. See package insert for dosing restrictions when used for Asians, patients with renal impairment, and patients taking cyclosporine, gemfibrozil, or protease inhibitor combinations that include ritonavir. [Trade only: Tabs unscored 5, 10, 20, 40 mg.] ▶L ♀X ▶– $$$

SIMCOR (simvastatin + niacin) <u>Hyperlipidemia:</u> 1 tab PO at bedtime with a low-fat snack. If niacin-naive or switching from immediate-release niacin, start: 20/500 mg PO q pm. If receiving extended-release niacin, do not start with more than 40/2000 mg PO every evening. Max 40/2000 mg/day. Aspirin or ibuprofen 30 min prior may decrease niacin flushing reaction. [Trade only: Tabs unscored extended-release simvastatin/niacin 20/500, 20/750, 20/1000 mg.] ▶LK ♀X ▶– $$$

SIMVASTATIN (*Zocor*) <u>Hyperlipidemia:</u> Start 20 to 40 mg PO q pm, max 80 mg/day. <u>Reduce cardiovascular mortality/events in high risk for coronary heart disease event:</u> Start 40 mg PO q pm, max 80 mg/day. See package insert for dosing restrictions when used for Chinese patients taking niacin, patients with severe renal impairment, and patients taking amiodarone, cyclosporine, danazol, diltiazem, gemfibrozil, or verapamil. [Generic/Trade: Tabs unscored 5, 10, 20, 40, 80 mg. Generic only: Tabs orally disintegrating 10, 20, 40, 80 mg.] ▶L ♀X ▶– $$$$

VYTORIN (ezetimibe + simvastatin) <u>Hyperlipidemia:</u> Start 10/20 mg PO q pm, max 10/80 mg/day. Start 10/40 mg if goal is > 55% LDL reduction. [Trade only: Tabs unscored ezetimibe/simvastatin 10/10, 10/20, 10/40, 10/80 mg.] ▶L ♀X ▶– $$$$

Anti-Hyperlipidemic Agents—Other

BEZAFIBRATE (*♦Bezalip*) Canada only. <u>Hyperlipidemia/hypertriglyceridemia:</u> 200 mg immediate-release PO bid to tid, or 400 mg of sustained-release PO daily. [Trade only: Tabs immediate-release 200 mg, sustained-release 400 mg.] ▶K ♀D ▶– $$$

EZETIMIBE (*Zetia, ✦Ezetrol*) <u>Hyperlipidemia:</u> 10 mg PO daily. [Trade only: Tabs unscored 10 mg.] ▶L ♀C ▶? $$$$

FENOFIBRATE (*TriCor, Antara, Lipofen, Triglide, ✦Lipidil Micro, Lipidil Supra, Lipidil EZ*) <u>Hypertriglyceridemia:</u> TriCor tabs: 48 to 145 mg PO daily, max 145 mg daily. Antara: 43 to 130 mg PO daily; max 130 mg daily. Fenoglide: 40 to 120 mg PO daily; max 120 mg daily. Lipofen: 50 to 150 mg PO daily, max 150 mg daily. Lofibra: 54 to 200 mg PO daily, max 200 mg daily. Triglide: 50 to 160 mg PO daily, max 160 mg daily. Generic caps: 54 to 160 mg, max 160 mg daily. Generic caps: 67 to 200 mg PO daily; max 200 mg daily. <u>Hypercholesterolemia/mixed dyslipidemia:</u> TriCor tabs: 145 mg PO daily. Antara: 130 mg PO daily. Fenoglide: 120 mg daily. Lipofen: 150 mg daily. Lofibra: 160 to 200 mg daily, max 200 mg daily. Triglide: 160 mg daily. Generic tabs: 160 mg daily. Generic caps 200 mg PO daily. All formulations, except Antara, TriCor, and Triglide, should be taken with food. [Generic only: Tabs unscored 54, 160 mg. Generic caps 67, 134, 200 mg. Trade only: Tabs (TriCor) unscored 48, 145 mg. Caps (Antara) 43, 130 mg. Tabs (Fenoglide) unscored 40, 120 mg. Tabs (Lipofen) unscored 50, 100, 150 mg. Tabs (Lofibra) unscored 54, 160 mg. Tabs (Triglide) unscored 50, 160 mg. Caps (Lofibra) 67, 134, 200 mg.] ▶LK ♀C ▶– $$$

FENOFIBRIC ACID (*Fibricor, TriLipix*) <u>In combination with statin for mixed dyslipidemia and CHD or CHD risk equivalent:</u> TriLipix: 135 mg PO daily. <u>Hypertriglyceridemia:</u> Fibricor: 35 to 105 mg PO daily, max 105 mg daily. TriLipix: 45 to 135 mg PO daily, max 135 mg daily. <u>Hypercholesterolemia/mixed dyslipidemia:</u> Fibricor: 105 mg PO daily. TriLipix: 135 mg PO daily. [Trade only: Caps (TriLipix) delayed-release 45, 135 mg. Tabs (Fibricor) 35, 105 mg.] ▶LK ♀C ▶– $$$

GEMFIBROZIL (*Lopid*) <u>Hypertriglyceridemia/primary prevention of CAD:</u> 600 mg PO bid 30 min before meals. [Generic/Trade: Tabs scored 600 mg.] ▶LK ♀C ▶? $$$

Antihypertensive Combinations (See component drugs for ▶ L ▶)

NOTE *Dosage should first be adjusted using each drug separately. See component drugs for further details.*

BY TYPE: ACE Inhibitor/Diuretic: Accuretic, Capozide, Inhibace Plus, Lotensin HCT, Monopril HCT, Prinzide, Uniretic, Vaseretic, Zestoretic. **ACE Inhibitor/Calcium Channel Blocker:** Lexxel, Lotrel, Tarka. **Angiotensin Receptor Blocker/Diuretic:** Atacand HCT, Avalide, Benicar HCT, Diovan HCT, Hyzaar, Micardis HCT, Teveten HCT. **Angiotensin Receptor Blocker/Calcium Channel Blocker:** Azor, Exforge, Twyn-sta. **Angiotensin Receptor Blocker/Calcium Channel Blocker/Diuretic:** Exforge HCT, Tribenzor. **Angiotensin Receptor Blocker/Direct renin inhibitor:** Valturna. **Beta-blocker/Diuretic:** Corzide, Inderide, Lopressor HCT, Tenoretic, Ziac. **Direct renin inhibitor/Calcium Channel Blocker:** Tekamlo. **Diuretic combinations:** Dyazide, Maxzide, Moduretic. **Diuretic/miscellaneous antihypertensive:** Aldactazide, Aldoril, Apresazide, Clor-pres, Minizide, Tekturna HCT. **Other:** BiDil.

BY NAME: *Accuretic* (quinapril + hydrochlorothiazide): Generic/Trade: Tabs, 10/12.5, 20/12.5, 20/25. *Aldactazide* (spironolactone + hydrochlorothiazide): Generic/Trade: Tabs, unscored 25/25.Trade only: Tabs, scored 50/50 mg. *Aldoril* (methyldopa + hydrochlorothiazide): Generic only: Tabs, unscored, 250/15, 250/25 mg. *Apresazide* (hydralazine + hydrochlorothiazide): Generic only: Caps 25/25, 50/50 mg. *Atacand HCT* (candesartan + hydrochlorothiazide, ✦*Atacand Plus*): Trade only: Tab, scored 16/12.5, 32/12.5, 32/25 mg. *Avalide* (irbesartan + hydrochlorothiazide): Trade only: Tabs, unscored 150/12.5, 300/12.5, 300/25 mg. *Azor* (olmesartan + amlodipine): Trade only: Tabs, unscored 5/20, 5/40, 10/20, 10/40 mg. *Benicar HCT* (olmesartan + hydrochlorothiazide): Trade only: Tabs, unscored 20/12.5, 40/12.5, 40/25 mg. *Capozide* (captopril + hydrochlorothiazide): Generic/Trade: Tabs, scored 25/15, 25/25, 50/15, 50/25 mg. *Clorpres* (clonidine + chlorthalidone): Trade only: Tabs, scored 0.1/15, 0.2/15, 0.3/15 mg. *Corzide* (nadolol + bendroflumethiazide): Generic/Trade: Tabs 40/5, 80/5 mg. *Diovan HCT* (valsartan + hydrochlorothiazide): Trade only: Tabs, unscored 80/12.5, 160/12.5, 160/25, 320/12.5, 320/25 mg. *Dyazide* (triamterene + hydrochlorothiazide): Generic/Trade: Caps, (Dyazide) 37.5/25, (generic only) 50/25 mg. *Exforge* (amlodipine + valsartan): Trade only: Tabs, unscored 5/160, 5/320, 10/160, 10/320 mg. *Exforge HCT* (amlodipine + valsartan + hydrocholrothiazide): Trade only: Tabs, unscored 5/160/12.5, 5/160/25, 10/160/12.5, 10/160/25, 10/320/25 mg. *Hyzaar* (losartan + hydrochlorothiazide): Trade only: Tabs, unscored 50/12.5, 100/12.5, 100/25 mg. *Inderide* (propranolol + hydrochlorothiazide): Generic/Trade: Tabs, scored 40/25, 80/25. *Inhibace Plus* (cilazapril + hydrochlorothiazide): Trade only: Scored tabs 5 mg cilazapril + 12.5 mg HCTZ. *Lexxel* (enalapril + felodipine): Trade only: Tabs, unscored 5/2.5, 5/5 mg. *Lopressor HCT* (metoprolol + hydrochlorothiazide): Generic/Trade: Tabs, scored 50/25, 100/25, 100/50 mg. *Lotensin HCT* (benazepril + hydrochlorothiazide): Generic/Trade: Tabs, scored 5/6.25, 10/12.5, 20/12.5, 20/25 mg. *Lotrel* (amlodipine + benazepril): Generic/Trade: Cap, 2.5/10, 5/10, 5/20, 10/20 mg. Trade only: Cap, 5/40, 10/40 mg. *Maxzide* (triamterene + hydrochlorothiazide, ✦*Triazide*): Generic/Trade: Tabs, scored 75/50 mg. *Maxzide-25* (triamterene + hydrochlorothiazide): Generic/Trade: Tabs, scored 37.5/25. *Micardis HCT* (telmisartan + hydrochlorothiazide, ✦*Micardis Plus*): Trade only: Tabs, unscored 40/12.5, 80/12.5, 80/25 mg. *Minizide* (prazosin + polythiazide): Trade only: Caps, 1/0.5, 2/0.5, 5/0.5 mg. *Moduretic* (amiloride + hydrochlorothiazide, ✦*Moduret*): Generic only: Tabs, scored 5/50 mg. *Monopril HCT* (fosinopril + hydrochlorothiazide): Generic/Trade: Tabs, unscored 10/12.5, scored 20/12.5 mg. *Prinzide* (lisinopril + hydrochlorothiazide): Generic/Trade: Tabs, unscored 10/12.5, 20/12.5, 20/25 mg. *Tarka* (trandolapril + verapamil): Trade only: Tabs, unscored 2/180, 1/240, 2/240, 4/240 mg. *Tekamlo* (aliskiren + amlodipine): Trade only: Tabs, unscored 150/5, 150/10, 300/5, 300/10 mg. *Tekturna HCT* (aliskiren + hydrochlorothiazide): Trade only: Tabs, unscored 150/12.5, 150/25, 300/12.5, 300/25 mg *Tenoretic* (atenolol + chlorthalidone): Generic/Trade: Tabs, scored 50/25, unscored 100/25 mg. *Teveten HCT* (eprosartan + hydrochlorothiazide): Trade only: Tabs, unscored 600/12.5, 600/25 mg. *Tribenzor* (olmesartan + amlodipine + hydrochlorothiazide): Trade only:

(cont.)

Tabs, unscored 20/5/12.5, 40/5/12.5, 40/5/25, 40/10/12.5, 40/10/25 mg. *Twynsta* (amlodipine + telmisartan): Trade: Tabs, 5/40, 5/80, 10/40, 10/80 mg. *Uniretic* (moexipril + hydrochlorothiazide): Generic/Trade: Tabs, scored 7.5/12.5, 15/12.5, 15/25 mg. *Valturna* (aliskiren + valsartan): Trade only: Tabs, unscored 150/160, 300/320 mg. *Vaseretic* (enalapril + hydrochlorothiazide): Generic/Trade: Tabs, unscored 5/12.5, 10/25 mg. *Zestoretic* (lisinopril + hydrochlorothiazide): Generic/Trade: Tabs, unscored 10/12.5, 20/12.5, 20/25 mg. *Ziac* (bisoprolol + hydrochlorothiazide): Generic/Trade: Tabs, unscored 2.5/6.25, 5/6.25, 10/6.25 mg.

Antihypertensives—Other

ALISKIREN (*Tekturna*) HTN: 150 mg PO daily, max 300 mg/day. [Trade only: Tabs unscored 150, 300 mg.] ▶LK ♀– ▶–? $$$

FENOLDOPAM (*Corlopam*) Severe HTN: 10 mg in 250 mL D5W (40 mcg/mL), start at 0.1 mcg/kg/min titrate q 15 min, usual effective dose 0.1 to 1.6 mcg/kg/min. ▶LK ♀B ▶? $$$

HYDRALAZINE (*Apresoline*) Hypertensive emergency: 10 to 50 mg IM or 10 to 20 mg IV, repeat prn. HTN: Start 10 mg PO bid to qid, max 300 mg/day. Headaches, peripheral edema, SLE syndrome. [Generic only: Tabs unscored 10, 25, 50, 100 mg.] ▶LK ♀C ▶+ $

NITROPRUSSIDE (*Nitropress*) Hypertensive emergency: Dilute 50 mg in 250 mL D5W (200 mcg/mL), rate of 6 mL/h for 70 kg adult delivers starting dose of 0.3 mcg/kg/min. Max 10 mcg/kg/min. Protect from light. Cyanide toxicity with high doses (10 mcg/kg/min), hepatic/renal impairment, and prolonged infusions (longer than 3 to 7 days); check thiocyanate levels. ▶RBCs ♀C ▶– $

STATINS

Minimum Dose for 30-40% LDL Reduction	LDL *	LFT Monitoring**
atorvastatin 10 mg	-39%	Baseline, 12 weeks, semiannually
fluvastatin 40 mg bid	-36%	Baseline, 12 weeks
fluvastatin XL 80 mg	-35%	Baseline, 12 weeks
lovastatin 40 mg	-31%	Baseline
pitavastatin 2 mg	-36%	Baseline, 12 weeks
pravastatin 40mg	-34%	Baseline
rosuvastatin 5 mg	-45%	Baseline, 12 weeks, semiannually
simvastatin 20 mg	-38%	Baseline for all doses; Get LFTs prior to & 3 months after dose increase to 80 mg, then semiannually for first year.

LDL=low-density lipoprotein, LFT=liver function tests. Will get ~6% decrease in LDL with every doubling of dose. National Lipid Association Statin Safety Task Force Report (*Am J Cardiol* 2006; 8A:89c-94c) schedule for LFT monitoring: baseline, ~12 weeks after starting/titrating therapy, when clinically indicated. Stop statin therapy if LFTs are >3 times upper limit of normal. *Adapted from *Circulation* 2004;110:227-239. **From Prescribing information

PHENTOLAMINE (_Regitine, Rogitine_) <u>Diagnosis of pheochromocytoma:</u> 5 mg increments IV/IM. Peds 0.05 to 0.1 mg/kg IV/IM up to 5 mg per dose. <u>Extravasation:</u> 5 to 10 mg in 10 mL NS inject 1 to 5 mL SC (in divided doses) around extravasation site. ▶Plasma ♀C ▶? $$$

Antiplatelet Drugs

ABCIXIMAB (_ReoPro_) <u>Platelet aggregation inhibition, percutaneous coronary intervention:</u> 0.25 mg/kg IV bolus via separate infusion line before procedure, then 0.125 mcg/kg/min (max 10 mcg/min) IV infusion for 12 h. ▶Plasma ♀C ▶? $$$$$

AGGRENOX (acetylsalicylic acid + dipyridamole) <u>Prevention of CVA after TIA/CVA:</u> 1 cap PO bid. [Trade only: Caps 25 mg aspirin/200 mg extended-release dipyridamole.] ▶LK ♀D ▶? $$$$

CLOPIDOGREL (_Plavix_) <u>Reduction of thrombotic events: Recent acute MI/CVA, established peripheral arterial disease:</u> 75 mg PO daily; <u>non-ST segment elevation acute coronary syndrome:</u> 300 mg loading dose, then 75 mg PO daily in combination with aspirin. <u>ST segment elevation MI:</u> Start with/without 300 mg loading dose, then 75 mg PO daily in combination with aspirin, with/without thrombolytic. [Trade: Tabs unscored 75, 300 mg.] ▶LK ♀B ▶? $$$$

LDL CHOLESTEROL GOALS[1]		Lifestyle Changes[2]	Also Consider Meds at LDL (mg/dL)[3]
Risk Category	**LDL Goal**		
High risk: CHD or equivalent risk,[4,5,6] 10-year risk >20%	<100 (optional <70)[7]	LDL ≥ 100[8]	≥100 (<100: consider Rx options)[9]
Moderately high risk: 2+ risk factors,[10] 10-year risk 10–20%	<130 (optional <100)	LDL ≥ 130[8]	≥130 (100–129: consider Rx options)[11]
Moderate risk: 2+ risk factors,[10] 10-year risk <10%	<130 mg/dL	LDL ≥ 130	≥160
Lower risk: 0 to 1 risk factor[5]	<160 mg/dL	LDL ≥ 160	≥190 (160–189: Rx optional)

1. CHD = coronary heart disease. LDL = low density lipoprotein. Adapted from NCEP: *JAMA* 2001; 285:2486; NCEP Report: *Circulation* 2004;110:227–239. All 10-year risks based upon Framingham stratification; calculator available at: http://www.nhlbi.nih.gov/atpiii/calculator.asp?usertype=prof. 2. Dietary modification, wt reduction, exercise. 3. When using LDL lowering therapy, achieve at least 30-40% LDL reduction. 4. Equivalent risk defined as diabetes, other atherosclerotic disease (peripheral artery disease, abdominal aortic aneurysm, symptomatic carotid artery disease,CKD or prior ischemic CVA/TIA), or ≥ 2 risk factors such that 10-year risk > 20%. 5. History of ischemic CVA or transient ischemic attack = CHD risk equivalents (*Stroke* 2006;37:577-617). 6. Chronic kidney disease = CHD risk equivalent [*Am J Kidney Dis* 2003 Apr;41 (4 suppl 3):I-IV,S1-S1]. 7. For any patient with atherosclerotic disease, may treat to LDL < 70 mg/dL (*Circulation* 2006;113:2363–72). 8. Regardless of LDL, lifestyle changes are indicated when lifestyle-related risk factors (obesity, physical inactivity, ↑TG, ↓HDL, or metabolic syndrome) are present. 9. If baseline LDL < 100, starting LDL lowering therapy is an option based on clinical trials. With ↑TG or ↓HDL, consider combining fibrate or nicotinic acid with LDL lowering drug. 10. Risk factors: Cigarette smoking, HTN (BP ≥ 140/90 mmHg or on antihypertensive meds), low HDL (< 40 mg/dL), family hx of CHD (1° relative: ♂ < 55 yo, ♀ < 65 yo), age (♂ ≥ 45 yo, ♀ ≥ 55 yo). 11. At baseline or after lifestyle changes - initiating therapy to achieve LDL < 100 is an option based on clinical trials.

DIPYRIDAMOLE (*Persantine*) Antithrombotic: 75 to 100 mg PO qid. [Generic/Trade: Tabs unscored 25, 50, 75 mg.] ▶L ♀B ▶? $$$

EPTIFIBATIDE (*Integrilin*) Acute coronary syndrome: Load 180 mcg/kg IV bolus, then infusion 2 mcg/kg/min for up to 72 h. Discontinue infusion prior to CABG. Percutaneous coronary intervention: Load 180 mcg/kg IV bolus just before procedure, followed by infusion 2 mcg/kg/min and a 2nd 180 mcg/kg IV bolus 10 min after the first bolus. Continue infusion for up to 18 to 24 h (minimum 12 h) after procedure. Reduce infusion dose to 1 mcg/kg/min with CrCl < 50 mL/min; contraindicated in dialysis patients. ▶K ♀B ▶? $$$$$

PRASUGREL (*Effient*) Reduction of thrombotic events after acute coronary syndrome managed with percutaneous coronary intervention (PCI): 60 mg loading dose, then 10 mg PO daily in combination with aspirin. For wt less than 60 kg consider lowering maintenance dose to 5 mg PO daily. [Trade: Tabs unscored 5, 10 mg.] ▶LK ♀B ▶? $$$$

TICLOPIDINE (*Ticlid*) Due to high incidence of neutropenia and thrombotic thrombocytopenia purpura, other drugs preferred. Platelet aggregation inhibition/reduction of thrombotic CVA: 250 mg PO bid with food. [Generic/Trade: Tabs unscored 250 mg.] ▶L ♀B ▶? $$$$

TIROFIBAN (*Aggrastat*) Acute coronary syndromes: Start 0.4 mcg/kg/min IV infusion for 30 min, then decrease to 0.1 mcg/kg/min for 48 to 108 h or until 12 to 24 h after coronary intervention. Half dose with CrCl <30 mL/min. Use concurrent heparin to keep PTT 2× normal. ▶K ♀B ▶? $$$$$

Beta-Blockers

NOTE *See also antihypertensive combinations. Not first line for HTN (unless to treat angina, post MI, LV dysfunction, or heart failure). Abrupt discontinuation may precipitate angina, MI, arrhythmias, or rebound HTN; discontinue by tapering over 1 to 2 weeks. Avoid use of nonselective beta-blockers in patients with asthma/COPD. For patients with asthma/COPD, use agents with beta-1 selectivity and monitor cautiously. Beta-1 selectivity diminishes at high doses. Avoid initiating beta-blocker therapy in acute decompensated heart failure, sick sinus syndrome without pacer, and severe peripheral artery disease.*

ACEBUTOLOL (*Sectral*, *✦Rhotral*) HTN: Start 400 mg PO daily or 200 mg PO bid, maximum 1200 mg/day. Beta-1 receptor selective. [Generic/Trade: Caps 200, 400 mg.] ▶LK ♀B ▶− $$

ATENOLOL (*Tenormin*) Acute MI: 50 to 100 mg PO daily or in divided doses; or 5 mg IV over 5 min, repeat in 10 min. HTN: Start 25 to 50 mg PO daily or divided bid, maximum 100 mg/day. Beta-1 receptor selective. [Generic/Trade: Tabs unscored 25, 100 mg; scored, 50 mg.] ▶K ♀D ▶− $

BETAXOLOL (*Kerlone*) HTN: Start 5 to 10 mg PO daily, max 20 mg/day. Beta-1 receptor selective. [Generic: Tabs scored 10 mg, unscored 20 mg.] ▶LK ♀C ▶? $$

BISOPROLOL (*Zebeta*, *✦Monocor*) HTN: Start 2.5 to 5 mg PO daily, max 20 mg/day. Beta-1 receptor selective. [Generic/Trade: Tabs scored 5 mg, unscored 10 mg.] ▶LK ♀C ▶? $$

CARVEDILOL (*Coreg, Coreg CR*) <u>Heart failure, immediate-release:</u> Start 3.125 mg PO bid, double dose every 2 weeks as tolerated up to max of 25 mg bid (for wt 85 kg or less) or 50 mg bid (for wt greater than 85 kg). <u>Heart failure, sustained-release:</u> Start 10 mg PO daily, double dose every 2 weeks as tolerated to max of 80 mg/day. <u>LV dysfunction following acute MI, immediate-release:</u> Start 3.125 to 6.25 mg PO bid, double dose q 3 to 10 days as tolerated to max of 25 mg bid. <u>LV dysfunction following acute MI, sustained-release:</u> Start 10 to 20 mg PO daily, double dose q 3 to 10 days as tolerated to max of 80 mg/day. <u>HTN, immediate-release:</u> Start 6.25 mg PO bid, double dose q 7 to 14 days as tolerated to max 50 mg/day. <u>HTN, sustained-release:</u> Start 20 mg PO daily, double dose q 7 to 14 days as tolerated to max 80 mg/day. Take with food to decrease orthostatic hypotension. Give Coreg CR in the morning. Alpha-1, beta-1, and beta-2 receptor blocker. [Generic/Trade: Tabs immediate-release unscored 3.125, 6.25, 12.5, 25 mg. Trade only: Caps extended-release 10, 20, 40, 80 mg.] ▶L ♀C ▷? $$$$

ESMOLOL (*Brevibloc*) <u>SVT/HTN emergency:</u> Load 500 mcg/kg over 1 min (dilute 5 g in 500 mL to make a solution of 10 mg/mL and give 3.5 mL to deliver 35 g bolus for 70 kg patient) then start infusion 50 to 200 mcg/kg/min (40 mL/h delivers 100 mcg/kg/min for 70 kg patient). Half-life is 9 min. Beta-1 receptor selective. ▶K ♀C ▷? $

LABETALOL (*Trandate*) <u>HTN:</u> Start 100 mg PO bid, max 2400 mg/day. <u>HTN emergency:</u> Start 20 mg IV slow injection, then 40 to 80 mg IV q 10 min prn up to 300 mg or IV infusion 0.5 to 2 mg/min. Peds: Start 0.3 to 1 mg/kg/dose (max 20 mg). Alpha-1, beta-1, and beta-2 receptor blocker. [Generic/Trade: Tabs scored 100, 200, 300 mg.] ▶LK ♀C ▷+ $$$

METOPROLOL (*Lopressor, Toprol-XL, ✦Betaloc*) <u>Acute MI:</u> 50 to 100 mg PO q 12 h; or 5 mg increments IV q 5 to 15 min up to 15 mg followed by oral therapy. <u>HTN (immediate-release):</u> Start 100 mg PO daily or in divided doses, increase prn up to 450 mg/day; may require multiple daily doses to maintain 24 h BP control. <u>HTN (extended-release):</u> Start 25 to 100 mg PO daily, increase prn up to 400 mg/day. <u>Heart failure:</u> Start 12.5 to 25 mg (extended-release) PO daily, double dose every 2 weeks as tolerated up to max 200 mg/day. <u>Angina:</u> Start 50 mg PO bid (immediate-release) or 100 mg PO daily (extended-release), increase prn up to 400 mg/day. Beta-1 receptor selective. IV to PO conversion: 1 mg IV is equivalent to 2.5 mg PO (divided qid). Immediate-release form is metoprolol tartrate; extended-release form is metoprolol succinate. Take with food. [Generic/Trade: Tabs scored 50, 100 mg, extended-release 25, 50, 100, 200 mg. Generic only: Tabs scored 25 mg.] ▶L ♀C ▷? $$

NADOLOL (*Corgard*) <u>HTN:</u> Start 20 to 40 mg PO daily, max 320 mg/day. Beta-1 and beta-2 receptor blocker. [Generic/Trade: Tabs scored 20, 40, 80, 120, 160 mg.] ▶K ♀C ▷− $$

NEBIVOLOL (*Bystolic*) <u>HTN:</u> Start 5 mg PO daily, maximum 40 mg/day. Beta-1 receptor selective at doses of 10 mg or less and in patients who extensively metabolize CYP2D6; otherwise, inhibits both beta-1 and beta-2 receptors. [Trade only: Tabs unscored 2.5, 5, 10, 20 mg.] ▶L ♀C ▷− $$$

OXPRENOLOL (✦*Trasicor, Slow-Trasicor*) Canada only. <u>HTN:</u> Regular-release: Initially 20 mg PO tid, titrate upwards prn to usual maintenance 120 to 320 mg/day divided bid to tid. Alternatively, may substitute an equivalent daily dose of sustained-release product; do not exceed 480 mg/day. [Trade only: Tabs regular-release 40, 80 mg. Tabs sustained-release 80, 160 mg.] ▶L ♀D ▶– $$

PINDOLOL (✦*Visken*) <u>HTN:</u> Start 5 mg PO bid, max 60 mg/day. Beta-1 and beta-2 receptor blocker. [Generic only: Tabs scored 5, 10 mg.] ▶K ♀B ▶? $$$

PROPRANOLOL (*Inderal, Inderal LA, InnoPran XL*) <u>HTN:</u> Start 20 to 40 mg PO bid or 60 to 80 mg PO daily, max 640 mg/day; extended-release (Inderal LA) max 640 mg/day; extended-release (InnoPran XL) 80 mg at bedtime (10 pm), max 120 mg at bedtime (chronotherapy). <u>Supraventricular tachycardia or rapid atrial fibrillation/flutter:</u> 1 mg IV q 2 min. Max of 2 doses in 4 h. <u>Migraine prophylaxis:</u> Start 40 mg PO bid or 80 mg PO daily (extended-release), max 240 mg/day. Beta-1 and beta-2 receptor blocker. [Generic/Trade: Tabs scored 40, 60, 80. Caps extended-release 60, 80, 120, 160 mg. Generic only: Soln 20, 40 mg/5 mL. Tabs 10, 20 mg. Trade only: (InnoPran XL at bedtime) 80, 120 mg.] ▶L ♀C ▶+ $$

Calcium Channel Blockers (CCBs)—Dihydropyridines

NOTE *See also antihypertensive combinations.*

AMLODIPINE (*Norvasc*) <u>HTN:</u> Start 5 mg PO daily, max 10 daily. Elderly, small, frail, or with hepatic insufficiency: Start 2.5 PO daily. [Generic/Trade: Tabs unscored 2.5, 5, 10 mg. Generic only: Orally disintegrating tabs 2.5, 5, 10 mg.] ▶L ♀C ▶? $$$

CLEVIDIPINE (*Cleviprex*) <u>HTN:</u> Start 1 to 2 mg/h IV, titrate q 1.5 to 10 min to BP response, usual maintenance dose 4 to 6 mg/h, max 32 mg/h IV. An increase of 1 to 2 mg/h will decrease SBP approximately 2 to 4 mmHg. ▶KL ♀C ▶? $$$

FELODIPINE (*Plendil, ✦Renedil*) <u>HTN:</u> Start 2.5 to 5 mg PO daily, maximum 10 mg/day. [Generic/Trade: Tabs extended-release, unscored 2.5, 5, 10 mg.] ▶L ♀C ▶? $$

ISRADIPINE (*DynaCirc, DynaCirc CR*) <u>HTN:</u> Start 2.5 mg PO bid, max 20 mg/day (max 10 mg/day in elderly). Controlled-release: 5 to 20 mg PO daily. [Trade only: Tabs controlled-release 5, 10 mg. Generic only: Immediate-release caps 2.5, 5 mg.] ▶L ♀C ▶? $$$$

NICARDIPINE (*Cardene, Cardene SR*) <u>HTN emergency:</u> Begin IV infusion at 5 mg/h, titrate to effect, max 15 mg/h. <u>HTN:</u> Start 20 mg PO tid, max 120 mg/day. Sustained-release: Start 30 mg PO bid, max 120 mg/day. [Generic/Trade: Caps immediate-release 20, 30 mg. Trade only: Caps sustained-release 30, 45, 60 mg.] ▶L ♀C ▶? $$$

NIFEDIPINE (*Procardia, Adalat, Procardia XL, Adalat CC, Afeditab CR, ✦Adalat XL, Adalat PA*) <u>HTN/Angina:</u> Extended-release: 30 to 60 mg PO

(cont.)

daily, max 120 mg/day. <u>Angina:</u> Immediate-release: Start 10 mg PO tid, max 120 mg/day. <u>Sublingual administration</u>, may cause excessive hypotension, acute MI, CVA. Do not use immediate-release caps for treating HTN. <u>Preterm labor:</u> Loading dose: 10 mg PO q 20 to 30 min if contractions persist, up to 40 mg within the first h. Maintenance dose: 10 to 20 mg PO q 4 to 6 h or 60 to 160 mg extended-release PO daily. [Generic/Trade: Caps 10, 20 mg. Tabs extended-release (Adalat CC, Afeditab CR, Procardia XL) 30, 60 mg, (Adalat CC, Procardia XL) 90 mg.] ▶L ♀C ▶– $$

NISOLDIPINE *(Sular)* <u>HTN:</u> Start 17 mg PO daily, max 34 mg/day. Take on an empty stomach. [Trade only: Tabs extended-release 8.5, 17, 25.5, 34 mg. These replace the former 10, 20, 30, 40 mg tabs. Generic only: Tabs extended-release 20, 30, 40 mg.] ▶L ♀C ▶? $$$

Calcium Channel Blockers (CCBs)—Non-Dihydropyridines

NOTE *See also antihypertensive combinations.*

DILTIAZEM *(Cardizem, Cardizem LA, Cardizem CD, Cartia XT, Dilacor XR, Diltiazem CD, Diltzac, Diltia XT, Tiazac, Taztia XT)* <u>Atrial fibrillation/ flutter, PSVT:</u> Bolus 20 mg (0.25 mg/kg) IV over 2 min. Rebolus 15 min later (if needed) 25 mg (0.35 mg/kg). Infusion 5 to 15 mg/h. <u>HTN, once daily, extended-release:</u> Start 120 to 240 mg PO daily, max 540 mg/day. <u>HTN, once daily, graded extended-release (Cardizem LA):</u> Start 180 to 240 mg PO daily, max 540 mg/day. <u>HTN, twice daily, sustained-release:</u> Start 60 to 120 mg PO bid, max 360 mg/day. <u>Angina, immediate-release:</u> Start 30 mg PO qid, max 360 mg/day divided tid to qid; <u>Angina, extended-release:</u> start 120 to 240 mg PO daily, max 540 mg/day. <u>Angina, once daily, graded extended-release (Cardizem LA):</u> start 180 mg PO daily, doses more than 360 mg may provide no additional benefit. [Generic/Trade: Tabs immediate-release, unscored (Cardizem) 30, scored 60, 90, 120 mg; Caps extended-release (Cardizem CD, Cartia XT daily) 120, 180, 240, 300, 360 mg, (Diltzac, Taztia XT, Tiazac daily) 120, 180, 240, 300, 360, 420 mg, (Dilacor XR, Diltia XT) 120, 180, 240 mg. Trade only: Tabs extended-release graded (Cardizem LA daily) 120, 180, 240, 300, 360, 420 mg.] ▶L ♀C ▶+ $$

VERAPAMIL *(Isoptin SR, Calan, Covera-HS, Verelan, Verelan PM, ✦Veramil)* <u>SVT adults:</u> 5 to 10 mg IV over 2 min; <u>SVT peds</u> (age 1 to 15 yo): 2 to 5 mg (0.1 to 0.3 mg/kg) IV, max dose 5 mg. <u>Angina:</u> Immediate-release, start 40 to 80 mg PO tid to qid, max 480 mg/day; sustained to release, start 120 to 240 mg PO daily, max 480 mg/day (use bid dosing for doses greater than 240 mg/day with Isoptin SR and Calan SR); (Covera-HS) 180 mg PO at bedtime, max 480 mg/day. <u>HTN:</u> Same as angina, except (Verelan PM) 100 to 200 mg PO at bedtime, max 400 mg/day; immediate-release tabs should be avoided in treating HTN. Use cautiously with impaired renal/hepatic function. [Generic/Trade: Tabs immediate-release, scored (Calan) 40, 80, 120 mg; Tabs sustained-release, unscored (Isoptin SR) 120 mg, scored 180, 240 mg; Caps sustained-release (Verelan) 120, 180, 240, 360 mg; Caps extended-release

(cont.)

(Verelan PM) 100, 200, 300 mg. Trade only: Tabs extended-release (Covera HS) 180, 240 mg.] ▶L ♀C ▶– $$

Diuretics—Carbonic Anhydrase Inhibitors

ACETAZOLAMIDE (*Diamox, Diamox Sequels*) <u>Glaucoma:</u> 250 mg PO up to qid (immediate-release) or 500 mg PO up to bid (sustained-release). Max 1 g/day. <u>Acute Glaucoma:</u> 250 mg IV q 4 h or 500 mg IV initially with 125 to 250 mg q 4 h, followed by oral therapy. <u>Mountain sickness prophylaxis:</u> 125 to 250 mg PO bid to tid, beginning 1 to 2 days prior to ascent and continuing at least 5 days at higher altitude. <u>Edema:</u> Rarely used, start 250 to 375 mg IV/PO q am given intermittently (every other day or 2 consecutive days followed by none for 1 to 2 days) to avoid loss of diuretic effect. [Generic only: Tabs 125, 250 mg. Generic/Trade: Caps extended-release 500 mg.] ▶LK ♀C ▶+ $

Diuretics—Loop

BUMETANIDE (*Bumex, ✦Burinex*) <u>Edema:</u> 0.5 to 1 mg IV/IM; 0.5 to 2 mg PO daily. 1 mg bumetanide is roughly equivalent to 40 mg furosemide. [Generic/Trade: Tabs scored 0.5, 1, 2 mg.] ▶K ♀C ▶? $

ETHACRYNIC ACID (*Edecrin*) Rarely used. May be useful in sulfa-allergic patients. <u>Edema:</u> 0.5 to 1 mg/kg IV, max 100 mg/dose; 25 to 100 mg PO daily to bid. [Trade only: Tabs scored 25 mg.] ▶K ♀B ▶? $$$

FUROSEMIDE (*Lasix*) <u>Edema:</u> Initial dose 20 to 80 mg IV/IM/PO, increase dose by 20 to 40 mg q 6 to 8 h until desired response is achieved, max 600 mg/day. Use lower doses in elderly. [Generic/Trade: Tabs unscored 20, scored 40, 80 mg. Generic only: Oral soln 10 mg/mL, 40 mg/5 mL.] ▶K ♀C ▶? $

TORSEMIDE (*Demadex*) <u>Edema:</u> 5 to 20 mg IV/PO daily. [Generic/Trade: Tabs scored 5, 10, 20, 100 mg.] ▶LK ♀B ▶? $

Diuretics—Thiazide Type

NOTE *See also antihypertensive combinations.*

CHLORTHALIDONE (*Thalitone*) <u>HTN:</u> 12.5 to 25 mg PO daily, max 50 mg/day. <u>Edema:</u> 50 to 100 mg PO daily, max 200 mg/day. <u>Nephrolithiasis</u> (unapproved use): 25 to 50 mg PO daily. [Trade only: Tabs unscored (Thalitone) 15 mg. Generic only: Tabs unscored 25, 50 mg.] ▶L ♀B, D if used in pregnancy-induced HTN ▶+ $

HYDROCHLOROTHIAZIDE (*HCTZ, Esidrix, Oretic, Microzide, HydroDiuril*) <u>HTN:</u> 12.5 to 25 mg PO daily, max 50 mg/day. <u>Edema:</u> 25 to 100 mg PO daily, max 200 mg/day. [Generic/Trade: Tabs scored 25, 50 mg; Caps 12.5 mg.] ▶L ♀B, D if used in pregnancy-induced HTN ▶+ $

INDAPAMIDE (*Lozol, ✦Lozide*) <u>HTN:</u> 1.25 to 5 mg PO daily, max 5 mg/day. <u>Edema:</u> 2.5 to 5 mg PO qam. [Generic only: Tabs unscored 1.25, 2.5 mg.] ▶L ♀B, D if used in pregnancy-induced HTN ▶? $

METOLAZONE (*Zaroxolyn*) <u>Edema:</u> 5 to 10 mg PO daily, max 10 mg/day in heart failure, 20 mg/day in renal disease. If used with loop diuretic, start with 2.5 mg PO daily. [Generic/Trade: Tabs 2.5, 5, 10 mg.] ▶L ♀B, D if used in pregnancy-induced HTN ▶? $$$

Nitrates

ISOSORBIDE DINITRATE (*Isordil, Dilatrate-SR, ✦Cedocard SR, Coronex*) <u>Angina prophylaxis:</u> 5 to 40 mg PO tid (7 am, noon, 5 pm), sustained-release: 40 to 80 mg PO bid (8 am, 2 pm). <u>Acute angina,</u> SL Tabs: 2.5 to 10 mg SL q 5 to 10 min prn, up to 3 doses in 30 min. [Generic/Trade: Tabs scored 5, 10, 20, 30 mg. Trade only: Tabs (Isordil) 40 mg, Caps extended-release (Dilatrate-SR) 40 mg. Generic only: Tabs sustained-release 40 mg, Tabs sublingual 2.5, 5 mg.] ▶L ♀C ▶? $

ISOSORBIDE MONONITRATE (*ISMO, Monoket, Imdur*) <u>Angina:</u> 20 mg PO bid (8 am and 3 pm). Extended-release: Start 30 to 60 mg PO daily, maximum 240 mg/day. [Generic/Trade: Tabs unscored (ISMO, bid dosing) 20 mg, scored (Monoket, bid dosing) 10, 20 mg extended-release, scored (Imdur, daily dosing) 30, 60, unscored 120 mg.] ▶L ♀C ▶? $$

NITROGLYCERIN INTRAVENOUS INFUSION (*Tridil*) <u>Perioperative HTN, acute MI/Heart failure, acute angina:</u> Mix 50 mg in 250 mL D5W (200 mcg/mL), start at 10 to 20 mcg/min (3 to 6 mL/h), then titrate upward by 10 to 20 mcg/min prn. [Brand name "Tridil" no longer manufactured but retained herein for name recognition.] ▶L ♀C ▶? $

NITROGLYCERIN OINTMENT (*Nitro-BID*) <u>Angina prophylaxis:</u> Start 0.5 inch q 8 h, maintenance 1 to 2 inch q 8 h, maximum 4 inch q 4 to 6 h; 15 mg/inch. Allow for a nitrate-free period of 10 to 14 h to avoid nitrate tolerance. 1 inch ointment is ~15 mg. [Trade only: Ointment, 2%, tubes 1, 30, 60 g (Nitro-BID).] ▶L ♀C ▶? $

NITROGLYCERIN SPRAY (*Nitrolingual, NitroMist*) <u>Acute angina:</u> 1 to 2 sprays under the tongue prn, max 3 sprays in 15 min. [Trade only: Nitrolingual soln, 4.9, 12 mL. 0.4 mg/spray (60 or 200 sprays/canister); NitroMist aerosol 0.4 mg/spray (230 sprays/canister).] ▶L ♀C ▶? $$$$

NITROGLYCERIN SUBLINGUAL (*Nitrostat, NitroQuick*) <u>Acute angina:</u> 0.4 mg SL under tongue, repeat dose q 5 min prn up to 3 doses in 15 min. [Generic/Trade: Sublingual tabs unscored 0.3, 0.4, 0.6 mg; in bottles of 100 or package of 4 bottles with 25 tabs each.] ▶L ♀C ▶? $

NITROGLYCERIN TRANSDERMAL (*Minitran, Nitro-Dur, ✦Trinipatch*) <u>Angina prophylaxis:</u> 1 patch 12 to 14 h each day. Allow for a nitrate-free period of 10 to 14 h each day to avoid nitrate tolerance. [Generic/Trade: Transdermal system 0.1, 0.2, 0.4, 0.6 mg/h. Trade only: (Nitro-Dur) 0.3, 0.8 mg/h.] ▶L ♀C ▶? $$

Pressors/Inotropes

DOBUTAMINE (*Dobutrex*) <u>Inotropic support:</u> 2 to 20 mcg/kg/min. Dilute 250 mg in 250 mL D5W (1 mg/mL), a rate of 21 mL/h delivers 5 mcg/kg/min for a 70 kg patient. ▶Plasma ♀D ▶– $

DOPAMINE (*Intropin*) Pressor: Start at 5 mcg/kg/min, increase prn by 5 to 10 mcg/kg/min increments at 10 min intervals, max 50 mcg/kg/min. Mix 400 mg in 250 mL D5W (1600 mcg/mL) a rate of 13 mL/h delivers 5 mcg/kg/min in a 70 kg patient. Doses in mcg/kg/min: 2 to 4 (traditional renal dose, apparently ineffective) dopaminergic receptors; 5 to 10 (cardiac dose) dopaminergic and beta-1 receptors; more than 10 dopaminergic, beta-1, and alpha-1 receptors. ▶Plasma ♀C ▶– $

EPHEDRINE Pressor: 10 to 25 mg slow IV, repeat q 5 to 10 min prn. [Generic only: Caps 50 mg.] ▶K ♀C ▶? $

EPINEPHRINE (*EpiPen, EpiPen Jr, Twinject, adrenalin*) Cardiac arrest: 1 mg IV q 3 to 5 min. Anaphylaxis: 0.1 to 0.5 mg SC/IM, may repeat SC dose q 10 to 15 min. Acute asthma and hypersensitivity reactions: Adults: 0.1 to 0.3 mg of 1:1000 soln SC or IM; Peds: 0.01 mg/kg up to 0.3 mg) of 1:1000 soln SC or IM. [Soln for injection: 1:1000 (1 mg/mL in 1 mL amps or 10 mL vial). Trade only: EpiPen Auto-injector delivers one 0.3 mg (1:1000, 0.3 mL) IM dose. EpiPen Jr. Autoinjector delivers one 0.15 mg (1:2000, 0.3 mL) IM dose. Twinject auto-injector delivers one 0.15 mg (1:1000, 0.15 mL) or 0.3 mg (1:1000, 0.3 mL) IM/SQ dose.] ▶Plasma ♀C ▶– $

INAMRINONE Heart failure: 0.75 mg/kg bolus IV over 2 to 3 min, then infusion 5 to 10 mcg/kg/min; mix 100 mg in 100 mL NS (1 mg/mL) a rate of 21 mL/h delivers 5 mcg/kg/min for a 70 kg patient. ▶K ♀C ▶? $$$$$

MIDODRINE (*Orvaten, ProAmatine, ✦Amatine*) Orthostatic hypotension: 10 mg PO tid while awake. [Generic/Trade: Tabs scored 2.5, 5, 10 mg.] ▶LK ♀C ▶? $$$$$

MILRINONE (*Primacor*) Systolic heart failure (NYHA class III, IV): Load 50 mcg/kg IV over 10 min, then begin IV infusion of 0.375 to 0.75 mcg/kg/min. ▶K ♀C ▶? $$

NOREPINEPHRINE (*Levophed*) Acute hypotension: start 8 to 12 mcg/min, adjust to maintain BP, average maintenance rate 2 to 4 mcg/min. Mix 4 mg in 500 mL D5W (8 mcg/mL), a rate of 22.5 mL/h delivers 3 mcg/min. Ideally through central line. ▶Plasma ♀C ▶– $

PHENYLEPHRINE—INTRAVENOUS (*Neo-Synephrine*) Severe hypotension: Infusion: 20 mg in 250 mL D5W (80 mcg/mL), start 100 to 180 mcg/min (75 to 135 mL/h), usual dose once BP is stabilized 40 to 60 mcg/min. ▶Plasma ♀C ▶– $

CARDIAC PARAMETERS AND FORMULAS
Cardiac output (CO) = heart rate × CVA volume [normal 4-8 l/min]
Cardiac index (CI) = CO/BSA [normal 2.8-4.2 l/min/m²]
MAP (mean arterial press) = [(SBP - DBP)/3] + DBP [normal 80-100 mmHg]
SVR (systemic vasc resis) = (MAP - CVP) x (80)/CO [normal 800-1200 dyne/sec/cm5]
PVR (pulm vasc resis) = (PAM - PCWP) x (80)/CO [normal 45-120 dyne/sec/cm5]
QTc = QT/square root of RR [normal 0.38-0.42]
Right atrial pressure (central venous pressure) [normal 0-8 mmHg]
Pulmonary artery systolic pressure (PAS) [normal 20-30 mmHg]
Pulmonary artery diastolic pressure (PAD) [normal 10-15 mmHg]
Pulmonary capillary wedge pressure (PCWP) [normal 8-12 mmHg (post-MI ~16 mmHg)]

Pulmonary Arterial Hypertension

SILDENAFIL (*Revatio*) <u>Pulmonary arterial hypertension:</u> 20 mg PO tid; or 10 mg IV tid. Contraindicated with nitrates. Coadministration is not recommended with ritonavir, potent CYP3A inhibitors, or other phosphodiesterase-5 inhibitors. Teach patients to seek medical attention for vision loss, hearing loss, or erections lasting longer than 4 h. [Trade only (Revatio): Tabs 20 mg.] ▶LK ♀B ▶– $$$$

TADALAFIL (*Adcirca*) <u>Pulmonary arterial hypertension:</u> 40 mg PO daily. Coadministration is not recommended with nitrates. Coadministration is not recommended with potent CYP3A inhibitors (itraconazole, ketoconazole), potent CYP3A inducers (rifampin), other phosphodiesterase-5 inhibitors. Caution with ritonavir, see PI for specific dose adjustments. Teach patients to seek medical attention for vision loss, hearing loss, or erections lasting longer than 4 h. [Trade only (Adcirca): Tabs 20 mg.] ▶L ♀B ▶– $$$$

Thrombolytics

ALTEPLASE (*tpa, t-PA, Activase, Cathflo, ✦Activase rt-PA*) <u>Acute MI:</u> (dose for wt 67 kg or less) give 15 mg IV bolus, then 0.75 mg/kg (max 50 mg) over 30 min, then 0.5 mg/kg (max 35 mg) over the next 60 min; (dose for wt greater than 67 kg) give 15 mg IV bolus, then 50 mg over 30 min, then 35 mg over the next 60; use concurrent heparin infusion. <u>Acute ischemic stroke with symptoms 3 h or less:</u> 0.9 mg/kg (max 90 mg); give 10% of total dose as an IV bolus, and the remainder IV over 60 min. Multiple exclusion criteria. <u>Acute pulmonary embolism:</u> 100 mg IV over 2 h, then restart heparin when PTT twice normal or less. <u>Occluded central venous access device:</u> 2 mg/mL in catheter for 2 h. May use second dose if needed. ▶L ♀C ▶? $$$$$

RETEPLASE (*Retavase*) <u>Acute MI:</u> 10 units IV over 2 min; repeat once in 30 min. ▶L ♀C ▶? $$$$$

THROMBOLYTIC THERAPY FOR ACUTE MI

Indications (if high-volume cath lab unavailable): Clinical history & presentation strongly suggestive of MI within 12 h plus at least 1 of the following: 1 mm ST elevation in at least 2 contiguous leads; new left BBB; or 2 mm ST depression in V1-4 suggestive of true posterior MI.

Absolute contraindications: Previous cerebral hemorrhage, known cerebral aneurysm or arteriovenous malformation, known intracranial neoplasm, recent (<3 months) ischemic CVA (except acute ischemic CVA < 3 h), aortic dissection, active bleeding or bleeding diathesis (excluding menstruation), significant closed head or facial trauma (<3 months).

Relative contraindications: Severe uncontrolled HTN (>180/110 mm Hg) on presentation or chronic severe HTN; prior ischemic CVA (>3 months), dementia, other intracranial pathology; traumatic/prolonged (>10 min) cardiopulmonary resuscitation; major surgery (<3 weeks); recent (within 2–4 weeks) internal bleeding; puncture of noncompressible vessel; pregnancy; active peptic ulcer disease; current use of anticoagulants. For streptokinase/anistreplase: prior exposure (>5 days ago) or prior allergic reaction.

Reference: *Circulation* 2004;110:588–636

STREPTOKINASE (*Streptase, Kabikinase*) <u>Acute MI:</u> 1.5 million units IV over 60 min. ▶L ♀C ▶? $$$$$

TENECTEPLASE (*TNKase*) <u>Acute MI:</u> Single IV bolus dose over 5 sec based on body wt; 30 mg for wt less than 60 kg, 35 mg for wt 60 to 69 kg, 40 mg for wt 70 to 79 kg, 45 mg for wt 80 to 89 kg, 50 mg for wt 90 kg or more. ▶L ♀C ▶? $$$$$

UROKINASE (*Kinlytic*) <u>PE:</u> 4400 units/kg IV loading dose over 10 min, followed by IV infusion 4400 units/kg/h for 12 h. <u>Occluded IV catheter:</u> 5000 units instilled into catheter, remove soln after 5 min. ▶L ♀B ▶? $$$$$

Volume Expanders

ALBUMIN (*Albuminar, Buminate, Albumarc, ✦Plasbumin*) <u>Shock, burns:</u> 500 mL of 5% soln IV infusion as rapidly as tolerated, repeat in 30 min if needed. ▶L ♀C ▶? $$$$$

DEXTRAN (*Rheomacrodex, Gentran, Macrodex*) <u>Shock/hypovolemia:</u> up to 20 mL/kg in first 24 h, then up to 10 mL/kg for 4 days. ▶K ♀C ▶? $$

HETASTARCH (*Hespan, Hextend*) <u>Shock/hypovolemia:</u> 500 to 1000 mL IV infusion, usually should not exceed 20 mL/kg/day (1500 mL) ▶K ♀C ▶? $$

PLASMA PROTEIN FRACTION (*Plasmanate, Protenate, Plasmatein*) <u>Shock/hypovolemia:</u> 5% soln 250 to 500 mL IV prn. ▶L ♀C ▶? $$$

Other

BIDIL (**hydralazine + isosorbide dinitrate**) <u>Heart failure</u> (adjunct to standard therapy in black patients): Start 1 tab PO tid, increase as tolerated to max 2 tabs tid. May decrease to ½ tab tid with intolerable side effects; try to increase dose when side effects subside. [Trade only: Tabs scored 37.5/20 mg.] ▶LK ♀C ▶? $$$$$

CILOSTAZOL (*Pletal*) <u>Intermittent claudication:</u> 100 mg PO bid on empty stomach. 50 mg PO bid with CYP 3A4 inhibitors (eg, ketoconazole, itraconazole, erythromycin, diltiazem) or CYP 2C19 inhibitors (eg, omeprazole). [Generic/Trade: Tabs 50, 100 mg.] ▶L ♀C ▶? $$$$

NESIRITIDE (*Natrecor*) <u>Hospitalized patients with decompensated heart failure with dyspnea at rest:</u> 2 mcg/kg IV bolus over 60 sec, then 0.01 mcg/kg/min IV infusion for up to 48 h. Do not initiate at higher doses. Limited experience with increased doses. Mix 1.5 mg vial in 250 mL D5W (for a 70 kg patient, a bolus of 23.3 mL is 2 mcg/kg for a 70 kg patient, infusion set at rate 7 mL/h delivers a 0.01 mcg/kg/min for a 70 kg patient. Symptomatic hypotension. May increase mortality. Not indicated for outpatient infusion, for scheduled repetitive use, to improve renal function, or to enhance diuresis. ▶K, plasma ♀C ▶? $$$$$

PENTOXIFYLLINE (*Trental*) 400 mg PO tid with meals. [Generic/Trade: Tabs extended-release 400 mg.] ▶L ♀C ▶? $$$

RANOLAZINE (*Ranexa*) <u>Chronic angina:</u> 500 mg PO bid, max 1000 mg bid. Baseline and follow-up ECGs; may prolong QT interval. Contraindicated with clinically significant hepatic impairment, potent CYP3A4 inhibitors, CYP3A inducers. Max 500 mg bid, if used with diltiazem, verapamil, or moderate CYP3A inhibitors. [Trade only: Tabs extended-release 500, 1000 mg.] ▶LK ♀C ▶? $$$$$

CONTRAST MEDIA

MRI Contrast—Gadolinium-based

NOTE *Avoid gadolinium-based contrast agents if severe renal insufficiency (GFR less than 30 mL/min/1.73 m2) due to risk of nephrogenic systemic fibrosis/nephrogenic fibrosing dermopathy. Similarly avoid in acute renal insufficiency of any severity due to hepatorenal syndrome or during the perioperative phase of liver transplant.*

GADOBENATE (*MultiHance*)   Non-iodinated, nonionic IV contrast for MRI. ▶K ♀C ▶? $$$$

GADODIAMIDE (*Omniscan*)   Non-iodinated, nonionic IV contrast for MRI. ▶K ♀C ▶? $$$$

GADOPENTETATE (*Magnevist*)   Non-iodinated IV contrast for MRI. ▶K ♀C ▶? $$$

GADOTERIDOL (*Prohance*)   Non-iodinated, nonionic IV contrast for MRI. ▶K ♀C ▶? $$$$

GADOVERSETAMIDE (*OptiMARK*)   Non-iodinated IV contrast for MRI. ▶K ♀C ▶− $$$$

MRI Contrast—Other

FERUMOXIDES (*Feridex*)   Non-iodinated, nonionic, iron-based IV contrast for hepatic MRI. ▶L ♀C ▶? $$$$

FERUMOXSIL (*GastroMARK*)   Non-iodinated, nonionic, iron-based, oral GI contrast for MRI. ▶L ♀B ▶? $$$$

MANGAFODIPIR (*Teslascan*)   Non-iodinated manganese-based IV contrast for MRI. ▶L ♀− ▶− $$$$

Radiography Contrast

NOTE *Beware of allergic or anaphylactoid reactions. Avoid IV contrast in renal insufficiency or dehydration. Hold metformin (Glucophage) prior to or at the time of iodinated contrast dye use and for 48 h after procedure. Restart after procedure only if renal function is normal.*

BARIUM SULFATE   Non-iodinated GI (eg, oral, rectal) contrast. ▶Not absorbed ♀? ▶+ $

DIATRIZOATE (*Cystografin, Gastrografin, Hypaque, MD-Gastroview, RenoCal, Reno-DIP, Reno-60, Renografin*)   Iodinated, ionic, high osmolality IV or GI contrast. ▶K ♀C ▶? $

IODIXANOL (*Visipaque*)   Iodinated, nonionic, iso-osmolar IV contrast. ▶K ♀B ▶? $$$

IOHEXOL (*Omnipaque*)   Iodinated, nonionic, low osmolality IV and oral/body cavity contrast. ▶K ♀B ▶? $$$

IOPAMIDOL (*Isovue*)   Iodinated, nonionic, low osmolality IV contrast. ▶K ♀? ▶? $$

IOPROMIDE (*Ultravist*) Iodinated, nonionic, low osmolality IV contrast. ▶K ♀B ▶? $$$

IOTHALAMATE (*Conray*, ✦*Vascoray*) Iodinated, ionic, high osmolality IV contrast. ▶K ♀B ▶– $

IOVERSOL (*Optiray*) Iodinated, nonionic, low osmolality IV contrast. ▶K ♀B ▶? $$

IOXAGLATE (*Hexabrix*) Iodinated, ionic, low osmolality IV contrast. ▶K ♀B ▶– $$$

IOXILAN (*Oxilan*) Iodinated, nonionic, low osmolality IV contrast. ▶K ♀B ▶– $$$

DERMATOLOGY

Acne Preparations

***ACANYA* (clindamycin + benzoyl peroxide)** Apply qd. [Trade only: Gel (clindamycin 1.2% + benzoyl peroxide 2.5%) 50 g.] ▶K ♀C ▶+ $$$$

ADAPALENE (*Differin*) Apply at bedtime. [Generic/Trade: Gel 0.1%. Cream 0.1% (45 g). Trade only: Gel 0.3% (45 g). Soln 0.1% (30 mL). Swabs 0.1% (60 ea).] ▶Bile ♀C ▶? $$$$

AZELAIC ACID (*Azelex, Finacea, Finevin*) Apply bid. [Trade only: Cream 20%, 30, 50 g (Azelex). Gel 15% 50 g (Finacea).] ▶K ♀B ▶? $$$$

***BENZACLIN* (clindamycin + benzoyl peroxide)** Apply bid. [Generic/Trade: Gel (clindamycin 1% + benzoyl peroxide 5%) 50 g (jar). Trade only: 25, 35 g (jar) and 50 g (pump).] ▶K ♀C ▶+ $$$$

***BENZAMYCIN* (erythromycin base + benzoyl peroxide)** Apply bid. [Generic/Trade: Gel (erythromycin 3% + benzoyl peroxide 5%) 23.3, 46.6 g. Trade only: Benzamycin Pak, #60 gel pouches.] ▶LK ♀C ▶? $$$

BENZOYL PEROXIDE (*Benzac, Benzagel 10%, Desquam, Clearasil, ✦Solugel, Benoxyl*) Apply daily; increase to bid to tid if needed. [OTC and Rx generic: Liquid 2.5, 5, 10%. Bar 5, 10%. Mask 5%. Lotion 4, 5, 8, 10%. Cream 5, 10%. Gel 2.5, 4, 5, 6, 10, 20%. Pad 3, 4, 6, 8, 9%. Other strengths available.] ▶LK ♀C ▶? $

***CLENIA* (sulfacetamide + sulfur)** Apply daily to tid. [Generic only: Lotion (sodium sulfacetamide 10%/sulfur 5%) 25, 30, 45, 60 g. Cream (sodium sulfacetamide 10%/sulfur 5%) 28 g. Generic/Trade: Foaming Wash 170, 340 g.] ▶K ♀C ▶? $$$

CLINDAMYCIN—TOPICAL (*Cleocin T, Clindagel, ClindaMax, Evoclin, ✦Dalacin T*) Apply daily (Evoclin, Clindagel, Clindamax) or bid (Cleocin T). [Generic/Trade: Gel 1% 30, 60 g. Lotion 1% 60 mL. Soln 1% 30, 60 mL. Trade only: Foam 1% 50, 100 g (Evoclin). Gel 1% 40, 75 mL (Clindagel).] ▶L ♀B ▶? $$$

***DIANE-35* (cyproterone + ethinyl estradiol)** Canada only. 1 tab PO daily for 21 consecutive days, stop for 7 days, repeat cycle. [Canada Generic/Trade: Blister pack of 21 tabs 2 mg cyproterone acetate/0.035 mg ethinyl estradiol.] ▶L ♀X ▶– $$

***DUAC* (clindamycin + benzoyl peroxide) (✦*Clindoxyl*)** Apply at bedtime. [Trade only: Gel (clindamycin 1% + benzoyl peroxide 5%) 45 g.] ▶K ♀C ▶+ $$$$

EPIDUO (adapalene + benzoyl peroxide) Apply daily. [Trade only: Gel (0.1% adapalene + benzoyl peroxide 2.5%) 45 g.] ▶Bile, K ♀C ▶? $$$$$

ERYTHROMYCIN—TOPICAL (*Eryderm, Erycette, Erygel, A/T/S, ✦Sans-Acne, Erysol*) Apply bid. [Generic/Trade: Soln 2% 60 mL. Pads 2%. Gel 2% 30, 60 g. Ointment 2% 25 g. Generic only: Soln 1.5% 60 mL.] ▶L ♀B ▶? $

ISOTRETINOIN (*Accutane, Amnesteem, Claravis, Sotret, ✦Clarus*) 0.5 to 2 mg/kg/day PO divided bid for 15 to 20 weeks. Typical target dose is 1 mg/kg/day. Potent teratogen; use extreme caution. Can only be prescribed by healthcare professionals who are registered with the iPLEDGE program. May cause depression. Not for long-term use. [Generic: Caps 10, 20, 40 mg. Generic only (Sotret and Claravis): Caps 30 mg.] ▶LK ♀X ▶– $$$$$

ROSULA (sulfacetamide + sulfur) Apply daily to tid. [Trade only: Gel (sodium sulfacetamide 10%/sulfur 5%) 45 g. Aqueous cleanser (sodium sulfacetamide 10%/sulfur 5%) 355 mL. Soap (sodium sulfacetamide 10%/sulfur 4%) 473 mL.] ▶K ♀C ▶? $$$$

SALICYLIC ACID (*Akurza, Clearasil Cleanser, Stridex Pads*) Apply/wash area up to tid. [OTC Generic/Trade: Pads, Gel, Lotion, Liquid, Mask scrub, 0.5%, 1%, 2%. Rx Trade only (Akurza): Cream 6% 340 g. Lotion 6%, 355 mL.] ▶Not absorbed ♀? ▶? $

SULFACETAMIDE—TOPICAL (*Klaron, Rosula NS*) Apply bid. [Generic/Trade (Klaron): Lotion 10% 118 mL. Trade only: Single-use pads 10%, 30 ea (Rosula NS).] ▶K ♀C ▶? $$$$

SULFACET-R (sulfacetamide + sulfur) Apply daily to tid. [Generic/Trade: Lotion (sodium sulfacetamide 10%/sulfur 5%) 25 g.] ▶K ♀C ▶? $$$

TAZAROTENE (*Tazorac, Avage*) Acne (Tazorac): Apply 0.1% cream at bedtime. Psoriasis: Apply 0.05% cream at bedtime, increase to 0.1% prn. [Trade only (Tazorac): Cream 0.05% and 0.1% 30, 60 g. Gel 0.05% and 0.1% 30, 100 g. Trade only (Avage): Cream 0.1% 15, 30 g.] ▶L ♀X ▶? $$$$

TRETINOIN—TOPICAL (*Retin-A, Retin-A Micro, Renova, Retisol-A, ✦Stieva-A, Rejuva-A, Vitamin A Acid Cream*) Apply at bedtime. [Generic/Trade: Cream 0.025% 20, 45 g; 0.05% 20, 45 g; 0.1% 20, 45 g. Gel 0.025% 15, 45 g, 0.1% 15, 45 g. Renova cream 0.02% 40, 60 g. Retin-A Micro gel 0.04%, 0.1% 20, 45, 50 g.] ▶LK ♀C ▶? $$$

ZIANA (clindamycin + tretinoin) Apply at bedtime. [Trade only: Gel clindamycin 1.2% + tretinoin 0.025% 30, 60 g.] ▶LK ♀C ▶? $$$$

Actinic Keratosis Preparations

DICLOFENAC—TOPICAL (*Solaraze, Voltaren*) Solaraze: Actinic/solar keratoses: Apply bid to lesions for 60 to 90 days. Voltaren: Osteoarthritis of areas amenable to topical therapy: 2 g (upper extremities) to 4 g (lower extremities) qid. [Trade only: Gel 3% 50 g (Solaraze), 100 g (Solaraze, Voltaren).] ▶L ♀B ▶? $$$$$

FLUOROURACIL—TOPICAL (*5-FU, Carac, Efudex, Fluoroplex*) Actinic keratoses: Apply bid for 2 to 6 weeks. Superficial basal cell carcinomas: Apply 5% cream/soln bid. [Trade only: Cream 0.5% 30 g (Carac), 5% 25 g (Efudex), 1% 30 g (Fluoroplex). Generic/Trade: Soln 2%, 5% 10 mL (Efudex). Cream 5% 40 g.] ▶L ♀X ▶– $$$

METHYLAMINOLEVULINATE (*Metvix, Metvixia*) Apply cream to <u>non-hyperkeratotic actinic keratoses</u> lesion and surrounding area on face or scalp; cover with dressing for 3 h; remove dressing and cream and perform illumination therapy. Repeat in 7 days. [Trade only: Cream 16.8%, 2 g tube.] ▶Not absorbed ♀C ▶? ?

Antibacterials (Topical)

BACITRACIN (✦*Baciguent*) Apply daily to tid. [OTC Generic/Trade: Ointment 500 units/g 1, 15, 30 g.] ▶Not absorbed ♀C ▶? $

FUSIDIC ACID—TOPICAL (✦*Fucidin*) Canada only. Apply tid to qid. [Canada trade only: Cream 2% fusidic acid 5, 15, 30 g. Ointment 2% sodium fusidate 5, 15, 30 g.] ▶L ♀? ▶? $

GENTAMICIN—TOPICAL (*Garamycin*) Apply tid to qid. [Generic only: Ointment 0.1% 15, 30 g. Cream 0.1% 15, 30 g.] ▶K ♀D ▶? $

MAFENIDE (*Sulfamylon*) Apply daily to bid. [Trade only: Cream 5% 57, 114, 454 g. Topical soln 50 g packets.] ▶LK ♀C ▶? $

METRONIDAZOLE—TOPICAL (*Noritate, MetroCream, MetroGel, MetroLotion, ✦Rosasol*) <u>Rosacea:</u> Apply daily (1%) or bid (0.75%). [Trade only: Gel (MetroGel) 1% 45. 60 g. Cream (Noritate) 1% 60 g. Generic/Trade: Gel 0.75% 45 g. Cream 0.75% 45 g. Lotion (MetroLotion) 0.75% 59 mL.] ▶KL ♀B(– in 1st trimester) ▶?

MUPIROCIN (*Bactroban, Centany*) <u>Impetigo/infected wounds:</u> Apply tid. <u>Nasal methicillin-resistant S. aureus eradication:</u> 0.5 g in each nostril bid for 5 days. [Generic/Trade: Ointment 2% 22 g. Nasal ointment 2% 1 g single-use tubes (for MRSA eradication). Trade only: Cream 2% 15, 30 g.] ▶Not absorbed ♀B ▶? $$

NEOSPORIN CREAM (neomycin + polymyxin + bacitracin) Apply daily to tid. [OTC Trade only: neomycin 3.5 mg/g + polymyxin 10,000 units/g 15 g and unit dose 0.94 g.] ▶K ♀C ▶? $

NEOSPORIN OINTMENT (bacitracin + neomycin + polymyxin) Apply daily to tid. [OTC Generic/Trade: bacitracin 400 units/g + neomycin 3.5 mg/g + polymyxin 5000 units/g 15, 30 g, and "to go" 0.9 g packets.] ▶K ♀C ▶? $

POLYSPORIN (bacitracin + polymyxin) (✦*Polytopic*) Apply daily to tid. [OTC Trade only: Ointment 15, 30 g, and unit dose 0.9 g. Powder 10 g.] ▶K ♀C ▶? $

RETAPAMULIN (*Altabax*) <u>Impetigo:</u> Apply bid for 5 days. [Trade only: Ointment 1% 5, 10, 15 g.] ▶Not absorbed ♀B ▶? $$$

SILVER SULFADIAZINE (*Silvadene, ✦Dermazin, Flamazine, SSD*) Apply daily to bid. [Generic/Trade: Cream 1% 20, 50, 85, 400, 1000 g.] ▶LK ♀B ▶– $$

Antifungals (Topical)

BUTENAFINE (*Lotrimin Ultra, Mentax*) Apply daily to bid. [Rx Trade only: Cream 1% 15, 30 g (Mentax). OTC Trade only: Cream 1% 12, 24 g (Lotrimin Ultra).] ▶L ♀B ▶? $

CICLOPIROX (*Loprox, Penlac, ✦Stieprox shampoo*) Cream, lotion: Apply bid. Nail soln: Apply daily to affected nails; apply over previous coat; remove with alcohol every 7 days. Seborrheic dermatitis (Loprox shampoo): Shampoo twice weekly for 4 weeks. [Trade only: Shampoo (Loprox) 1% 120 mL. Generic/Trade: Gel 0.77% 30, 45, 100 g. Nail soln (Penlac) 8% 6.6 mL. Cream (Loprox) 0.77% 15, 30, 90 g. Lotion (Loprox TS) 0.77% 30, 60 mL.] ▶K ♀B ▶? $$$$

CLOTRIMAZOLE—TOPICAL (*Lotrimin AF, Mycelex, ✦Canesten, Clotrimaderm*) Apply bid. [Note that Lotrimin brand cream, lotion, soln are clotrimazole, while Lotrimin powders and liquid spray are miconazole. Rx Generic only: Cream 1% 15, 30, 45 g. Soln 1% 10, 30, 60 mL. OTC Trade only (Lotrimin AF): Cream 1% 12, 24 g. Soln 1% 10 mL.] ▶L ♀B ▶? $

ECONAZOLE Tinea pedis, cruris, corporis, tinea versicolor: Apply daily. Cutaneous candidiasis: Apply bid. [Generic only: Cream 1% 15, 30, 85 g.] ▶Not absorbed ♀C ▶? $$

KETOCONAZOLE—TOPICAL (*Extina, Nizoral, Xolegel, ✦Ketoderm*) Tinea/candidal infections: Apply daily. Seborrheic dermatitis: Apply cream daily to bid for 4 weeks or gel daily for 2 weeks or foam bid for 4 weeks. Dandruff: Apply 1% shampoo twice a week. Tinea versicolor: Apply shampoo to affected area, leave on for 5 min, rinse. [Generic/Trade: Cream 2% 15, 30, 60 g. Shampoo 2% 120 mL. Trade only: Shampoo 1% 120, 210 mL (OTC Nizoral). Gel 2% 15 g (Xolegel). Foam 2% 50, 100 g (Extina).] ▶L ♀C ▶? $$

MICONAZOLE—TOPICAL (*Micatin, Lotrimin AF, ZeaSorb AF*) Tinea, candida: Apply bid. [Note that Lotrimin brand cream, lotion, soln are clotrimazole, while Lotrimin powders and liquid spray are miconazole. OTC Trade only: Powder 2% 70, 160 g. Spray powder 2% 90, 100, 140 g. Spray liquid 2% 90, 105 mL. Gel 2% 24 g.] ▶L ♀+ ▶? $

NAFTIFINE (*Naftin*) Tinea: Apply daily (cream) or bid (gel). [Trade only: Cream 1% 15, 30, 60, 90 g. Gel 1% 20, 40, 60, 90 g.] ▶LK ♀B ▶? $$$

NYSTATIN—TOPICAL (*Mycostatin, ✦Nilstat, Nyaderm, Candistatin*) Candidiasis: Apply bid to tid. [Generic/Trade: Cream, Ointment 100,000 units/g 15, 30 g. Powder 100,000 units/g 15, 30, 60 g.] ▶Not absorbed ♀C ▶? $

OXICONAZOLE (*Oxistat, Oxizole*) Tinea pedis, cruris, and corporis: Apply daily to bid. Tinea versicolor (cream only): Apply daily. [Trade only: Cream 1% 15, 30, 60 g. Lotion 1% 30 mL.] ▶? ♀B ▶? $$$

SERTACONAZOLE (*Ertaczo*) Tinea pedis: Apply bid. [Trade only: Cream 2% 30, 60 g.] ▶Not absorbed ♀C ▶? $$$

TERBINAFINE—TOPICAL (*Lamisil, Lamisil AT*) Tinea: Apply daily to bid. [OTC Trade only: Cream 1% 12, 24 g. Spray pump soln 1% 30 mL. Gel 1% 6, 12 g.] ▶L ♀B ▶? $$

TOLNAFTATE (*Tinactin*) Apply bid. [OTC Generic/Trade: Cream 1% 15, 30 g. Soln 1% 10 mL. Powder 1% 45 g. OTC Trade only: Gel 1% 15 g. Powder 1% 90 g. Spray powder 1% 100, 133, 150 g. Spray liquid 1% 100, 113 mL.] ▶? ♀? ▶? $

Antiparasitics (Topical)

A-200 (*pyrethrins + piperonyl butoxide*) (*✦R&C*) Lice: Apply shampoo, wash after 10 min. Reapply in 5 to 7 days. [OTC Generic/Trade: Shampoo (0.33% pyrethrins, 4% piperonyl butoxide) 60, 120 mL.] ▶L ♀C ▶? $

CROTAMITON (*Eurax*) <u>Scabies:</u> Apply cream/lotion topically from chin to feet, repeat in 24 h, bathe 48 h later. <u>Pruritus:</u> Massage prn. [Trade only: Cream 10% 60 g. Lotion 10% 60, 480 mL.] ▶? ♀C ▶? $$

LINDANE (✦*Hexit*) Other drugs preferred. <u>Scabies:</u> Apply 30 to 60 mL of lotion, wash after 8 to 12 h. <u>Lice:</u> 30 to 60 mL of shampoo, wash off after 4 min. Can cause seizures in epileptics or if overused/misused in children. Not for infants. [Generic only: Lotion 1% 60, 480 mL. Shampoo 1% 60, 480 mL.] ▶? ♀B ▶? $

MALATHION (*Ovide*) Apply to dry hair, let dry naturally, wash off in 8 to 12 h. [Generic/Trade only: Lotion 0.5% 59 mL.] ▶? ♀B ▶? $$$$

PERMETHRIN (*Elimite, Acticin, Nix, ✦Kwellada-P*) <u>Scabies:</u> Apply cream from head (avoid mouth/nose/eyes) to soles of feet and wash after 8 to 14 h. 30 g is typical adult dose. <u>Lice:</u> Saturate hair and scalp with 1% rinse, wash after 10 min. Do not use in age younger than 2 mo. May repeat therapy in 7 days, as necessary. [Generic/Trade: Cream (Elimite, Acticin) 5% 60 g. OTC Generic/Trade: Liquid creme rinse (Nix) 1% 60 mL.] ▶L ♀B ▶? $$

RID **(pyrethrins + piperonyl butoxide)** <u>Lice:</u> Apply shampoo/mousse, wash after 10 min. Reapply in 7 to 10 days. [OTC Generic/Trade: Shampoo 60, 120, 240 mL. OTC Trade only: Mousse 5.5 oz.] ▶? ♀C ▶? $

Antipsoriatics

ACITRETIN (*Soriatane*) 25 to 50 mg PO daily. Avoid pregnancy during therapy and for 3 years after discontinuation. [Trade only: Caps 10, 25 mg.] ▶L ♀X ▶– $$$$$

ALEFACEPT (*Amevive*) 7.5 mg IV or 15 mg IM once a week for 12 doses. May repeat with 1 additional 12-week course after 12 weeks have elapsed since last dose. ▶? ♀B ▶? $$$$$

ANTHRALIN (*Drithocreme, ✦Anthrascalp, Anthranol, Anthraforte, Dithranol*) Apply daily. Short contact periods (ie, 15 to 20 min) followed by removal may be preferred. [Trade only: Cream 0.5, 1% 50 g.] ▶? ♀C ▶– $$$

CALCIPOTRIENE (*Dovonex*) Apply bid. [Trade only: Ointment 0.005% 30, 60, 100 g. Cream 0.005% 30, 60, 100 g. Generic/Trade: Scalp soln 0.005% 60 mL.] ▶L ♀C ▶? $$$$

TACLONEX **(calcipotriene + betamethasone)** Apply daily for up to 4 weeks. [Trade only: Ointment (calcipotriene 0.005% + betamethasone dipropionate 0.064%) 15, 30, 60, 100 g. Topical susp 15, 30, 60 g.] ▶L ♀C ▶? $$$$$

USTEKINUMAB (*Stelara*) <u>Severe plaque psoriasis:</u> wt less than 100 kg, use 45 mg initially and again 4 weeks later, followed by 45 mg every 12 weeks. For wt greater than 100 kg, use 90 mg initially and again 4 weeks later, followed by 90 mg every 12 weeks. [Trade only: 45 and 90 mg prefilled syringe and vial.] ▶L – ♀B ▶? $$$$$

Antivirals (Topical)

ACYCLOVIR—TOPICAL (*Zovirax*) <u>Herpes genitalis:</u> Apply ointment q 3 h (6 times per day) for 7 days. <u>Recurrent herpes labialis:</u> Apply cream 5 times per day for 4 days. [Trade only: Ointment 5% 15 g. Cream 5% 2, 5 g.] ▶K ♀C ▶? $$$$$

DOCOSANOL (*Abreva*) <u>Oral-facial herpes</u> (cold sores): Apply 5 times per day until healed. [OTC Trade only: Cream 10% 2 g.] ▶Not absorbed ♀B ▶? $

IMIQUIMOD (*Aldara*) <u>Genital/perianal warts:</u> Apply 3 times per week overnight for up to 16 weeks. Wash off after 8 h. <u>Non-hyperkeratotic, non-hypertrophic actinic keratoses on face/scalp in immunocompetent adults:</u> Apply twice a week overnight for 16 weeks. Wash off after 8 h. <u>Primary superficial basal cell carcinoma:</u> Apply 5 times a week for 6 weeks. Wash off after 8 h. [Generic/Trade: Cream 5% single-use packets.] ▶Not absorbed ♀C ▶? $$$$$

PENCICLOVIR (*Denavir*) <u>Herpes labialis</u> (cold sores): Apply cream q 2 h while awake for 4 days. [Trade only: Cream 1% tube 1.5 g.] ▶Not absorbed ♀B ▶? $$

PODOFILOX (*Condylox*, ✦*Condyline, Wartec*) <u>External genital warts</u> (gel and soln) and <u>perianal warts</u> (gel only): Apply bid for 3 consecutive days of the week and repeat for up to 4 weeks. [Generic/Trade: Soln 0.5% 3.5 mL. Trade only: Gel 0.5% 3.5 g.] ▶? ♀C ▶? $$$$

PODOPHYLLIN (*Podocon-25*, *Podofin*, *Podofilm*) <u>Warts:</u> Apply by physician. [Not to be dispensed to patients. For hospital/clinic use; not intended for outpatient prescribing. Trade only: Liquid 25% 15 mL.] ▶? ♀– ▶– $$$

SINECATECHINS (*Veregen*) Apply tid to <u>external genital warts</u> for up to 16 weeks. [Trade only: Ointment 15% 15, 30 g.] ▶Unknown ♀C ▶? $$$$$

Atopic Dermatitis Preparations

PIMECROLIMUS (*Elidel*) <u>Atopic dermatitis:</u> Apply bid. [Trade only: Cream 1% 30, 60, 100 g.] ▶L ♀C ▶? $$$$

TACROLIMUS—TOPICAL (*Protopic*) <u>Atopic dermatitis:</u> Apply bid. [Trade only: Ointment 0.03%, 0.1% 30, 60, 100 g.] ▶Minimal absorption ♀C ▶? $$$$$

Corticosteroid/Antimicrobial Combinations

CORTISPORIN (neomycin + polymyxin + hydrocortisone) Apply bid to qid. [Trade only: Cream 7.5 g. Ointment 15 g.] ▶LK ♀C ▶? $$$

FUCIDIN H (fusidic acid + hydrocortisone) Canada only. Apply tid. [Canada Trade only: Cream (2% fusidic acid, 1% hydrocortisone acetate) 30 g.] ▶L ♀? ▶? $$

LOTRISONE (clotrimazole + betamethasone) (✦*Lotriderm*) Apply bid. Do not use for diaper rash. [Generic/Trade: Cream (clotrimazole 1% + betamethasone 0.05%) 15, 45 g. Lotion (clotrimazole 1% + betamethasone 0.05%) 30 mL.] ▶L ♀C ▶? $$$

MYCOLOG II (nystatin + triamcinolone) Apply bid. [Generic only: Cream, Ointment 15, 30, 60, 120, 454 g.] ▶L ♀C ▶? $

Hemorrhoid Care

DIBUCAINE (*Nupercainal*) Apply cream/ointment tid to qid prn. [OTC Trade only: Ointment 1% 30, 60 g.] ▶L ♀? ▶? $

CORTICOSTEROIDS—TOPICAL

Potency*	Generic	Trade Name	Forms	Frequency
Low	alclometasone dipropionate	Aclovate	0.05% C/O	bid-tid
Low	clocortolone pivalate	Cloderm	0.1% C	tid
Low	desonide	DesOwen, Tridesilon	0.05% C/L/O	bid-tid
Low	hydrocortisone	Hytone, others	0.5% C/L/O; 1% C/L/O; 2.5% C/L/O	bid-qid
Low	hydrocortisone acetate	Cortaid, Corticaine	0.5% C/O; 1% C/O/Sp	bid-qid
Medium	betamethasone valerate	Luxiq	0.1% C/L/O; 0.12% F (Luxiq)	qd-bid
Medium	desoximetasone‡	Topicort	0.05% C	bid
Medium	fluocinolone	Synalar	0.01% C/S; 0.025% C/O	bid-qid
Medium	flurandrenolide	Cordran	0.025% C/O; 0.05% C/L/O/T	bid-qid
Medium	fluticasone propionate	Cutivate	0.005% O; 0.05% C/L	qd-bid
Medium	hydrocortisone butyrate	Locoid	0.1% C/O/S	bid-tid
Medium	hydrocortisone valerate	Westcort	0.2% C/O	bid-tid
Medium	mometasone furoate	Elocon	0.1% C/L/O	qd
Medium	triamcinolone‡	Aristocort, Kenalog	0.025% C/L/O; 0.1% C/L/O/S	bid-tid
High	amcinonide	Cyclocort	0.1% C/L/O	bid-tid
High	betamethasone dipropionate‡	Maxivate, others	0.05% C/L/O (non-Diprolene)	qd-bid
High	desoximetasone‡	Topicort	0.05% G; 0.25% C/O	bid
High	diflorasone diacetate‡	Maxiflor	0.05% C/O	bid
High	fluocinonide	Lidex	0.05% C/G/O/S	bid-qid
High	halcinonide	Halog	0.1% C/O/S	bid-tid
High	triamcinolone‡	Aristocort, Kenalog	0.5% C/O	bid-tid
Very high	betamethasone dipropionate‡	Diprolene, Diprolene AF	0.05% C/G/L/O	qd-bid
Very high	clobetasol	Temovate, Cormax, Olux	0.05% C/G/O/L/S/Sp/F (Olux)	bid
Very high	diflorasone diacetate‡	Psorcon	0.05% C/O	qd-tid
Very high	halobetasol propionate	Ultravate	0.05% C/O	qd-bid

*Potency based on vasoconstrictive assays, which may not correlate with efficacy. Not all available products are listed, including those lacking potency ratings. ‡These drugs have formulations in more than once potency category. C, cream; O, ointment; L, lotion; T, tape; F, foam; S, solution; G, gel; Sp, spray

PRAMOXINE (*Tucks Hemorrhoidal Ointment, Fleet Pain Relief, Proctofoam NS*) Ointment/pads/foam up to 5 times per day prn. [OTC Trade only: Ointment (Tucks Hemorrhoidal Ointment) 30 g. Pads (Fleet Pain Relief) 100 ea. Aerosol foam (ProctoFoam NS) 15 g.] ▶Not absorbed ♀+ ▶+ $

STARCH (*Tucks Suppositories*) 1 suppository up to 6 times per day prn. [OTC Trade only: Suppository (51% topical starch; vegetable oil, tocopheryl acetate) 12, 24 ea.] ▶Not absorbed ♀+ ▶+ $

WITCH HAZEL (*Tucks*) Apply to anus/perineum up to 6 times per day prn. [OTC Generic/Trade: Pads 50% 12, 40, 100 ea, generically available in various quantities.] ▶? ♀+ ▶+ $

Other Dermatologic Agents

ALITRETINOIN (*Panretin*) Apply bid to qid to cutaneous Kaposi's lesions [Trade only: Gel 0.1% 60 g] ▶Not absorbed ♀D ▶– $$$$$

ALUMINUM CHLORIDE (*Drysol, Certain Dri*) Apply at bedtime. [Rx Trade only: Soln 20% 37.5 mL bottle, 35, 60 mL bottle with applicator. OTC Trade only (Certain Dri): Soln 12.5% 36 mL bottle.] ▶K ♀? ▶? $

BECAPLERMIN (*Regranex*) Diabetic ulcers: Apply daily. [Trade only: Gel 0.01%, 2, 15 g.] ▶Minimal absorption ♀C ▶? $$$$$

CALAMINE Apply tid to qid prn for poison ivy/oak or insect bite itching. [OTC Generic only: Lotion 120, 240, 480 mL.] ▶? ♀? ▶? $

CAPSAICIN (*Zostrix, Zostrix-HP*) Arthritis, post-herpetic or diabetic neuralgia: Apply tid to qid. [OTC Generic/Trade: Cream 0.025% 60 g, 0.075% (HP) 60 g. OTC Generic only: Lotion 0.025% 59 mL, 0.075% 59 mL.] ▶? ♀? ▶? $

COAL TAR (*Polytar, Tegrin, Cutar, Tarsum*) Apply shampoo at least twice a week, or for psoriasis apply daily to qid. [OTC Generic/Trade: Shampoo, cream, ointment, gel, lotion, liquid, oil, soap.] ▶? ♀? ▶? $

DOXEPIN—TOPICAL (*Zonalon*) Pruritus: Apply qid for up to 8 days. [Trade only: Cream 5% 30, 45 g.] ▶L ♀B ▶– $$$$

EFLORNITHINE (*Vaniqa*) Reduction of facial hair: Apply to face bid. [Trade only: Cream 13.9% 30 g.] ▶K ♀C ▶? $$$

EMLA (*prilocaine + lidocaine—topical*) Topical anesthesia: Apply 2.5 g cream or 1 disc to region at least 1 h before procedure. Cover with occlusive dressing. [Generic/Trade: Cream (2.5% lidocaine + 2.5% prilocaine) 5, 30 g.] ▶LK ♀B ▶? $$

HYALURONIC ACID (*Bionect, Restylane, Perlane*) Moderate to severe facial wrinkles: Inject into wrinkle/fold (Restylane). Protection of dermal ulcers: Apply gel/cream/spray bid or tid (Bionect). [OTC Trade only: Cream 2% 15, 30 g. Rx Generic/Trade: Soln 3% 30 mL. Gel 4% 30 g. Cream 4% 15, 30, 60 g.] ▶? ♀? ▶? $$$

HYDROQUINONE (*Eldopaque, Eldoquin, Eldoquin Forte, EpiQuin Micro, Esoterica, Glyquin, Lustra, Melanex, Solaquin, Claripel, ✦Ultraquin*) Hyperpigmentation: Apply bid. [OTC Trade only: Cream 2% 15, 30 g. Rx Generic/Trade: Soln 3% 30 mL. Gel 4% 30 g. Cream 4% 15, 30, 60 g.] ▶? ♀C ▶? $

LACTIC ACID (*Lac-Hydrin, Amlactin, ✚Dermalac*) Apply bid. [Trade only: Lotion 12% 150, 360 mL. Generic/OTC: Cream 12% 140, 385 g. AmLactin AP is lactic acid (12%) with pramoxine (1%).] ▶? ♀? ▶? $$

LIDOCAINE—TOPICAL (*Xylocaine, ELA-Max, Lidoderm, Numby Stuff, LMX, Zingo, ✚Maxilene*) Apply prn. Dose varies with anesthetic procedure, degree of anesthesia required, and individual patient response. Postherpetic neuralgia: Apply up to 3 patches to affected area at once for up to 12 h within a 24-h period. Apply 30 min prior to painful procedure (ELA-Max 4%). Discomfort with anorectal disorders: Apply prn (ELA-Max 5%). Intradermal powder injection for venipuncture/IV cannulation, 3 to 18 yo (Zingo): 0.5 mg to site 1 to 10 min prior. [For membranes of mouth and pharynx: Spray 10%. Ointment 5%. Liquid 5%. Soln 2%, 4%, Dental patch. For urethral use: Jelly 2%. Patch (Lidoderm) 5%. Intradermal powder injection system: 0.5 mg (Zingo). OTC Trade only: Liposomal lidocaine 4% (ELA-Max).] ▶LK ♀B ▶+ $$

MINOXIDIL—TOPICAL (*Rogaine, Women's Rogaine, Rogaine Extra Strength, Minoxidil for Men, Theroxidil Extra Strength, ✚Minox, Apo-Gain*) Androgenetic alopecia in men or women: 1 mL to dry scalp bid. [OTC Generic/Trade: Soln 2% 60 mL (Rogaine, Womens Rogaine). Soln 5% 60 mL (Rogaine Extra Strength, Theroxidil Extra Strength - for men only). Foam 5% 60 g (Rogaine Extra Strength).] ▶K ♀C ▶– $

MONOBENZONE (*Benoquin*) Extensive vitiligo: Apply bid to tid. [Trade only: Cream 20% 35.4 g.] ▶Minimal absorption ♀C ▶? $$$

OATMEAL (*Aveeno*) Pruritus from poison ivy/oak, varicella: Apply lotion qid prn. Also bath packets for tub. [OTC Generic/Trade: Lotion. Bath packets.] ▶Not absorbed ♀? ▶? $

PANAFIL (papain + urea + chlorophyllin copper complex) Debridement of acute or chronic lesions: Apply to clean wound and cover daily to bid. [Trade only: Ointment 6, 30 g. Spray 33 mL.] ▶? ♀? ▶? $$$

PLIAGIS (tetracaine + lidocaine—topical) Apply 20 to 30 min prior to superficial dermatological procedure (60 min for tattoo removal). [Trade only: Cream lidocaine 7% + tetracaine 7%.] ▶Minimal absorption ♀B ▶? $$

PRAMOSONE (pramoxine + hydrocortisone) (*✚Pramox HC*) Inflammatory and pruritic manifestations of corticosteroid-responsive dermatoses: Apply tid to qid. [Trade only: Cream 1% pramoxine/1% hydrocortisone acetate 30, 60 g. Ointment 30 g, Lotion 60, 120, 240 mL. Cream 1% pramoxine/2.5% hydrocortisone acetate 30, 60 g. Ointment 30 g, Lotion 60, 120 mL.] ▶Not absorbed ♀C ▶? $$$

SELENIUM SULFIDE (*Selsun, Exsel, Versel*) Dandruff, seborrheic dermatitis: Apply 5 to 10 mL lotion/shampoo twice per week for 2 weeks then less frequently, thereafter. Tinea versicolor: Apply 2.5% lotion/shampoo to affected area daily for 7 days. [OTC Generic/Trade: Lotion/Shampoo 1% 120, 210, 240, 325 mL, 2.5% 120 mL. Rx Generic/Trade: Lotion/Shampoo 2.5% 120 mL.] ▶? ♀C ▶? $

SOLAG (mequinol + tretinoin) (*✚Solage*) Apply to solar lentigines bid. [Trade only: Soln 30 mL (mequinol 2% + tretinoin 0.01%).] ▶Not absorbed ♀X ▶? $$$$

SYNERA (*tetracaine + lidocaine—topical*) Apply 20 to 30 min prior to superficial dermatological procedure. [Trade only: Topical patch (lidocaine 70 mg + tetracaine 70 mg.] ▶Minimal absorption ♀B ▶? $$

TRI-LUMA (*fluocinolone + hydroquinone + tretinoin*) Melasma of the face: Apply qhs for 4 to 8 weeks. [Trade only: Cream 30 g (fluocinolone 0.01% + hydroquinone 4% + tretinoin 0.05%).] ▶Minimal absorption ♀C ▶? $$$$

VUSION (*miconazole - topical + zinc oxide + white petrolatum*) Apply to affected diaper area with each change for 7 days. [Trade only: Ointment 50 g.] ▶Minimal absorption ♀C ▶? $$$$$

ENDOCRINE & METABOLIC

Androgens/Anabolic Steroids

NOTE *Monitor LFTs and lipids. See OB/GYN section for other hormones.*

METHYLTESTOSTERONE (*Android, Methitest, Testred, Virilon*) Advancing inoperable breast cancer in women who are 1 to 5 years postmenopausal: 50 to 200 mg/day PO in divided doses. Hypogonadism in men: 10 to 50 mg PO daily. [Trade/Generic: Caps 10 mg, Tabs 10, 25 mg.] ▶L ♀X ▶? ©III $$$

NANDROLONE (*♦Deca-Durabolin*) Anemia of renal disease: Women 50 to 100 mg IM once a week, men 100 to 200 mg IM once a week. [Generic only: Injection 50, 100, 200 mg/mL.] ▶L ♀X ▶— ©III $$

OXANDROLONE (*Oxandrin*) Weight gain: 2.5 mg/day to 20 mg/day PO divided bid to qid for 2 to 4 weeks. [Generic/Trade: Tabs 2.5, 10 mg.] ▶L ♀X ▶? ©III $$$$$

TESTOSTERONE (*Androderm, AndroGel, Delatestryl, Depo-Testosterone, Striant, Testim, Testopel, Testro AQ, ♦Andriol*) Injectable enanthate or cypionate: 50 to 400 mg IM q 2 to 4 weeks. Transdermal: Androderm: 5 mg patch to nonscrotal skin at bedtime. AndroGel 1%: Apply 5 g from gel pack or 4 pumps (5 g) from dispenser daily to shoulders/upper arms/abdomen. Testim: 1 tube (5 g) daily to shoulders/upper arms. Pellet: Testopel: 2 to 6 (150 to 450 mg testosterone) pellets SC q 3 to 6 months. Buccal: Striant: 30 mg q 12 h on upper gum above the incisor tooth; alternate sides for each application. [Trade only: Patch 2.5, 5 mg/24 h (Androderm). Gel 1% 2.5, 5 g packet, 75 g multidose pump (AndroGel). Gel 1%, 5 g tube (Testim). Pellet 75 mg (Testopel). Buccal: Blister packs: 30 mg (Striant). Generic/Trade: Injection 100, 200 mg/mL (cypionate), 200 mg/mL (ethanate).] ▶L ♀X ▶? ©III $$$

Bisphosphonates

ALENDRONATE (*Fosamax, Fosamax Plus D, ♦Fosavance*) Postmenopausal osteoporosis prevention (5 mg PO daily or 35 mg PO weekly) and treatment (10 mg daily, 70 mg PO weekly, 70 mg/vit D3 2800 international units PO

(cont.)

weekly, or 70 mg/vit D3 5600 international units PO weekly). Treatment of <u>glucocorticoid-induced osteoporosis:</u> 5 mg PO daily in men and women or 10 mg PO daily in postmenopausal women not taking estrogen. Treatment of <u>osteoporosis in men:</u> 10 mg PO daily, 70 mg PO weekly, or 70 mg/vit D3 2800 international units PO weekly, or 70 mg/vit D3 5600 international units PO weekly. <u>Paget's disease</u> in men and women: 40 mg PO daily for 6 months. [Generic/Trade (Fosamax): Tabs 5, 10, 35, 40, 70 mg. Trade only: Oral soln 70 mg/75 mL (single-dose bottle). Fosamax Plus D: 70 mg + either 2800 or 5600 units of vitamin D3.] ▶K ♀C ▶– $$

CLODRONATE (✦*Clasteon, Bonefos*) Canada only. <u>Hypercalcemia of malignancy; management of osteolysis resulting from bone metastases of malignant tumors:</u> IV single dose, 1500 mg slow infusion over at least 4 h. IV multiple dose, 300 mg slow infusion daily over 2 to 5 h up to 10 days. Oral, following IV therapy, maintenance 1600 to 2400 mg/day in single or divided doses. Max PO dose 3200 mg/day; duration of therapy is usually 6 months. [Generic/Trade: Caps 400 mg.] ▶K ♀D ▶? $$$$$

ETIDRONATE (*Didronel*) <u>Paget's disease:</u> 5 to 10 mg/kg PO daily for 6 months or 11 to 20 mg/kg daily for 3 months. [Generic/Trade: Tabs 400 mg. Generic only: Tabs 200 mg] ▶K ♀C ▶? $$$$$

IBANDRONATE (*Boniva*) Treatment/Prevention of <u>postmenopausal osteoporosis:</u> Oral: 2.5 mg PO daily or 150 mg PO once a month. IV: 3 mg IV q 3 months. [Trade only: Tabs 2.5, 150 mg.] ▶K ♀C ▶? $$$$

PAMIDRONATE (*Aredia*) <u>Hypercalcemia of malignancy:</u> 60 to 90 mg IV over 2 to 24 h. Wait at least 7 days before considering retreatment. ▶K ♀D ▶? $$$$$

RISEDRONATE (*Actonel, Actonel Plus Calcium*) Prevention and treatment of <u>postmenopausal osteoporosis:</u> 5 mg PO daily, 35 mg PO weekly, or 150 mg once a month. Treatment of <u>osteoporosis in men:</u> 35 mg PO weekly. Prevention and treatment of <u>glucocorticoid-induced osteoporosis:</u> 5 mg PO daily. <u>Paget's disease:</u> 30 mg PO daily for 2 months. [Trade only: Tabs 5, 30, 35, 150 mg. Trade only (Actonel + Calcium): Tabs 35/1250 mg.] ▶K ♀C ▶? $$$$

ZOLEDRONIC ACID (*Reclast, Zometa, ✦Aclasta*) Treatment of <u>osteoporosis:</u> 5 mg (Reclast) once yearly IV infusion over 15 min or longer. Prevention and treatment of <u>glucocorticoid-induced osteoporosis:</u> 5 mg (Reclast) once a year IV infusion over 15 min or longer. <u>Hypercalcemia</u> (Zometa): 4 mg IV infusion over 15 min or longer. Wait at least 7 days before considering retreatment. <u>Paget's disease</u> (Reclast): 5 mg IV single dose infused over 15 min or longer. <u>Multiple myeloma and metastatic bone lesions from solid tumors</u> (Zometa): 4 mg IV infusion over 15 min or longer q 3 to 4 weeks. ▶K ♀D ▶? $$$$$

Corticosteroids

NOTE *See also dermatology, ophthalmology.*

BETAMETHASONE (*Celestone, Celestone Soluspan, ✦Betaject*) <u>Anti-inflammatory/Immunosuppressive:</u> 0.6 to 7.2 mg/day PO divided bid to qid; up to 9 mg/day IM. <u>Fetal lung maturation, maternal antepartum:</u> 12 mg IM q 24 h for 2 doses. [Trade only: Syrup 0.6 mg/5 mL.] ▶L ♀C ▶– $$$$$

CORTISONE (*Cortone*) 25 to 300 mg PO daily. [Generic only: Tabs 25 mg.] ▶L ♀D ▶– $

DEXAMETHASONE (*Decadron, Dexpak, ✦Dexasone*) Anti-inflammatory/Immunosuppressive: 0.5 to 9 mg/day PO/IV/IM, divided bid to qid. Cerebral edema: 10 to 20 mg IV load, then 4 mg IM q 6 h (off-label IV use common) or 1 to 3 mg PO tid. Bronchopulmonary dysplasia in preterm infants: 0.5 mg/kg PO/IV divided q 12 h for 3 days, then taper. Croup: 0.6 mg/kg PO or IM for one dose. Acute asthma: age older than 2 yo: 0.6 mg/kg to max 16 mg PO daily for 2 days. Fetal lung maturation, maternal antepartum: 6 mg IM q 12 h for 4 doses. Antiemetic, prophylaxis: 8 mg IV or 12 mg PO prior to chemotherapy; 8 mg PO daily for 2 to 4 days. Antiemetic, treatment: 10 to 20 mg PO/IV q 4 to 6 h. [Generic/Trade: Tabs 0.5, 0.75. Generic only: Tabs 0.25, 1.0, 1.5, 2, 4, 6 mg; elixir 0.5 mg/5 mL; Soln 0.5 mg/5 mL, 1 mg/1 mL (concentrate). Trade only: Dexpak 13 day (51 total 1.5 mg tabs for a 13-day taper), Dexpak 10 day (35 total 1.5 mg tabs for 10-day taper), Dexpak 6 days (21 total 1.5 mg tabs for 6-day taper).] ▶L ♀C ▶– $

FLUDROCORTISONE (*Florinef*) Mineralocorticoid activity: 0.1 mg PO 3 times a week to 0.2 mg PO daily. [Generic only: Tabs 0.1 mg.] ▶L ♀C ▶? $

HYDROCORTISONE (*Cortef, Cortenema, Solu-Cortef*) 100 to 500 mg IV/IM q 2 to 6 h prn (sodium succinate) or 20 to 240 mg/day PO divided tid to qid. Ulcerative colitis: 100 mg retention enema at bedtime (laying on side for 1 h or longer) for 21 days. [Generic/Trade: Tabs 5, 10, 20 mg; Enema 100 mg/60 mL.] ▶L ♀C ▶– $

METHYLPREDNISOLONE (*Solu-Medrol, Medrol, Depo-Medrol*) Oral (Medrol): Dose varies, 4 to 48 mg PO daily. Medrol Dosepak tapers 24 to 0 mg PO over 7 days. IM/Joints (Depo-Medrol): Dose varies, 4 to 120 mg IM q 1 to 2 weeks. Parenteral (Solu-Medrol): Dose varies, 10 to 250 mg IV/IM. Peds: 0.5 to 1.7 mg/kg PO/IV/IM divided q 6 to 12 h. Acute spinal cord injury: 30 mg/kg IV over 15 min, then 45 min by a 5.4 mg/kg/h IV infusion for 23 to 47 h. [Trade only: Tabs 2, 16, 32 mg. Generic/Trade: Tabs 4, 8 mg. Medrol Dosepak (4 mg, 21 tabs).] ▶L ♀C ▶– $

CORTICO-STEROIDS	Approximate Equivalent Dose (mg)	Relative Anti-inflammatory Potency	Relative Mineralocorticoid Potency	Biological Half-life (h)
betamethasone	0.6–0.75	20–30	0	36–54
cortisone	25	0.8	2	8–12
dexamethasone	0.75	20–30	0	36–54
fludrocortisone	n.a.	10	125	18–36
hydrocortisone	20	1	2	8–12
methylprednisolone	4	5	0	18–36
prednisolone	5	4	1	18–36
prednisone	5	4	1	18–36
triamcinolone	4	5	0	12–36

n.a., not available.

PREDNISOLONE (*Flo-Pred, Prelone, Pediapred, Orapred, Orapred ODT*) 5 to 60 mg PO daily. [Generic/Trade: Syrup 15 mg/5 mL (Prelone; wild cherry flavor). Soln 5 mg/5 mL (Pediapred, raspberry flavor), 15 mg/5 mL (Orapred; grape flavor). Trade only: Orally disintegrating tabs 10, 15, 30 mg (Orapred ODT); Susp 5 mg/5 mL, 15 mg/5 mL (Flo-Pred; cherry flavor). Generic only: Tabs 5 mg. Syrup 5 mg/5 mL.] ▶L ♀C ▶+ $$

PREDNISONE (*Deltasone, Sterapred, ✦Winpred*) 1 to 2 mg/kg or 5 to 60 mg PO daily. [Trade only: Sterapred (5 mg tabs: Tapers 30 to 5 mg PO over 6 days or 30 to 10 mg over 12 days), Sterapred DS (10 mg tabs: Tapers 60 to 10 mg over 6 days, or 60 to 20 mg PO over 12 days) taper packs. Generic only: Tabs 1, 2.5, 5, 10, 20, 50 mg. Soln 5 mg/5 mL, 5 mg/mL (Prednisone Intensol).] ▶L ♀C ▶+ $

TRIAMCINOLONE (*Aristospan, Kenalog, Trivaris*) 4 to 48 mg PO/IM daily. Intra-articular 2.5 to 40 mg (Kenalog, Trivaris), 2 to 20 mg (Aristospan). [Trade only: Injection 10 mg/mL, 40 mg/mL (Kenalog), 5 mg/mL, 20 mg/mL (Aristospan), 8 mg (80 mg/mL) syringe (Trivaris).] ▶L ♀C ▶– $

Diabetes-Related—Alpha-Glucosidase Inhibitors

ACARBOSE (*Precose, ✦Glucobay*) Start 25 mg PO tid with meals, and gradually increase as tolerated to maintenance, 50 to 100 mg tid. [Generic/Trade: Tabs 25, 50, 100 mg.] ▶Gut/K ♀B ▶– $$$

MIGLITOL (*Glyset*) Start 25 mg PO tid with meals, maintenance 50 to 100 tid. [Trade only: Tabs 25, 50, 100 mg.] ▶K ♀B ▶– $$$

Diabetes-Related—Combinations

ACTOPLUS MET (pioglitazone + metformin) 1 tab PO daily or bid. If inadequate control with metformin monotherapy, start 15/500 or 15/850 PO daily or bid. If inadequate control with pioglitazone monotherapy, start 15/500 bid or 15/850 daily. Max 45/2550 mg/day. Extended release, start 1 tab (15/100 mg or 30/1000 mg) daily with evening meal. Max: 45/2000 mg/day. Obtain LFTs before therapy and periodically thereafter. [Trade only: Tabs 15/500, 15/850 mg, Extended release, tabs: 15/1000 mg, 30/1000 mg.] ▶KL ♀C ▶? $$$$$

AVANDAMET (rosiglitazone + metformin) Initial therapy (drug-naive): Start 2/500 mg PO daily or bid. If inadequate control with metformin alone, select tab strength based on adding 4 mg/day rosiglitazone to existing metformin dose. If inadequate control with rosiglitazone alone, select tab strength based on adding 1000 mg/day metformin to existing rosiglitazone dose. Max 8/2000 mg/day. Obtain LFTs before therapy and periodically thereafter. [Trade only: Tabs 2/500, 4/500, 2/1000, 4/1000 mg.] ▶KL ♀C ▶? $$$$$

AVANDARYL (rosiglitazone + glimepiride) Initial therapy (drug-naive): Start 4/1 mg PO daily. If switching from monotherapy with a sulfonylurea or glitazone, consider 4/2 mg PO daily. Max 8/4 mg/day. Obtain LFTs before therapy and periodically thereafter. [Trade only: Tabs 4/1, 4/2, 4/4, 8/2, 8/4 mg rosiglitazone/glimepiride.] ▶LK ♀C ▶? $$$$

DIABETES NUMBERS*

Criteria for diagnosis:	Self-monitoring glucose goals

Criteria for diagnosis:
Pre-diabetes: Fasting glucose 100–125 mg/dL
Diabetes:† A1C ≥ 6.5%
Fasting glucose ≥ 126 mg/dL, random glucose
with symptoms: ≥ 200 mg/dL, or ≥ 200 mg/dL
2 h after 75 g oral glucose load

Self-monitoring glucose goals

Preprandial	70–130 mg/dL
Postprandial	< 180 mg/dL
A1C goal	< 7%

Critically ill glucose goal: 140–180 mg/dl
Non-critically ill glucose goal (hospitalized patients): premeal blood glucose < 140 mg/dL, random < 180 mg/dL. May consider stricter targets in stable patients.

Estimated average glucose (eAG): eAG (mg/dL) = (28.7 × A1C) – 46.7

Complications prevention & management: ASA‡ (75–162 mg/day) in Type 1 & 2 adults for primary prevention if 10-year cardiovascular risk > 10% (includes most men > 50 yo or women > 60 yo with at least one other major risk factor) and secondary prevention (those with vascular disease); statin therapy to achieve 30–40% LDL reduction regardless of baseline LDL (for those with vascular disease, those > 40 yo and additional risk factor, or those < 40 yo but LDL > 100 mg/dL); ACE inhibitor or ARB if hypertensive or micro-/macro-albuminuria; pneumococcal vaccine (revaccinate one time if age ≥ 65 and previously received vaccine at age < 65 and > 5 yr ago). *Every visit:* Measure wt & BP (goal < 130/80 mm Hg); visual foot exam; review self-monitoring glucose record; review/adjust meds; review self-mgmt skills, dietary needs, and physical activity; smoking cessation counseling. *Twice a year:* A1C in those meeting treatment goals with stable glycemia (quarterly if not); dental exam. *Annually:* Fasting lipid profile** [goal LDL < 100 mg/dL; cardiovascular disease consider LDL < 70mg/dL, HDL > 40 mg/dL (> 50 mg/dL in women), TG < 150 mg/dL], q 2 yr with low-risk lipid values; creatinine; albumin to creatinine ratio spot collection; dilated eye exam; flu vaccine.

*See recommendations at: care.diabetesjournals.org. Reference: *Diabetes Care* 2010;33(Suppl 1):S11-61. Glucose values are plasma. †In the absence of symptoms, confirm diagnosis with glucose testing on subsequent day. ‡Avoid ASA if < 21 yo due to Reye's Syndrome risk; use if < 30 yo has not been studied. **LDL is primary target of therapy.

DUETACT (pioglitazone + glimepiride) Start 30/2 mg PO daily. Start up to 30/4 mg PO daily if prior glimepiride therapy, or 30/2 mg PO daily if prior pioglitazone therapy; max 30/4 mg/day. Obtain LFTs before therapy and periodically thereafter. [Trade only: Tabs 30/2, 30/4 mg pioglitazone/glimepiride.] ▶LK ♀C ▶– $$$$

GLUCOVANCE (glyburide + metformin) Initial therapy (drug-naive): Start 1.25/250 mg PO daily or bid with meals; max 10/2000 mg daily. Inadequate control with a sulfonylurea or metformin alone: Start 2.5/500 or 5/500 mg PO bid with meals; max 20/2000 mg daily. [Generic/Trade: Tabs 1.25/250, 2.5/500, 5/500 mg.] ▶KL ♀B ▶? $$$

JANUMET (sitagliptin + metformin) 1 tab PO bid. Individualize based on patient's current therapy. If inadequate control with metformin monotherapy, start 50/500 or 50/1000 mg based on current metformin dose. If inadequate control on sitagliptin, start 50/500 bid. Max 100/2000 mg/day. Give with meals. [Trade only: Tabs 50/500, 50/1000 mg sitagliptin/metformin.] ▶K ♀B ▶? $$$$

METAGLIP (glipizide + metformin) Initial therapy (drug-naive): Start 2.5/250 mg PO daily to 2.5/500 mg PO bid with meals; max 10/2000 mg daily. Inadequate control with a sulfonylurea or metformin alone: Start 2.5/500 or 5/500 mg PO bid with meals; max 20/2000 mg daily. [Generic/Trade: Tabs 2.5/250, 2.5/500, 5/500 mg.] ▶KL ♀C ▶? \$\$\$

PRANDIMET (repaglinide + metformin) Initial therapy (drug-naive): Start 1/500 mg PO daily before meals; max 10/2500 mg daily or 4/1000 mg/meal. May start higher if already taking higher coadministered doses of repaglinide and metformin. [Trade: Tabs 1/500, 2/500 mg.] ▶KL ♀C ▶? \$\$\$

Diabetes-Related—"Glitazones" (Thiazolidinediones)

PIOGLITAZONE (Actos) Start 15 to 30 mg PO daily, max 45 mg/day. Monitor LFTs. [Trade only: Tabs 15, 30, 45 mg.] ▶L ♀C ▶– \$\$\$\$\$

ROSIGLITAZONE (Avandia) Diabetes monotherapy or in combination with metformin or sulfonylurea: Start 4 mg PO daily or divided bid, max 8 mg/day. Obtain LFTs before therapy and periodically thereafter. [Trade only (restricted access): Tabs 2, 4, 8 mg.] ▶L ♀C ▶– \$\$\$\$

Diabetes-Related—Insulins

INSULIN—INJECTABLE COMBINATIONS (Humalog Mix 75/25, Humalog Mix 50/50, Humulin 70/30, Humulin 50/50, Novolin 70/30, NovoLog Mix 70/30, NovoLog Mix 50/50) Diabetes: Doses vary, but typically total insulin 0.3 to 1 unit/kg/day SC in divided doses (Type 1), and 0.5 to 1.5 unit/kg/day SC in divided doses (Type 2). Administer rapid-acting insulin mixtures (Humalog, NovoLog) within 15 min before or immediately after a meal. Administer regular insulin mixtures 30 min before meals. [Trade only: Insulin lispro protamine susp/insulin lispro (Humalog Mix 75/25, Humalog Mix 50/50). Insulin aspart protamine/insulin aspart (NovoLog Mix 70/30, NovoLog Mix 50/50). NPH and regular mixtures (Humulin 70/30, Novolin 70/30 or Humulin 50/50). Insulin available in pen form: Novolin 70/30 InnoLet, NovoLog Mix 70/30, NovoLog Mix 50/50, FlexPen, Humulin 70/30, Humalog Mix 75/25 KwikPen, Humalog Mix 50/50 KwikPen.] ▶LK ♀B/C ▶+ \$\$\$\$

INSULIN—INJECTABLE INTERMEDIATE/LONG-ACTING (Novolin N, Humulin N, Lantus, Levemir) Diabetes: Doses vary, but typically total insulin 0.3 to 0.5 unit/kg/day SC in divided doses (Type 1), and 1 to 1.5 unit/kg/day SC in divided doses (Type 2). Generally, 50 to 70% of insulin requirements are provided by rapid or short-acting insulin and the remainder from intermediate- or long-acting insulin. Lantus: Start 10 units SC daily (same time everyday) in insulin-naive patients. Levemir: Type 2 DM (inadequately controlled on oral meds): Start 0.1 to 0.2 units/kg once daily in evening or 10 units SC daily or BID. [Trade only: Injection NPH (Novolin N, Humulin N). Insulin glargine (Lantus). Insulin detemir (Levemir). Insulin available in pen form: Novolin N InnoLet, Humulin N Pen, Lantus OptiClik (reusable), Lantus SoloStar (prefilled-disposable), Levemir InnoLet, Levemir FlexPen. Premixed preparations of NPH and regular insulin also available.] ▶LK ♀B/C ▶+ \$\$\$\$

INJECTABLE INSULINS*		Onset (h)	Peak (h)	Duration (h)
Rapid/short-acting:	Insulin aspart (NovoLog)	<0.2	1–3	3–5
	Insulin glulisine (Apidra)	0.30–0.4	1	4–5
	Insulin lispro (Humalog)	0.25–0.5	0.5–2.5	≤5
	Regular (Novolin R, Humulin R)	0.5–1	2–3	3–6
Intermediate/long-acting:	NPH (Novolin N, Humulin N)	2–4	4–10	10–16
	Insulin detemir (Levemir)	n.a.	flat action profile	up to 23†
	Insulin glargine (Lantus)	2–4	peakless	24
Mixtures:	Insulin aspart protamine susp/ aspart (NovoLog Mix 70/30, NovoLog Mix 50/50)	0.25	1–4 (biphasic)	up to 24
	Insulin lispro protamine susp/ insulin lispro (HumaLog Mix 75/25, HumaLog Mix 50/50)	<0.25	1–3 (biphasic)	10–20
	NPH/Reg (Humulin 70/30, Humulin 50/50, Novolin 70/30)	0.5–1	2–10 (biphasic)	10–20

*These are general guidelines, as onset, peak, and duration of activity are affected by the site of injection, physical activity, body temperature, and blood supply. † Dose dependent duration of action, range from 6 to 23 h., n.a., not available.

INSULIN—INJECTABLE SHORT/RAPID-ACTING (*Apidra, Novolin R, NovoLog, Humulin R, Humalog, ◆NovoRapid*) Diabetes: Doses vary, but typically total insulin 0.3 to 0.5 unit/kg/day SC in divided doses (Type 1), and 1 to 1.5 unit/kg/day SC in divided doses (Type 2). Generally, 50 to 70% of insulin requirements are provided by rapid or short-acting insulin and the remainder from intermediate- or long-acting insulin. Administer rapid-acting insulin (Humalog, NovoLog, Apidra) within 15 min before or immediately after a meal. Administer regular insulin 30 min before meals. Severe hyperkalemia: 5 to 10 units regular insulin plus concurrent dextrose IV. Profound hyperglycemia (eg, DKA): 0.1 unit regular/kg IV bolus, then initial infusion 100 units regular in 100 mL NS (1 unit/mL), at 0.1 units/kg/h. 70 kg: 7 units/h (7 mL/h). [Trade only: Injection regular (Novolin R, Humulin R). Insulin glulisine (Apidra). Insulin lispro (Humalog). Insulin aspart (NovoLog). Insulin available in pen form: Novolin R InnoLet, Humulin R, Apidra OptiClik, Humalog KwikPen, NovoLog FlexPen.] ▶LK ♀B/C ▶+ $$$

Diabetes-Related—Meglitinides

NATEGLINIDE (*Starlix*) 120 mg PO tid within 30 min before meals; use 60 mg PO tid in patients who are near goal A1C. [Generic/Trade: Tabs 60, 120 mg.] ▶L ♀C ▶? $$$

REPAGLINIDE (*Prandin, ◆Gluconorm*) Start 0.5 to 2 mg PO tid before meals, maintenance 0.5 to 4 mg tid to qid, max 16 mg/day. [Trade only: Tabs 0.5, 1, 2 mg.] ▶L ♀C ▶? $$$$$

Diabetes-Related—Sulfonylureas—2nd Generation

GLICLAZIDE (*★Diamicron, Diamicron MR*) Canada only. Immediate-release: Start 80 to 160 mg PO daily, max 320 mg PO daily (160 mg or more per day should be in divided doses. Modified-release: Start 30 mg PO daily, max 120 mg PO daily. [Generic/Trade: Tabs 80 mg (Diamicron). Trade only: Tabs modified-release 30 mg (Diamicron MR).] ▶KL ♀C ▶? $

GLIMEPIRIDE (*Amaryl*) Start 1 to 2 mg PO daily, usual 1 to 4 mg/day, max 8 mg/day. [Generic/Trade: Tabs 1, 2, 4 mg. Generic only: Tabs 3, 6, 8 mg.] ▶LK ♀C ▶– $$

GLIPIZIDE (*Glucotrol, Glucotrol XL*) Start 5 mg PO daily, usual 10 to 20 mg/day, max 40 mg/day (divide bid if more than 15 mg/day). Extended-release: Start 5 mg PO daily, usual 5 to 10 mg/day, max 20 mg/day. [Generic/Trade: Tabs 5, 10 mg; Extended-release tabs 2.5, 5, 10 mg.] ▶LK ♀C ▶? $

GLYBURIDE (*DiaBeta, Glynase PresTab, ★Euglucon*) Start 1.25 to 5 mg PO daily, usual 1.25 to 20 mg daily or divided bid, max 20 mg/day. Micronized tabs: Start 1.5 to 3 mg PO daily, usual 0.75 to 12 mg/day divided bid, max 12 mg/day. [Generic/Trade: Tabs (scored) 1.25, 2.5, 5 mg. Micronized Tabs (scored) 1.5, 3, 4.5, 6 mg.] ▶LK ♀B ▶? $

Diabetes-Related—Other

A1C HOME TESTING (*A1CNow*) For home A1C testing [Fingerstick blood.] ▶None ♀+ ▶+ $

DEXTROSE (*Glutose, B-D Glucose, Insta-Glucose, Dex-4*) Hypoglycemia: 0.5 to 1 g/kg (1 to 2 mL/kg) up to 25 g (50 mL) of 50% soln IV. Dilute to 25% for pediatric administration. [OTC Generic/Trade: Chewable tabs 4 g (Dex-4), 5 g (Glutose). Trade only: Oral gel 40%.] ▶L ♀C ▶? $

EXENATIDE (*Byetta*) Type 2 DM adjunctive therapy when inadequate control on metformin, a sulfonylurea, or a glitazone (alone or in combination): 5 mcg SC bid (within 1 h before the morning and evening meals, or 1 h before the two main meals of the day at least 6 h apart). May increase to 10 mcg SC bid after 1 month. [Trade only: Prefilled pen (60 doses each) 5 mcg/dose, 1.2 mL; 10 mcg/dose, 2.4 mL.] ▶K ♀C ▶? $$$$$

GLUCAGON (*GlucaGen*) Hypoglycemia: 1 mg IV/IM/SC, onset 5 to 20 min. Diagnostic aid: 1 mg IV/IM/SC. [Trade only: Injection 1 mg.] ▶LK ♀B ▶? $$$

GLUCOSE HOME TESTING (*Accu-Chek Active, Accu-Check Advantage, Accu-Check Aviva, Accu-Check Compact, Accu-Check Compact Plus, Accu-Check Complete, Accu-Check Voicemate, FreeStyle Flash, FreeStyle Freedom, FreeStyle Freedom Lite, FreeStyle Lite, OneTouch Ultra, OneTouch UltraMin*) Use for home glucose monitoring. [Plasma: Accu-Chek meters, FreeStyle meters, OneTouch meters, Precision Xtra, ReliOn, Sidekick, True Track. Urine: Clinistix, Clinitest, Diastix, Tes-Tape.] ▶None ♀+ ▶+ $$

LIRAGLUTIDE (*Victoza*) Type 2 DM: Start 0.6 mg SC daily for 1 week, then increase to 1.2 mg SC daily. May increase to 1.8 mg SC daily. [Trade only: Multidose pen (18 mg/3ml) delivers doses of 0.6 mg, 1.2 mg or 1.8 mg.] ▶endogenous ♀C ▶? $$$$$

METFORMIN (*Glucophage, Glucophage XR, Glumetza, Fortamet, Riomet*) <u>Diabetes, type 2:</u> Immediate-release: Start 500 mg PO daily to bid or 850 mg PO daily with meals, may gradually increase to max 2550 mg/day. Extended-release: Glucophage XR: 500 mg PO daily with evening meal; increase by 500 mg once a week to max 2000 mg/day (may divide bid). Glumetza: 1000 mg PO daily with evening meal; increase by 500 mg once a week to max 2000 mg/day (may divide bid). Fortamet: 500 to 1000 mg daily with evening meal; increase by 500 mg once a week to max 2500 mg/day. <u>Polycystic ovary syndrome</u> (unapproved, immediate-release): 500 mg PO tid. [Generic/Trade: Tabs 500, 850, 1000 mg, extended-release: Fortamet 500, 750 mg. Trade only, extended-release: Fortamet 500, 1000 mg; Glumetza 500, 1000 mg. Trade only: Oral soln 500 mg/5 mL (Riomet).] ▶K ♀B ▶? $

PRAMLINTIDE (*Symlin, Symlinpen*) <u>Type 1 DM</u> with mealtime insulin therapy: Initiate 15 mcg SC immediately before major meals and titrate by 15 mcg increments (if significant nausea has not occurred for at least 3 day) to maintenance 30 to 60 mcg as tolerated. <u>Type 2 DM</u> with mealtime insulin therapy: Initiate 60 mcg SC immediately before major meals and increase to 120 mcg as tolerated (if significant nausea has not occurred for 3 to 7 days). [Trade only: 600 mcg/mL in 5 mL vials, 1000 mcg/mL pen injector (Symlinpen) 1.5, 2.7 mL.] ▶K ♀C ▶? $$$$

SAXAGLIPTIN (*Onglyza*) <u>Type 2 DM:</u> 2.5 or 5 mg PO daily. [Trade only: Tabs 2.5, 5 mg.] ▶K ♀B ▶? $$$$$

SITAGLIPTIN (*Januvia*) <u>Type 2 DM:</u> 100 mg PO daily. [Trade only: Tabs 25, 50, 100 mg.] ▶K ♀B ▶? $$$$

Diagnostic Agents

COSYNTROPIN (*Cortrosyn*, ✦*Synacthen*) <u>Rapid screen for adrenocortical insufficiency:</u> 0.25 mg (0.125 mg if age younger than 2 yo) IM/IV over 2 min; measure serum cortisol before and 30 to 60 min after. ▶L ♀C ▶? $

Gout-Related

ALLOPURINOL (*Aloprim, Zyloprim*) <u>Mild gout or recurrent calcium oxalate stones:</u> 200 to 300 mg PO daily to bid, max 800 mg/day. [Generic/Trade: Tabs 100, 300 mg.] ▶K ♀C ▶+ $

COLBENEMID (colchicine + probenecid) 1 tab PO daily for 1 week, then 1 tab PO bid. [Generic only: Tabs 0.5 mg colchicine + 500 mg probenecid.] ▶KL ♀C ▶? $

COLCHICINE (*Colcrys*) <u>Rapid treatment of acute gouty arthritis:</u> 1.2 mg (2 tab) PO at signs of attack then 0.6 mg (1 tab) 1h after initial administration. <u>Gout prophylaxis:</u> 0.6 mg PO bid if CrCl ≥ 50 mL/min, 0.6 mg PO daily if CrCl 35 to 49 mL/min, 0.6 mg PO q 2 to 3 days if CrCl 10 to 34 mL/min. <u>Familial Mediterranean Fever:</u> 1.2 to 2.4 mg PO daily or divided bid. [Generic/Trade: Tabs 0.6 mg.] ▶L ♀C ▶? $

FEBUXOSTAT (*Uloric*) <u>Hyperuricemia with gout:</u> Start 40 mg PO daily, max 80 mg daily. [Trade only: Tabs 40, 80 mg.] ▶LK ♀C ▶? $$$$

PROBENECID (*Benuryl*) <u>Gout:</u> 250 mg PO bid for 7 days, then 500 mg bid. <u>Adjunct to penicillin injection:</u> 1 to 2 g PO in divided doses. [Generic only: Tabs 500 mg.] ▶KL ♀B ▶? $

Minerals

CALCIUM ACETATE (*PhosLo*) <u>Hyperphosphatemia:</u> Initially 2 tabs/caps PO with each meal. [Generic/Trade: Gelcaps 667 mg (169 mg elemental Ca).] ▶K ♀+ ▶? $$$$

CALCIUM CARBONATE (*Caltrate, Mylanta Children's, Os-Cal, Oyst-Cal, Tums, Surpass, Viactiv, ✦Calsan*) <u>Supplement:</u> 1 to 2 g elemental Ca/day or more PO with meals divided bid to qid. <u>Antacid:</u> 1000 to 3000 mg PO q 2 h prn or 1 to 2 pieces gum chewed prn, max 7000 mg/day. [OTC Generic/Trade: Tabs 500, 650, 750, 1000, 1250, 1500 mg, Chewable tabs 400, 500, 750, 850, 1000, 1177, 1250 mg, Caps 1250 mg, Gum 300, 450 mg, Susp 1250 mg/5 mL. Calcium carbonate is 40% elemental Ca and contains 20 mEq of elemental Ca/g calcium carbonate. Not more than 500 to 600 mg elemental Ca/dose. Available in combination with sodium fluoride, vitamin D and/or vitamin K. Trade examples: Caltrate 600 + D is equivalent to 600 mg elemental Ca/200 units vit D, Os-Cal 500 + D is equivalent to 500 mg elemental Ca/400 units vit D, Os-Cal Extra D is equivalent to 500 mg elemental Ca/400 units vit D, Tums (regular strength) is equivalent to 200 mg elemental Ca, Tums (ultra) is equivalent to 400 mg elemental Ca, Viactiv (chewable) 500 mg elemental Ca+ 500 units vit D + 40 mcg vit K.] ▶K ♀– (? 1st trimester) ▶? $

CALCIUM CHLORIDE 500 to 1000 mg slow IV q 1 to 3 days. [Generic only: Injectable 10% (1000 mg/10 mL) 10 mL ampules, vials, syringes.] ▶K ♀+ ▶+ $

CALCIUM CITRATE (*Citracal*) 1 to 2 g elemental Ca/day or more PO with meals divided bid to qid. [OTC Trade only (mg elemental Ca): 200, 250 mg with 200 units vitamin D and 250 mg with 125 units vitamin D and 80 mg of magnesium. Chewable tabs 500 mg with 200 units vitamin D. OTC Generic/Trade: Tabs 200 mg, 315 mg with 200 units vitamin D.] ▶K ♀+ ▶+ $

CALCIUM GLUCONATE 2.25 to 14 mEq slow IV. 500 to 2000 mg PO bid to qid. [Generic only: Injectable 10% (1000 mg/10 mL, 4.65 mEq/10 mL) 1, 10, 50, 100, 200 mL. OTC Generic only: Tabs 50, 500, 650, 975, 1000 mg. Chewable tabs 650 mg.] ▶K ♀+ ▶+ $

FERRIC GLUCONATE COMPLEX (*Ferrlecit*) 125 mg elemental iron IV over 10 min or diluted in 100 mL NS IV over 1 h. Peds age 6 yo or older: 1.5 mg/kg (max 125 mg) elemental iron diluted in 25 mL NS and administered IV over 1 h. ▶KL ♀B ▶? $$$

FERROUS GLUCONATE (*Fergon*) 800 to 1600 mg ferrous gluconate PO divided tid. [OTC Generic/Trade: Tabs (ferrous gluconate) 240 mg (27 mg elemental iron). Generic only: Tabs 324, 325 mg.] ▶K ♀+ ▶+ $

FERROUS SULFATE (*Fer-in-Sol, Feosol, Slow FE, ✦Ferodan, Slow-Fe*) 500 to 1000 mg ferrous sulfate (100 to 200 mg elemental iron) PO divided tid. [OTC Generic/Trade (mg ferrous sulfate): Tabs extended-release 160 mg. Tabs 200, 324, 325 mg. OTC Generic only (mg ferrous sulfate): Soln 75 mg/0.6 mL, Elixir 220 mg/5 mL.] ▶K ♀+ ▶+ $

FERUMOXYTOL (*Feraheme*) Iron deficiency in chronic kidney disease: Give 510 mg IV push, followed by 510 mg IV push once given 3 to 8 days after initial injection. ▶KL ♀C ▶? $$$$$

FLUORIDE (*Luride, ✦Fluor-A-Day, Fluotic*) Adult dose: 10 mL of topical rinse swish and spit daily. Peds daily dose based on fluoride content of drinking water (table). [Generic only: Chewable tabs 0.5, 1 mg; Tabs 1 mg, gtts 0.125 mg, 0.25 mg, and 0.5 mg/ dropperful, Lozenges 1 mg, Soln 0.2 mg/mL, Gel 0.1%, 0.5%, 1.23%, Rinse (sodium fluoride) 0.05, 0.1, 0.2%).] ▶K ♀? ▶? $

IRON DEXTRAN (*InFed, DexFerrum, ✦Dexiron, Infufer*) 25 to 100 mg IM daily prn. Equations available to calculate IV dose based on wt and Hb. ▶KL ♀C ▶? $$$$

IRON POLYSACCHARIDE (*Niferex, Niferex-150, Nu-Iron 150, Ferrex 150*) 50 to 200 mg PO divided daily to tid. [OTC Trade only: Caps 60 mg (Niferex). OTC Generic/Trade: Caps 150 mg (Niferex-150, Nu-Iron 150, Ferrex-150), Elixir 100 mg/5 mL (Niferex). 1 mg iron polysaccharide is equivalent to 1 mg elemental iron.] ▶K ♀+ ▶+ $$

IRON SUCROSE (*Venofer*) Iron deficiency with hemodialysis: 5 mL (100 mg elemental iron) IV over 5 min or diluted in 100 mL NS IV over 15 min or longer. Iron deficiency in nondialysis chronic kidney disease: 10 mL (200 mg elemental iron) IV over 5 min. ▶KL ♀B ▶? $$$$$

MAGNESIUM CHLORIDE (*Slow-Mag*) 2 tabs PO daily. [OTC Trade only: Enteric coated tab 64 mg. 64 mg tab Slow-Mag is equivalent to 64 mg elemental magnesium.] ▶K ♀A ▶+ $

FLUORIDE SUPPLEMENTATION

Age	<0.3 ppm in drinking water	0.3–0.6 ppm in drinking water	>0.6 ppm in drinking water
0–0.5 yo	none	none	none
0.5–3 yo	0.25 mg PO daily	none	none
3–6 yo	0.5 mg PO daily	0.25 mg PO daily	none
6–16 yo	1 mg PO daily	0.5 mg PO daily	none

IV SOLUTIONS

Solution	Dextrose	Calories/Liter	Na*	K*	Ca*	Cl*	Lactate*	Osm*
0.9 NS	0 g/L	0	154	0	0	154	0	310
LR	0 g/L	9	130	4	3	109	28	273
D5 W	50 g/L	170	0	0	0	0	0	253
D5 0.2 NS	50 g/L	170	34	0	0	34	0	320
D5 0.45 NS	50 g/L	170	77	0	0	77	0	405
D5 0.9 NS	50 g/L	170	154	0	0	154	0	560
D5 LR	50 g/L	179	130	4	2.7	109	28	527

* All given in mEq/L

MAGNESIUM GLUCONATE (*Almora, Magtrate, Maganate, ✦Maglucate*) 500 to 1000 mg PO divided tid. [OTC Generic only: Tabs 500 mg (27 mg elemental Mg), liquid 54 mg elemental Mg/5 mL.] ▶K ♀A ▶+ $

MAGNESIUM OXIDE (*Mag-200, Mag-Ox 400*) 400 to 800 mg PO daily. [OTC Generic/Trade: Caps - 140 (84.5 mg elemental Mg), 250 (elemental), 400 (240 mg elemental Mg), 420 (253 mg elemental Mg), 500 mg (elemental).] ▶K ♀A ▶+ $

MAGNESIUM SULFATE <u>Hypomagnesemia:</u> 1 g of 20% soln IM q 6 h for 4 doses, or 2 g IV over 1 h (monitor for hypotension). Peds: 25 to 50 mg/kg IV/IM q 4 to 6 h for 3 to 4 doses, max single dose 2 g. <u>Eclampsia:</u> 4 to 6 g IV over 30 min, then 1 to 2 g/h. Drip: 5 g in 250 mL D5W (20 mg/mL), 2 g/h is a rate of 100 mL/h. <u>Preterm labor:</u> 6 g IV over 20 min, then 1 to 3 g/h titrated to decrease contractions. Monitor respirations and reflexes. If needed, may reverse toxic effects with calcium gluconate 1 g IV. <u>Torsades de pointes:</u> 1 to 2 g IV in D5W over 5 to 60 min. ▶K ♀A ▶+ $

PHOSPHORUS (*Neutra-Phos, K-Phos*) 1 cap/packet PO qid. 1 to 2 tabs PO qid. <u>Severe hypophosphatemia</u> (eg, <1 mg/dL): 0.08 to 0.16 mmol/kg IV over 6 h. [OTC Trade only: (Neutra-Phos, Neutra-Phos K) tab/cap/packet 250 mg (8 mmol) phosphorus. Rx: Trade only: (K-Phos) tab 250 mg (8 mmol) phosphorus.] ▶K ♀C ▶? $

POTASSIUM (*Cena-K, Effer-K, K+8, K+10, Kaochlor, Kaon, Kaon Cl, Kay Ciel, Kaylixir, K+Care, K+Care ET, K-Dur, K-G Elixir, K-Lease, K-Lor, Klor-con, Klorvess Effervescent, Klotrix, K-Lyte, K-Lyte Cl, K-Norm, Kolyum, K-Tab, K-vescent, Micro-K, Micro-K LS, Sl*) IV infusion 10 mEq/h (diluted). 20 to 40 mEq PO daily or bid. [Injectable, many different products in a variety of salt forms (ie, chloride, bicarbonate, citrate, acetate, gluconate), available in tabs, caps, liquids, effervescent tabs packets. Potassium gluconate is available OTC.] ▶K ♀C ▶? $

ZINC ACETATE (*Galzin*) <u>Dietary supplement:</u> 8 to 12 mg (elemental) daily. <u>Zinc deficiency:</u> 25 to 50 mg (elemental) daily. <u>Wilson's disease:</u> 25 to 50 mg (elemental) PO tid. [Trade only: Caps 25, 50 mg elemental zinc.] ▶Minimal absorption ♀A ▶– $$$

ZINC SULFATE (*Orazinc, Zincate*) <u>Dietary supplement:</u> 8 to 12 mg (elemental) daily. <u>Zinc deficiency:</u> 25 to 50 mg (elemental) PO daily. [OTC Generic/Trade: Tabs 66, 110, 200 mg. Rx Generic/Trade: Caps 220 mg.] ▶Minimal absorption ♀A ▶– $

POTASSIUM (oral forms)

Effervescent Granules:	<u>20 mEq:</u> Klorvess Effervescent, K-vescent
Effervescent Tabs:	<u>10 mEq:</u> Effer-K 20 mEq: Effer-K <u>25 mEq:</u> Effer-K, K+Care ET, K-Lyte, K-Lyte/Cl, Klor-Con/EF <u>50 mEq:</u> K-Lyte DS, K-Lyte/Cl 50
Liquids:	<u>20 mEq/15 mL:</u> Cena-K, Kaochlor S-F, K-G Elixir, Kaochlor 10%, Kay Ciel, Kaon, Kaylixir, Kolyum, Potasalan, Twin-K <u>30 mEq/15 mL:</u> Rum-K 40 mEq/15 mL: Cena-K, Kaon-Cl 20% <u>45 mEq/15 mL:</u> Tri-K
Powders:	<u>15 mEq/pack:</u> K+Care <u>20 mEq/pack:</u> Gen-K, K+Care, Kay Ciel, K-Lor, Klor-Con <u>25 mEq/pack:</u> K+Care, Klor-Con 25
Tabs/Caps:	<u>8 mEq:</u> K+8, Klor-Con 8, Slow-K, Micro-K <u>10 mEq:</u> K+10, K-Norm, Kaon-Cl 10 Klor-Con M10 Klotrix, K-Tab, K-Dur 10, Micro-K 10 <u>20 mEq:</u> Klor-Con M20, K-Dur 20

Nutritionals

BANANA BAG, RALLY PACK   Alcoholic malnutrition (one formula): Add thiamine 100 mg + folic acid 1 mg + IV multivitamins to 1 liter NS and infuse over 4 h. Magnesium sulfate 2 g may be added. "Banana bag" and "rally pack" are jargon and not valid drug orders. Specify individual components. ▶KL ♀+ ▶+ $

FAT EMULSION (*Intralipid, Liposyn*)   Dosage varies. ▶L ♀C ▶? $$$$$

FORMULAS—INFANT (*Enfamil, Similac, Isomil, Nursoy, Prosobee, Soyalac, Alsoy, Nutramigen Lipil*)   Infant meals. [OTC: Milk-based (Enfamil, Similac, SMA) or soy-based (Isomil, Nursoy, ProSobee, Soyalac, Alsoy).] ▶L ♀+ ▶+ $

LEVOCARNITINE (*Carnitor*)   10 to 20 mg/kg IV at each dialysis session. [Generic/Trade: Tabs 330 mg, Oral soln 1 g/10 mL.] ▶KL ♀B ▶? $$$$$

OMEGA-3-ACID ETHYL ESTERS (*Lovaza, fish oil, omega 3 fatty acids*)   Hypertriglyceridemia: 4 caps PO daily or divided bid. [Trade only: (Lovaza) 1 g cap (total 840 mg EPA + DHA).] ▶L ♀C ▶? $

Phosphate Binders

LANTHANUM CARBONATE (*Fosrenol*)   Hyperphosphatemia in end stage renal disease: Start 1500 mg/day PO in divided doses with meals. Titrate dose q 2 to 3 weeks in increments of 750 mg/day until acceptable serum phosphate is reached. Most will require 1500 to 3000 mg/day to reduce phosphate <6.0 mg/dL. [Trade only: Chewable tabs 500, 750, 1000 mg.] ▶Not absorbed ♀C ▶? $$$$$

SEVELAMER (*Renagel, Renvela*)   Hyperphosphatemia: 800 to 1600 mg PO tid with meals. [Trade only (Renagel - sevelamer hydrochloride): Tabs 400, 800 mg. (Renvela - sevelamer carbonate): Tabs 800 mg; Powder: 800, 2400 mg packets.] ▶Not absorbed ♀C ▶? $$$$$

Thyroid Agents

LEVOTHYROXINE (*L-Thyroxine, Levolet, Levo-T, Levothroid, Levoxyl, Novothyrox, Synthroid, Thyro-Tabs, Tirosint, Unithroid, T4, ✦Eltroxin, Euthyrox*)   Start 100 to 200 mcg PO daily (healthy adults) or 12.5 to 50 mcg PO daily (elderly or CV disease), increase by 12.5 to 25 mcg/day at 3 to 8 week intervals. Usual maintenance dose 100 to 200 mcg/day, max 300 mcg/day. [Generic/Trade: Tabs 25, 50, 75, 88, 100, 112, 125, 137, 150, 175, 200, 300 mcg. Trade only: Caps: 25, 50, 75, 100, 125, 150 mcg in 7 days blister packs, Tabs: 13 mcg (Tirosint).] ▶L ♀A ▶+ $

LIOTHYRONINE (*T3, Cytomel, Triostat*)   Start 25 mcg PO daily, max 100 mcg/day. [Generic/Trade: Tabs 5, 25, 50 mcg.] ▶L ♀A ▶? $$

METHIMAZOLE (*Tapazole*)   Start 5 to 20 mg PO tid or 10 to 30 mg PO daily, then adjust. [Generic/Trade: Tabs 5, 10. Generic only: Tabs 15, 20 mg.] ▶L ♀D ▶+ $$$

PROPYLTHIOURACIL (*PTU, ✦Propyl Thyracil*)   Start 100 mg PO tid, then adjust. Thyroid storm: 200 to 300 mg PO qid, then adjust. [Generic only: Tabs 50 mg.] ▶L ♀D (but preferred over methimazole in first trimester) ▶+ $

PEDIATRIC REHYDRATION SOLUTIONS

Brand	Glucose	Calories/Liter	Na*	K*	Cl*	Citrate*	Phos*	Ca*	Mg*
CeraLyte 50†	0 g/L	160	50	20	40	30	0	0	0
CeraLyte 70†	0 g/L	160	70	20	60	30	0	0	0
CeraLyte 90†	0 g/L	160	90	20	80	30	0	0	0
Infalyte	30 g/L	140	50	25	45	34	0	0	0
Kao Lectrolyte†	20 g/L	90	50	20	40	30	0	0	0
Lytren (Canada)	20 g/L	80	50	25	45	30	0	0	0
Naturalyte	25 g/L	100	45	20	35	48	0	0	0
Pedialyte and Pedialyte Freezer Pops	25 g/L	100	45	20	35	30	0	0	0
Rehydralyte	25 g/L	100	75	20	65	30	0	0	0
Resol	20 g/L	80	50	20	50	34	5	4	4

* All given in mEq/L
† Premeasured powder packet

SODIUM IODIDE I-131 (*Hicon, Iodotope, Sodium Iodide I-131 Therapeutic*) Specialized dosing for hyperthyroidism and thyroid carcinoma. [Generic/Trade: Caps Oral soln: Radioactivity range varies at the time of calibration. Hicon is a kit containing caps and a concentrated oral soln for dilution and cap preparation.] ▶K ♀X ▶– $$$$$

Vitamins

ASCORBIC ACID (*vitamin C, ◆Redoxon*) 70 to 1000 mg PO daily. [OTC Generic only: Tabs 25, 50, 100, 250, 500, 1000 mg, Chewable tabs 100, 250, 500 mg, Timed-release tabs 500, 1000, 1500 mg, Timed-release caps 500 mg, Lozenges 60 mg, Liquid 35 mg/0.6 mL, Oral soln 100 mg/mL, Syrup 500 mg/5 mL.] ▶K ♀C ▶? $

CALCITRIOL (*Rocaltrol, Calcijex*) 0.25 to 2 mcg PO daily. [Generic/Trade: Caps 0.25, 0.5 mcg. Oral soln 1 mcg/mL. Injection 1, 2 mcg/mL.] ▶L ♀C ▶? $$

CYANOCOBALAMIN (*vitamin B12, CaloMist, Nascobal*) Deficiency states: 100 to 200 mcg IM once a month or 1000 to 2000 mcg PO daily for 1 to 2 weeks followed by 1000 mcg PO daily, 500 mcg intranasal weekly (Nascobal: 1 spray 1 nostril once a week), or 50 to 100 mcg intranasal daily (CaloMist: 1 to 2 sprays each nostril daily). [OTC Generic only: Tabs 100, 500, 1000 mcg; Lozenges 100, 250, 500 mcg. Rx Trade only: Nasal spray 500 mcg/spray (Nascobal 2.3 mL), 25 mcg/spray (CaloMist, 18 mL).] ▶K ♀C ▶+ $

DOXERCALCIFEROL (*Hectorol*) Secondary hyperparathyroidism on dialysis: Oral: 10 mcg PO 3 times a week. May increase every 8 weeks by 2.5 mcg/dose; max 60 mcg/week. IV: 4 mcg IV 3 times a week. May increase dose every 8 weeks by 1 to 2 mcg/dose; max 18 mcg/week. Secondary hyperparathyroidism not on dialysis: Start 1 mcg PO daily, may increase by 0.5 mcg/dose q 2 weeks. Max 3.5 mcg/day. [Trade only: Caps 0.5, 2.5 mcg.] ▶L ♀B ▶? $$$$$

ERGOCALCIFEROL (*vitamin D2, Calciferol, Drisdol, ✦Osteoforte*) Osteoporosis prevention and treatment (age 50 or older): 800 to 1000 units daily. Familial hypophosphatemia (Vitamin D Resistant Rickets): 12,000 to 500,000 units PO daily. Hypoparathyroidism: 50,000 to 200,000 units PO daily. Adequate daily intake adults: 19 to 50 yo: 5 mcg (200 units) ergocalciferol; 51 to 70 yo: 10 mcg (400 units); older than 70 yo: 15 mcg (600 units). [OTC Generic only: Caps 400, 1000, 5000 units, Soln 8000 units/mL (Calciferol). Rx Generic/Trade: Caps 50,000 units. Rx Generic only: Caps 25,000 units.] ▶L ♀A (C if exceed RDA) ▶+ $

FOLIC ACID (*folate, Folvite*) 0.4 to 1 mg IV/IM/PO/SC daily. [OTC Generic only: Tabs 0.4, 0.8 mg. Rx Generic 1 mg.] ▶K ♀A ▶+ $

MULTIVITAMINS (*MVI*) Dose varies with product. Tabs come with and without iron. [OTC and Rx: Many different brands and forms available with and without iron (Tabs Caps chewable; Tabs Gtts liquid).] ▶LK ♀+ ▶+ $

NEPHROCAP (ascorbic acid + folic acid + niacin + thiamine + riboflavin + pyridoxine + pantothenic acid + biotin + cyanocobalamin) 1 cap PO daily. If on dialysis, take after treatment. [Generic/Trade: Vitamin C 100 mg/folic acid 1 mg/niacin 20 mg/thiamine 1.5 mg/riboflavin 1.7 mg/pyridoxine 10 mg/pantothenic acid 5 mg/biotin 150 mcg/cyanocobalamin 6 mcg.] ▶K ♀? ▶? $

NEPHROVITE (ascorbic acid + folic acid + niacin + thiamine + riboflavin + pyridoxine + pantothenic acid + biotin + cyanocobalamin) 1 tab PO daily. If on dialysis, take after treatment. [Generic/Trade: Vitamin C 60 mg/folic acid 1 mg/niacin 20 mg/thiamine 1.5 mg/riboflavin 1.7 mg/pyridoxine 10 mg/pantothenic acid 10 mg/biotin 300 mcg/cyanocobalamin 6 mcg.] ▶K ♀? ▶? $

NIACIN (*vitamin B3, nicotinic acid, Niacor, Nicolar, Slo-Niacin, Niaspan*) Niacin deficiency: 10 to 500 mg PO daily. Hyperlipidemia: Start 50 to 100 mg PO bid to tid with meals, increase slowly, usual maintenance range 1.5 to 3 g/day, max 6 g/day. Extended-release (Niaspan): Start 500 mg at bedtime, increase monthly pm up to max 2000 mg. Extended-release formulations not listed here may have greater hepatotoxicity. Titrate slowly and use aspirin or NSAID 30 min before niacin doses to decrease flushing reaction. [OTC Generic only: Tabs 50, 100, 250, 500 mg; Timed-release cap 125, 250, 400 mg; Timed-release tab 250, 500 mg; Liquid 50 mg/5 mL. Rx only: Timed-release: 250, 500, 750 mg (Slo-Niacin). Rx: Trade only: Tabs 500 mg (Niacor), Timed-release caps 500 mg, Timed-release tabs 500, 750, 1000 mg (Niaspan, $$$$).] ▶K ♀C ▶? $

PARICALCITOL (*Zemplar*) Prevention/treatment of secondary hyperparathyroidism with renal insufficiency: 1 to 2 mcg PO daily or 2 to 4 mcg PO 3 times

(cont.)

a week; increase dose by 1 mcg/day or 2 mcg/week until desired PTH level is achieved. Prevention/treatment of <u>secondary hyperparathyroidism with renal failure</u> (CrCl <15 mL/min): PO: To calculate initial dose divide baseline iPTH by 80 and then administer this dose in mcg 3 times a week. To titrate dose based on response, divide recent iPTH by 80 then administer this dose in mcg 3 times a week. IV: 0.04 to 0.1 mcg/kg (2.8 to 7 mcg) IV 3 times a week at dialysis; increase dose by 2 to 4 mcg q 2 to 4 weeks until desired PTH level is achieved. Max dose 0.24 mcg/kg (16.8 mcg). [Trade only: Caps 1, 2, 4 mcg.] ▶L ♀C ▶? $$$$$

PHYTONADIONE (*vitamin K, Mephyton, AquaMephyton*) Single dose of 0.5 to 1 mg IM within 1 h after birth. <u>Excessive oral anticoagulation:</u> Dose varies based on INR. INR 5 to 9: 1 to 2.5 mg PO (up to 5 mg PO may be given if rapid reversal necessary); INR >9 with no bleeding: 5 to 10 mg PO; Serious bleeding and elevated INR: 10 mg slow IV infusion. <u>Adequate daily intake:</u> 120 mcg (males) and 90 mcg (females). [Trade only: Tabs 5 mg.] ▶L ♀C ▶+ $

PYRIDOXINE (*vitamin B6*) 10 to 200 mg PO daily. <u>Prevention of deficiency due to isoniazid in high-risk patients:</u> 10 to 25 mg PO daily. Treatment of neuropathies due to INH: 50 to 200 mg PO daily. [OTC Generic only: Tabs 25, 50, 100 mg; Timed-release tab 100 mg.] ▶K ♀A ▶+ $

RIBOFLAVIN (*vitamin B2*) 5 to 25 mg PO daily. [OTC Generic only: Tabs 25, 50, 100 mg.] ▶K ♀A ▶+ $

THIAMINE (*vitamin B1*) 10 to 100 mg IV/IM/PO daily. [OTC Generic only: Tabs 50, 100, 250, 500 mg; Enteric-coated tab 20 mg.] ▶K ♀A ▶+ $

TOCOPHEROL (*vitamin E, ✦Aquasol E*) RDA is 22 units (natural, d-alpha-tocopherol) or 33 units (synthetic, d,l-alpha-tocopherol) or 15 mg (alpha-tocopherol). Max recommended 1000 mg alpha-tocopherol (1500 units) daily. <u>Antioxidant:</u> 400 to 800 units PO daily. [OTC Generic only: Tabs 200, 400 units; Caps 73.5, 100, 147, 165, 200, 330, 400, 500, 600, 1000 units; Gtts 50 mg/mL.] ▶L ♀A ▶? $

VITAMIN A RDA: 900 mcg RE (retinol equivalents) (males), 700 mcg RE (females). <u>Treatment of deficiency states:</u> 100,000 units IM daily for 3 days, then 50,000 units IM daily for 2 weeks. 1 RE is equivalent to 1 mcg retinol or 6 mcg beta-carotene. Max recommended daily dose 3000 mcg. [OTC Generic only: Caps 10,000, 15,000 units. Trade only: Tabs 5000 units. Rx: Generic: 25,000 units. Trade only: Soln 50,000 units/mL.] ▶L ♀A (C if exceed RDA, X in high doses) ▶+ $

VITAMIN D3 (*cholecalciferol, DDrops*) <u>Osteoporosis prevention and treatment</u> (age 50 or older): 800 to 1000 units daily. <u>Familial hypophosphatemia</u> (Vitamin D Resistant Rickets): 12,000 to 500,000 units PO daily. <u>Hypoparathyroidism:</u> 50,000 to 200,000 units PO daily. Adequate daily intake adults: 19 to 50 yo: 200 units; 51 to 70 yo: 400 units; older than 70 yo: 600 units. [OTC Generic: Caps/Tabs 200 units, 400 units, 800 units, 1000 units, 2000 units, 5000 units. Caps: 10,000 units, 50,000 units. Trade only: Soln 400 units/drop, 1000 units/drop, 2000 units/drop.] ▶L ▶+ $

Other

BROMOCRIPTINE (*Cycloset, Parlodel*) Type 2 DM: 0.8 mg PO qam (within 2 h of waking), may increase weekly by 0.8 mg to max tolerated dose of 1.6 to 4.8 mg. Hyperprolactinemia: Start 1.25 to 2.5 mg PO at bedtime, then increase every 3 to 7 days to usual effective dose of 2.5 to 15 mg/day, max 40 mg/day. Acromegaly: Usual effective dose is 20 to 30 mg/day, max 100 mg/day. Doses greater than 20 mg/day can be divided bid. Also approved for Parkinson's disease, but rarely used. Take with food to minimize dizziness and nausea. [Generic/Trade: Tabs 2.5 mg. Caps 5 mg.] ▶L ♀B ▶– $$$$$

CABERGOLINE (*Dostinex*) Hyperprolactinemia: 0.25 to 1 mg PO twice a week. [Generic/Trade: Tabs 0.5 mg.] ▶L ♀B ▶– $$$$$

CALCITONIN (*Miacalcin, Fortical, ✦Calcimar, Caltine*) Skin test before using injectable calcitonin: 1 unit intradermally and observe for local reaction. Osteoporosis: 100 units SC/IM every other day or 200 units (1 spray) intranasal daily (alternate nostrils). Paget's disease: 50 to 100 units SC/IM daily. Hypercalcemia: 4 units/kg SC/IM q 12 h. May increase after 2 days to max of 8 units/kg q 6 h. [Generic/Trade: Nasal spray 200 units/activation in 3.7 mL bottle (minimum of 30 doses/bottle).] ▶Plasma ♀C ▶? $$$$

DENOSUMAB (*Prolia*) Postmenopausal osteoporosis: 60 mg SC q6 months. [Trade only: 60 mg/1 mL vial, prefilled syringe.] ▶? ♀C ▶? $$$$$

DESMOPRESSIN (*DDAVP, Stimate, ✦Minirin, Octostim*) Diabetes insipidus: 10 to 40 mcg intranasally daily or divided bid to tid, 0.05 to 1.2 mg/day PO or divided bid to tid, or 0.5 to 1 mL/day SC/IV in 2 divided doses. Hemophilia A, von Willebrand's disease: 0.3 mcg/kg IV over 15 to 30 min, or 150 to 300 mcg intranasally. Enuresis: 0.2 to 0.6 mg PO at bedtime. Not for children younger than 6 yo. [Trade only: Stimate nasal spray 150 mcg/0.1 mL (1 spray), 2.5 mL bottle (25 sprays). Generic/Trade (DDAVP nasal spray): 10 mcg/0.1 mL (1 spray), 5 mL bottle (50 sprays). Note difference in concentration of nasal soln. Rhinal Tube: 2.5 mL bottle with 2 flexible plastic tube applicators with graduation marks for dosing. Generic only: Tabs 0.1, 0.2 mg.] ▶LK ♀B ▶? $$$$

SODIUM POLYSTYRENE SULFONATE (*Kayexalate*) Hyperkalemia: 15 g PO daily to qid or 30 to 50 g retention enema (as opposed to diarrhea) q 6 h prn. Retain for 30 min to several hours. Irrigate with tap water after enema to prevent necrosis. [Generic only: Susp 15 g/60 mL. Powdered resin.] ▶Fecal excretion ♀C ▶? $$$$

SOMATROPIN (*human growth hormone, Genotropin, Humatrope, Norditropin, Norditropin NordiFlex, Nutropin, Nutropin AQ, Nutropin Depot, Omnitrope, Protropin, Serostim, Serostim LQ, Saizen, Tev-Tropin, Valtropin, Zorbtive*) Dosages vary by indication and product. [Single-dose vials (powder for injection with diluent). Tev-Tropin: 5 mg vial (powder for injection with diluent, stable for 14 days when refrigerated). Genotropin: 1.5, 5.8, 13.8 mg cartridges. Humatrope: 6, 12, 24 mg cartridges; 5 mg vial (powder for injection with diluent, stable for 14 days when refrigerated). Nutropin AQ: 10 mg multidose vial, 5, 10, 20 mg/pen cartridges. Norditropin: 5, 10, 15 mg pen cartridges. Norditropin NordiFlex: 5, 10, 15 mg prefilled pens. Omnitrope: 1.5, 5.8 mg

(cont.)

vial (powder for injection with diluent). Saizen: **Preassembled reconstitution device** with autoinjector pen. Serostim: 4, 5, 6 mg single-dose vials; 4, 8.8 mg multidose vials; and 8.8 mg cartridges for autoinjector. Valtropin: 5 mg single-dose vials, 5 mg prefilled syringe. Zorbtive: 8.8 mg vial (powder for injection with diluent, stable for 14 days when refrigerated).] ▶LK ♀B/C ▶? $$$$$

TERIPARATIDE (Forteo) Treatment of <u>postmenopausal osteoporosis</u>, treatment of men and women with <u>glucocorticoid-induced osteoporosis</u> or to <u>increase bone mass in men with primary or hypogonadal osteoporosis and high risk for fracture:</u> 20 mcg SC daily in thigh or abdomen for no longer than 2 years. [Trade only: 28 dose pen injector (20 mcg/dose).] ▶LK ♀C ▶? $$$$$

VASOPRESSIN (Pitressin, ADH, ✦Pressyn AR) <u>Diabetes insipidus:</u> 5 to 10 units IM/SC bid to qid prn. <u>Cardiac arrest:</u> 40 units IV; may repeat if no response after 3 min. <u>Septic shock:</u> 0.01 to 0.1 units/min IV infusion, usual dose less than 0.04 units/min. <u>Variceal bleeding:</u> 0.2 to 0.4 units/min initially (max 0.8 units/min). ▶LK ♀C ▶? $$$$$

ENT

Antihistamines—Non-Sedating

DESLORATADINE (Clarinex, ✦Aerius) 5 mg PO daily for age older than 12 yo. Peds: 2 mL (1 mg) PO daily for age 6 to 11 mo, ½ teaspoonful (1.25 mg) PO daily for age 12 mo to 5 yo, 1 teaspoonful (2.5 mg) PO daily for age 6 to 11 yo. [Trade only: Tabs 5 mg. Fast-dissolve RediTabs 2.5, 5 mg. Syrup 0.5 mg/mL.] ▶LK ♀C ▶+ $$$

FEXOFENADINE (Allegra) 60 mg PO bid or 180 mg daily. Peds: 30 mg PO bid for age 2 to 11 yo. [Generic/Trade: Tabs 30, 60, 180 mg, Caps 60 mg. Trade only: Susp 30 mg/5 mL, orally disintegrating tab 30 mg.] ▶LK ♀C ▶+ $$$

LORATADINE (Claritin, Claritin Hives Relief, Claritin RediTabs, Alavert, Tavist ND) 10 mg PO daily for age older than 6 yo, 5 mg PO daily for age 2 to 5 yo. [OTC Generic/Trade: Tabs 10 mg. Fast-dissolve tabs (Alavert, Claritin RediTabs) 5, 10 mg. Syrup 1 mg/mL. Rx Trade only (Claritin): Chewable tabs 5 mg, Liqui-gel caps 10 mg.] ▶LK ♀B ▶+ $

Antihistamines—Other

CETIRIZINE (Zyrtec, ✦Reactine, Aller-Relief) 5 to 10 mg PO daily for age older than 6 yo. Peds: give 2.5 mg PO daily for age 6 to 23 mo, give 2.5 mg PO daily to bid for age 2 to 5 yo. [OTC Generic/Trade: Tabs 5, 10 mg. Syrup 5 mg/5 mL. Chewable tabs, grape-flavored 5, 10 mg.] ▶LK ♀B ▶– $$$

CHLORPHENIRAMINE (Chlor-Trimeton, Aller-Chlor) 4 mg PO q 4 to 6 h. Max 24 mg/day. Peds: give 2 mg PO q'4 to 6 h for age 6 to 11 yo. Max 12 mg/day. [OTC Trade only: Tabs extended-release 12 mg. Generic/Trade: Tabs 4 mg. Syrup 2 mg/5 mL. Tabs extended-release 8 mg.] ▶LK ♀B ▶– $

CLEMASTINE (Tavist-1) 1.34 mg PO bid. Max 8.04 mg/day. [OTC Generic/Trade: Tabs 1.34 mg. Rx: Generic/Trade: Tabs 2.68 mg, Syrup 0.67 mg/5 mL. Rx: Generic only: Syrup 0.5 mg/5 mL.] ▶LK ♀B ▶– $

CYPROHEPTADINE (*Periactin*) Start 4 mg PO tid. Max 32 mg/day. [Generic only: Tabs 4 mg. Syrup 2 mg/5 mL.] ▶LK ♀B ▶– $

DEXCHLORPHENIRAMINE (*Polaramine*) 2 mg PO q 4 to 6 h. Timed-release tabs: 4 or 6 mg PO at bedtime or q 8 to 10 h. [Generic only: Tabs immediate-release 2 mg, timed-release 4, 6 mg. Syrup 2 mg/5 mL.] ▶LK ♀? ▶– $$

DIPHENHYDRAMINE (*Benadryl, Banophen, Allermax, Diphen, Diphenhist, Dytan, Siladryl, Sominex, ✦Allerdryl, Nytol*) <u>Allergic rhinitis, urticaria, hypersensivity reactions:</u> 25 to 50 mg IV/IM/PO q 4 to 6 h. Peds: 5 mg/kg/day divided q 4 to 6 h. <u>EPS:</u> 25 to 50 mg PO tid to qid or 10 to 50 mg IV/IM tid to qid. <u>Insomnia:</u> 25 to 50 mg PO at bedtime. [OTC Trade only: Tabs 25, 50 mg, Chewable tabs 12.5 mg. OTC and Rx: Generic only: Caps 25, 50 mg, softgel cap 25 mg. OTC Generic/Trade: Soln 6.25 or 12.5 mg per 5 mL. Rx: Trade only: (Dytan) Susp 25 mg/mL, Chewable tabs 25 mg.] ▶LK ♀B ▶– $

HYDROXYZINE (*Atarax, Vistaril*) 25 to 100 mg IM/PO daily to qid or prn. [Generic only: Tabs 10, 25, 50, 100 mg; Caps 100 mg; Syrup 10 mg/5 mL. Generic/Trade: Caps 25, 50 mg, Susp 25 mg/5 mL (Vistaril). (Caps = Vistaril, Tabs = Atarax).] ▶L ♀C ▶– $$

LEVOCETIRIZINE (*Xyzal*) 5 mg PO daily for age 12 yo or older. Peds: give 2.5 mg PO daily for age 6 to 11 yo. [Trade only: Tabs scored 5 mg; Oral soln 2.5 mg/5 mL (148 mL).] ▶K ♀B ▶– $$$

MECLIZINE (*Antivert, Bonine, Medivert, Meclicot, Meni-D, ✦Bonamine*) <u>Motion sickness:</u> 25 to 50 mg PO 1 h prior to travel, then 25 to 50 mg PO daily. <u>Vertigo:</u> 25 mg PO q 6 h prn. [Rx/OTC/Generic/Trade: Tabs 12.5, 25 mg; Chewable tabs 25 mg. Rx/Trade only: Tabs 50 mg.] ▶L ♀B ▶? $

Antitussives/Expectorants

BENZONATATE (*Tessalon, Tessalon Perles*) 100 to 200 mg PO tid. Swallow whole. Do not chew. Numbs mouth; possible choking hazard. [Generic/Trade: Softgel caps: 100, 200 mg.] ▶L ♀C ▶? $$

DEXTROMETHORPHAN (*Benylin, Delsym, DexAlone, Robitussin Cough, Vick's 44 Cough*) 10 to 20 mg PO q 4 h or 30 mg PO q 6 to 8 h. Sustained action liquid 60 mg PO q 12 h. [OTC Trade only: Caps 15 mg (Robitussin), 30 mg (DexAlone), Susp, extended-release 30 mg/5 mL (Delsym). Generic/Trade: Syrup 5, 7.5, 10, 15 mg/5 mL. Generic only: Lozenges 5, 10 mg.] ▶L ♀+ ▶+ $

GUAIFENESIN (*Robitussin, Hytuss, Guiatuss, Mucinex*) 100 to 400 mg PO q 4 h. 600 to 1200 mg PO q 12 h (extended-release). Peds: 50 to 100 mg/dose for age 2 to 5 yo, give 100 to 200 mg/dose for age 6 to 11 yo. [Rx Generic/Trade: Extended-release tabs 600, 1200 mg. OTC Generic/Trade: Liquid, Syrup 100 mg/5 mL. OTC Trade only: Caps 200 mg (Hytuss), Extended-release tabs 600 mg (Mucinex). OTC Generic only: Tabs 100, 200, 400 mg.] ▶L ♀C ▶+ $

Decongestants

NOTE *See ENT—Nasal Preparations for nasal spray decongestants (oxymetazoline, phenylephrine). Deaths have occurred in children younger than 2 yo attributed to toxicity from cough and cold medications; the FDA does not recommend their use in this age group.*

ENT COMBINATIONS (selected)	Decon-gestant	Antihis-tamine	Anti-tussive	Typical Adult Doses
OTC				
Actifed Cold & Allergy	PE	CH	-	1 tab q 4–6 h
Actifed Cold & Sinus‡	PS	CH	-	2 tabs q 6 h
Allerfrim, Aprodine	PS	TR	-	1 tab or 10 mL q 4–6 h
Benadryl Allergy/Cold‡	PE	DPH	-	2 tabs q 4 h
Benadryl-D Allergy/Sinus Tablets	PE	DPH	-	1 tab q 4 h
Claritin-D 12-h, Alavert D-12	PS	LO	-	1 tab q 12 h
Claritin-D 24-h	PS	LO	-	1 tab daily
Dimetapp Cold & Allergy Elixir	PE	BR	-	20 mL q 4 h
Dimetapp DM Cold & Cough	PE	BR	DM	20 mL q 4 h
Drixoral Cold & Allergy	PS	DBR	-	1 tab q 12 h
Mucinex-DM Extended-Release	-	-	GU,DM	1-2 tab q 12 h
Robitussin CF	PE	-	GU, DM	10 mL q 4 h*
Robitussin DM, Mytussin DM	-	-	GU, DM	10 mL q 4 h*
Robitussin PE, Guiatuss PE	PE	-	GU	10 mL q 4 h*
Triaminic Cold & Allergy	PE	CH	-	10 mL q 4 h
Rx Only				
Allegra-D 12-h	PS	FE	-	1 tab q 12 h
Allegra-D 24-h	PS	FE	-	1 tab daily
Bromfenex	PS	BR	-	1 cap q 12 h
Clarinex-D 24-h	PS	DL	-	1 tab daily
Deconamine	PS	CH	-	1 tab or 10 mL tid-qid
Deconamine SR, Chlordrine SR	PS	CH	-	1 tab q 12 h
Deconsal I	PE	-	GU	1-2 tabs q 12 h
Dimetane-DX	PS	BR	DM	10 mL PO q 4 h
Duratuss	PE	-	GU	1 tab q 12 h
Duratuss HD©III	PE	-	GU, HY	5-10 mL q 4–6 h
Entex PSE, Guaifenex PSE 120	PS	-	GU	1 tab q 12 h
Histussin D ©III	PS	-	HY	5 mL qid
Histussin HC ©III	PE	CH	HY	10 mL q 4 h
Humibid DM	-	-	GU, DM	1 tab q 12 h
Hycotuss ©III	-	-	GU, HY	5 mL pc & qhs
Phenergan/Dextromethorphan	-	PR	DM	5 mL q 4–6 h
Phenergan VC	PE	PR	-	5 mL q 4–6 h
Phenergan VC w/codeine©V	PE	PR	CO	5 mL q 4–6 h
Robitussin AC ©V (generic only)	-	-	GU, CO	10 mL q 4 h*
Robitussin DAC ©V (generic only)	PS	-	GU, CO	10 mL q 4 h*
Rondec Syrup	PE	CH	-	5 mL qid†
Rondec DM Syrup	PE	CH	DM	5 mL qid†
Rondec Oral Drops	PE	CH	-	0.75 to 1 mL qid
Rondec DM Oral Drops	PE	CH	DM	0.75 to 1 mL qid
Rynatan	PE	CH	-	1-2 tabs q 12 h
Rynatan-P Pediatric	PE	CH	-	2.5–5 mL q 12 h*
Semprex-D	PS	AC	-	1cap q 4–6 h
Tanafed (generic only)	PS	CH	-	10–20 mL q 12 h*
Tussionex ©III	-	CH	HY	5 mL q 12 h

AC=acrivastine	DL= desloratadine	FE=fexofenadine	PE=phenylephrine
BR=brompheniramine	DM=dextromethorphan	GU=guaifenesin	PR=promethazine
CH=chlorpheniramine	DBR=dexbrompheniramine	HY=hydrocodone	PS=pseudoephedrine
CO=codeine	DPH=diphenhydramine	LO=loratadine	TR=triprolidine

*5 mL/dose if 6–11 yo. 2.5 mL if 2–5 yo. †2.5 mL/dose if 6–11 yo. 1.25 mL if 2–5 yo. ‡Also contains acetaminophen.

PHENYLEPHRINE (*Sudafed PE*) 10 mg PO q 4 h. [OTC Trade only: Tabs 10 mg.] ▶L ♀C ▶+ $

PSEUDOEPHEDRINE (*Sudafed, Sudafed 12 Hour, Efidac/24, Dimetapp Decongestant Infant Drops, PediaCare Infants' Decongestant Drops, Triaminic Oral Infant Drops, ✦Pseudofrin*) Adult: 60 mg PO q 4 to 6 h. Extended release tabs: 120 mg PO bid or 240 mg PO daily. Peds: give 15 mg PO q 4 to 6 h for age 2 to 5 yo, give 30 mg PO q 4 to 6 h for age 6 to 12 yo. [OTC Generic/Trade: Tabs 30, 60 mg, Tabs extended-release 120 mg (12 h), Soln 15, 30 mg/5 mL. Trade only: Chewable tabs 15 mg, Tabs extended-release 240 mg (24 h).] ▶L ♀C ▶+ $

Ear Preparations

AURALGAN (benzocaine + antipyrine) 2 to 4 gtts in ear(s) tid to qid prn. [Generic/Trade: Otic soln 10, 15 mL.] ▶Not absorbed ♀C ▶? $

CARBAMIDE PEROXIDE (*Debrox, Murine Ear*) 5 to 10 gtts in ear(s) bid for 4 days. [OTC Generic/Trade: Otic soln 6.5%, 15, 30 mL.] ▶Not absorbed ♀? ▶? $

CIPRO HC OTIC (ciprofloxacin + hydrocortisone) 3 gtts in ear(s) bid for 7 days for age 1 yo to adult. [Trade only: Otic susp 10 mL.] ▶Not absorbed ♀C ▶– $$$$

CIPRODEX OTIC (ciprofloxacin + dexamethasone) 4 gtts in ear(s) bid for 7 days for age 6 mo to adult. [Trade only: Otic susp 5, 7.5 mL.] ▶Not absorbed ♀C ▶– $$$$

CIPROFLOXACIN (*Cetraxal*) 1 single-use container in ear(s) bid for 7 days for age 1 yo to adult. [Trade only: 0.25 mL single-use containers with 0.2% ciprofloxacin soln, #14.] ▶Not absorbed ♀C ▶– $$$$

CORTISPORIN OTIC (hydrocortisone + polymyxin + neomycin, Pediotic) 4 gtts in ear(s) tid to qid up to 10 days of soln or susp. Peds: 3 gtts in ear(s) tid to qid up to 10 days. Caution with perforated TMs or tympanostomy tubes as this increases the risk of neomycin ototoxicity, especially if use prolonged or repeated. Use susp rather than acidic soln. [Generic only: Otic soln or susp 7.5, 10 mL.] ▶Not absorbed ♀? ▶? $

CORTISPORIN TC OTIC (hydrocortisone + neomycin + thonzonium + colistin) 4 to 5 gtts in ear(s) tid to qid up to 10 days. [Trade only: Otic susp, 10 mL.] ▶Not absorbed ♀? ▶? $$$

DOMEBORO OTIC (acetic acid + aluminum acetate) 4 to 6 gtts in ear(s) q 2 to 3 h. Peds: 2 to 3 gtts in ear(s) q 3 to 4 h. [Generic only: Otic soln 60 mL.] ▶Not absorbed ♀? ▶? $

FLUOCINOLONE—OTIC (*DermOtic*) 5 gtts in affected ear(s) bid for 7 to 14 days for age 2 yo to adult. [Trade only: Otic oil 0.01% 20 mL.] ▶L ♀C ▶? $$

OFLOXACIN – OTIC (*Floxin Otic*) Otitis externa: 5 gtts in ear(s) daily for age 1 to 12 yo, 10 gtts in ear(s) daily for age 12 yo or older. [Generic/Trade: Otic soln 0.3% 5, 10 mL. Trade only: "Singles": Single-dispensing containers 0.25 mL (5 gtts), 2 per foil pouch.] ▶Not absorbed ♀C ▶– $$$

SWIM-EAR (isopropyl alcohol + anhydrous glycerins) 4 to 5 gtts in ears after swimming. [OTC Trade only: Otic soln 30 mL.] ▶Not absorbed ♀? ▶? $

VOSOL HC (acetic acid + propylene glycol + hydrocortisone) 5 gtts in ear(s) tid to qid. Peds age older than 3 yo: 3 to 4 gtts in ear(s) tid to qid. [Generic/Trade: Otic soln 2%/3%/1% 10 mL.] ▶Not absorbed ♀? ▶? $

Mouth & Lip Preparations

AMLEXANOX (*Aphthasol, OraDisc A*) <u>Aphthous ulcers:</u> Apply ¼ inch paste or mucoadhesive patch to affected area qid after oral hygiene for up to 10 days. Up to 3 patches may be applied at one time. [Trade only: Oral paste 5% (Aphthasol), 3, 5 g tube. Mucoadhesive patch (OraDisc) 2 mg, #20.] ▶LK ♀B ▶? $

CEVIMELINE (*Evoxac*) <u>Dry mouth due to Sjogren's syndrome:</u> 30 mg PO tid. [Trade only: Caps 30 mg.] ▶L ♀C ▶– $$$$$

CHLORHEXIDINE GLUCONATE (*Peridex, Periogard, ◆Denticare*) Rinse with 15 mL of undiluted soln for 30 sec bid. Do not swallow. Spit after rinsing. [Generic/Trade: Oral rinse 0.12% 473 to 480 mL bottles.] ▶Fecal excretion ♀B ▶? $

DEBACTEROL (sulfuric acid + sulfonated phenolics) <u>Aphthous stomatitis, mucositis:</u> Apply to dry ulcer. Rinse with water. [Trade only: 1 mL prefilled, single-use applicator.] ▶Not absorbed ♀C ▶+ $$

GELCLAIR (maltodextrin + propylene glycol) <u>Aphthous ulcers, mucositis, stomatitis:</u> Rinse mouth with 1 packet tid or prn. Do not eat or drink for 1 h after treatment. [Trade only: 15 packets/box.] ▶Not absorbed ♀+ ▶+ $$$

LIDOCAINE—VISCOUS (*Xylocaine*) <u>Mouth or lip pain in adults only:</u> 15 to 20 mL topically or swish and spit q 3 h. [Generic/Trade: Soln 2%, 20 mL unit dose, 100 mL bottle.] ▶LK ♀B ▶+ $

MAGIC MOUTHWASH (diphenhydramine + Mylanta + sucralfate) 5 mL PO swish and spit or swish and swallow tid before meals and prn. [Compounded susp. A standard mixture is 30 mL diphenhydramine liquid (12.5 mg/5 mL)/60 mL Mylanta or Maalox/4 g Carafate.] ▶LK ♀B(– in first trimester) ▶– $$$

PILOCARPINE (*Salagen*) <u>Dry mouth due to radiation of head and neck or Sjogren's syndrome:</u> 5 mg PO tid to qid. [Generic/Trade: Tabs 5, 7.5 mg.] ▶L ♀C ▶– $$$$

Nasal Preparations—Corticosteroids

BECLOMETHASONE (*Vancenase, Vancenase AQ Double Strength, Beconase AQ*) Vancenase: 1 spray per nostril tid to qid. Beconase AQ: 1 to 2 spray(s) per nostril bid. Vancenase AQ Double Strength: 1 to 2 spray(s) per nostril daily. [Trade only: Vancenase 42 mcg/spray, 80 or 200 sprays/bottle. Beconase AQ 42 mcg/spray, 200 sprays/bottle. Vancenase AQ Double Strength 84 mcg/spray, 120 sprays/bottle.] ▶L ♀C ▶? $$$$

BUDESONIDE—NASAL (*Rhinocort Aqua*) 1 to 4 sprays per nostril daily. [Trade only: Nasal inhaler 120 sprays/bottle.] ▶L ♀B ▶? $$$$

CICLESONIDE (*Omnaris*) 2 sprays per nostril daily. [Trade only: Nasal spray, 50 mcg/spray, 120 sprays/bottle.] ▶L ♀C ▶? $$$

FLUNISOLIDE (*Nasalide, Nasarel, ◆Rhinalar*) Start 2 sprays per nostril bid. Max 8 sprays/nostril/day. [Generic/Trade: Nasal soln 0.025%, 200 sprays/bottle. Nasalide with pump unit. Nasarel with meter pump and nasal adapter.] ▶L ♀C ▷? $$$

FLUTICASONE—NASAL (*Flonase, Veramyst*) 2 sprays per nostril daily. [Generic/Trade: Flonase: Nasal spray 0.05%, 120 sprays/bottle. Trade only: (Veramyst): Nasal spray susp: 27.5 mcg/spray, 120 sprays/bottle.] ▶L ♀C ▷? $$$

MOMETASONE—NASAL (*Nasonex*) Adult: 2 sprays/nostril daily. Peds 2 to 11 yo: 1 spray/nostril daily. [Trade only: Nasal spray, 120 sprays/bottle.] ▶L ♀C ▷? $$$$

TRIAMCINOLONE—NASAL (*Nasacort AQ, Nasacort HFA, Tri-Nasal, AllerNaze*) Nasacort HFA, Tri-Nasal, AllerNaze: 2 sprays per nostril daily to bid. Max 4 sprays/nostril/day. Nasacort AQ: 1 to 2 sprays per nostril daily. [Trade only: Nasal inhaler 55 mcg/spray, 100 sprays/bottle (Nasacort HFA). Nasal spray, 55 mcg/spray, 120 sprays/bottle (Nasacort AQ). Nasal spray 50 mcg/spray, 120 sprays/bottle (Tri-Nasal, AllerNaze).] ▶L ♀C ▷– $$$$

Nasal Preparations—Other

AZELASTINE—NASAL (*Astelin, Astepro*) 1 to 2 sprays per nostril bid. [Generic: Nasal spray, 200 sprays/bottle.] ▶L ♀C ▷? $$$$

CROMOLYN—NASAL (*NasalCrom*) 1 spray per nostril tid to qid. [OTC Generic/Trade: Nasal inhaler (100 sprays/13 mL), 13 and 26 mL bottle.] ▶LK ♀B ▷+ $

IPRATROPIUM—NASAL (*Atrovent Nasal Spray*) 2 sprays per nostril bid to qid. [Generic/Trade: Nasal spray 0.03%, 345 sprays/bottle, 0.06%, 165 sprays/bottle.] ▶L ♀B ▷? $$

LEVOCABASTINE—NASAL (*◆Livostin Nasal Spray*) Canada only. 2 sprays per nostril bid, increase prn to tid to qid. [Trade only: Nasal spray 0.5 mg/mL, plastic bottles of 15 mL. 50 mcg/spray.] ▶L (but minimal absorption) ♀C ▷– $$

OLOPATADINE—NASAL (*Patanase*) 2 sprays per nostril bid. [Trade only: Nasal spray, 240 sprays/bottle.] ▶L ♀C ▷? $$$

OXYMETAZOLINE (*Afrin, Dristan 12 Hr Nasal, Nostrilla, Vicks Sinex 12 Hr*) 2 to 3 gtts/sprays per nostril bid prn nasal congestion for no more than 3 days. [OTC Generic/Trade: Nasal spray 0.05% 15, 30 mL; Nose gtts 0.025%, 0.05% 20 mL with dropper.] ▶L ♀C ▷? $

PHENYLEPHRINE—NASAL (*Neo-Synephrine, Vicks Sinex*) 2 to 3 sprays or gtts per nostril q 4 h prn × 3 days. [OTC Generic/Trade: Nasal gtts/spray 0.25, 0.5, 1% (15 mL).] ▶L ♀C ▷? $

SALINE NASAL SPRAY (*SeaMist, Entsol, Pretz, NaSal, Ocean, ◆HydraSense*) Nasal dryness: 1 to 3 sprays or gtts per nostril prn. [Generic/Trade: Nasal spray 0.4, 0.5, 0.65, 0.75%, Nasal gtts 0.4, 0.65%. Trade only: Preservative-free nasal spray 3% (Entsol).] ▶Not metabolized ♀A ▷+ $

Other

CETACAINE (benzocaine + tetracaine + butamben) Topical anesthesia of mucous membranes: Spray: Apply for no more than 1 sec. Liquid or gel: Apply with cotton applicator directly to site. [Trade only: (14%/2%/2%) Spray 56 mL. Topical liquid 56 mL. Topical gel 5, 29 g.] ▶LK ♀C ▷? $$

GASTROENTEROLOGY

Antidiarrheals

BISMUTH SUBSALICYLATE (*Pepto-Bismol, Kaopectate*) 2 tabs or caplets or 30 mL (262 mg/15 mL) PO q 30 min to 1 h up to 8 doses per day for up to 2 days. Peds: 5 mL (262 mg/15 mL) or 1/3 tab or caplet PO for age 3 to 6 yo, 10 mL (262 mg/15 mL) or 2/3 tab or caplet PO for age 6 to 9 yo. Risk of Reye's syndrome in children. [OTC Generic/Trade: Chewable tabs 262 mg. Susp 262, 525, 750 mg/15 mL. OTC Trade only: Caplets 262 mg (Pepto-Bismol). Susp 87 mg/5 mL (Kaopectate Children's Liquid).] ▶K ♀D ▶? $

***IMODIUM MULTI-SYMPTOM RELIEF* (loperamide + simethicone)** 2 tabs or caplets PO initially, then 1 tab or caplet PO after each unformed stool to a max of 4 tabs/caplets per day. Peds: 1 tab or caplet PO initially, then ½ caplet PO after each unformed stool (up to 2 tabs or caplets PO per day for age 6 to 8 yo or wt 48 to 59 lbs or up to 3 tabs or caplets PO per day for age 9 to 11 yo or wt 60 to 95 lbs). [OTC Generic/Trade: Caplets, Chewable tabs 2 mg loperamide/125 mg simethicone.] ▶L ♀C ▶– $

***LOMOTIL* (diphenoxylate + atropine)** 2 tabs or 10 mL PO qid. [Generic/Trade: Oral soln or tab 2.5 mg/ 0.025 mg diphenoxylate/atropine per 5 mL or tab.] ▶L ♀C ▶–

***LOPERAMIDE* (*Imodium, Imodium AD, ◆Loperacap, Diarr-eze*)** 4 mg PO initially, then 2 mg PO after each unformed stool to a maximum of 16 mg per day. Peds: 1 mg PO tid for wt 13 to 20 kg, 2 mg PO bid for wt 21 to 30 kg, 2 mg PO tid for wt greater than 30 kg. [OTC Generic/Trade: Tabs 2 mg. Oral soln 1 mg/5 mL. OTC Trade only: Oral soln 1 mg/7.5 mL.] ▶L ♀C ▶+ $

***MOTOFEN* (difenoxin + atropine)** 2 tabs PO initially, then 1 tab after each loose stool q 3 to 4 h prn (up to 8 tabs per day). [Trade only: Tabs difenoxin 1 mg + atropine 0.025 mg.] ▶L ♀C ▶– ©IV $$

***OPIUM* (*opium tincture, paregoric*)** 5 to 10 mL paregoric PO daily (up to qid) or 0.6 mL (range 0.3 to 1 mL) opium tincture PO every 2 to 6 hours, prn, to a max of 6 mL per day. [Trade only: Opium tincture 10% (deodorized opium tincture, 10 mg morphine equivalent/mL). Generic only: Paregoric (camphorated opium tincture, 2 mg morphine equivalent/5 mL).] ▶L ♀B (D with long-term use) ▶? ©II (opium tincture), III (paregoric) $$

Antiemetics—5-HT3 Receptor Antagonists

DOLASETRON (*Anzemet*) <u>Nausea with chemo:</u> 1.8 mg/kg (up to 100 mg) IV/PO single dose. <u>Post-op nausea:</u> 12.5 mg IV in adults and 0.35 mg/kg in children as single dose. Alternative for prevention: 100 mg (adults) PO or 1.2 mg/kg (children) PO 2 h before surgery. [Trade only: Tabs 50, 100 mg.] ▶LK ♀B ▶? $$$

GRANISETRON (*Kytril, Sancuso*) <u>Nausea with chemo:</u> 10 mcg/kg IV over 5 min, 30 min prior to chemo. Oral: 1 mg PO bid or 2 mg PO qd for 1 day only. <u>Radiation-induced nausea and vomiting:</u> 2 mg PO 1 h before first irradiation fraction of

(cont.)

each day. Transdermal (Sancuso): 1 patch to upper outer arm at least 24 h (but up to 48 h) before chemotherapy. Remove 24 h after completion of chemotherapy. Can be worn up to 7 days depending on the duration of chemo. [Generic/Trade: Tabs 1 mg. Oral soln 2 mg/10 mL (30 mL). Trade only (Sancuso): Transdermal patch 34.3 mg of granisetron delivering 3.1 mg/24 h.] ▶L ♀B ▶? $$$$

ONDANSETRON (*Zofran*) Nausea with chemo: IV: 32 mg IV over 15 min, or 0.15 mg/kg dose 30 min prior to chemo and repeated at 4 and 8 h after first dose for age 6 mo or older. PO: 4 mg PO 30 min prior to chemo and repeat at 4 and 8 hrs for age 4 to 11 yo, 8 mg PO and repeated 8 h later for age 12 yo or older. Prevention of post-op nausea: 4 mg IV over 2 to 5 min or 4 mg IM or 16 mg PO 1 h before anesthesia. Give 0.1 mg/kg IV over 2 to 5 min as a single dose for age 1 mo to 12 yo if wt 40 kg or less; 4 mg IV over 2 to 5 min as a single dose if wt greater than 40 kg. Prevention of N/V associated with radiotherapy: 8 mg PO tid. [Generic/Trade: Tabs 4, 8, 24 mg. Orally disintegrating tab 4, 8 mg. Oral soln 4 mg/5 mL. Generic only: Tabs 16 mg.] ▶L ♀B ▶? $$$$$

PALONOSETRON (*Aloxi*) Nausea with chemo: 0.25 mg IV over 30 sec, 30 min prior to chemo or 0.5 mg PO 1 h before start of chemotherapy. Prevention of post-op N/V: 0.075 mg IV over 10 sec just prior to anesthesia. [Trade only: Caps 0.5 mg.] ▶L ♀B ▶? $$$$$

Antiemetics—Other

APREPITANT (*Emend, fosaprepitant*) Prevention of nausea with moderately to highly emetogenic chemo, in combination with a corticosteroid and a 5-HT3 antagonist: 125 mg PO on day 1 (1 h prior to chemo), then 80 mg PO qam on day 2 and 3. Alternative for first dose only is 115 mg IV (fosaprepitant form) over 15 min given 30 min prior to chemo. Prevention of post-op N/V: 40 mg PO within 3 h prior to anesthesia. [Trade only (aprepitant): Caps 40, 80, 125 mg. IV prodrug form is fosaprepitant.] ▶L ♀B ▶? $$$$$

DICLECTIN (*doxylamine + pyridoxine*) Canada only. 2 tabs PO at bedtime. May add 1 tab in am and 1 tab in afternoon, if needed. [Canada Trade only: Delayed-release tabs doxylamine 10 mg + pyridoxine 10 mg.] ▶LK ♀A ▶? $

DIMENHYDRINATE (*Dramamine, +Gravol*) 50 to 100 mg PO/IM/IV q 4 to 6 h prn (max 400 mg/24 h PO, 600 mg/day IV/IM). [OTC Generic/Trade: Tabs 50 mg. Trade only: Chewable tabs 50 mg. Generic only: Oral soln 12.5 mg/5 mL. Canada only: Suppository 25, 50, 100 mg.] ▶LK ♀B ▶– $

DOMPERIDONE (*+Motilium*) Canada only. Postprandial dyspepsia: 10 to 20 mg PO tid to qid, 30 min before a meal. Nausea and vomiting: 20 mg PO tid to qid. [Canada only. Trade/generic: Tabs 10, 20 mg.] ▶L ♀? ▶– $$

DOXYLAMINE (*Unisom Nighttime Sleep Aid, others*) 12.5 mg PO bid to qid; often used in combination with pyridoxine. [Generic/Trade: Tabs 10 mg.] ▶L ♀A ▶? $

DRONABINOL (*Marinol*) Nausea with chemo: 5 mg/m2 PO 1 to 3 h before chemo then 5 mg/m2/dose q 2 to 4 h after chemo for 4 to 6 doses/day. Anorexia associated with AIDS: initially 2.5 mg PO bid before lunch and dinner. [Generic/Trade: Caps 2.5, 5, 10 mg.] ▶L ♀C ▶– ©III $$$$$

DROPERIDOL (*Inapsine*) 0.625 to 2.5 mg IV or 2.5 mg IM. May cause fatal QT prolongation, even in patients with no risk factors. Monitor ECG before. ▶L ♀C ▷? $

METOCLOPRAMIDE (*Reglan, Metozolv ODT, ✦Maxeran*) 10 mg IV/IM q 2 to 3 h prn. 10 to 15 mg PO qid, 30 min before meals and at bedtime. Caution with long-term (more than 3 months) use. [Generic/Trade: Tabs 5, 10 mg. Trade: Orally disintegrating tablets 5, 10 mg (Metozolv). Generic only: Oral soln 5 mg/5 mL.] ▶K ♀B ▷? $

NABILONE (*Cesamet*) 1 to 2 mg PO bid, 1 to 3 h before chemotherapy. [Trade only: Caps 1 mg.] ▶L ♀C ▷– ©II $$$$$

PHOSPHORATED CARBOHYDRATES (*Emetrol*) 15 to 30 mL PO q 15 min prn, max 5 doses. Peds: 5 to 10 mL per dose. [OTC Generic/Trade: Soln containing dextrose, fructose, and phosphoric acid.] ▶L ♀A ▷+ $

PROCHLORPERAZINE (*Compazine, ✦Stemetil*) 5 to 10 mg IV over at least 2 min. 5 to 10 mg PO/IM tid to qid. 25 mg PR q 12 h. Sustained-release: 15 mg PO q am or 10 mg PO q 12 h. Peds: 0.1 mg/kg/dose PO/PR tid to qid or 0.1 to 0.15 mg/kg/dose IM tid to qid. [Generic only: Tabs 5, 10, 25 mg. Suppository 25 mg.] ▶LK ♀C ▷? $

PROMETHAZINE (*Phenergan*) Adults: 12.5 to 25 mg PO/IM/PR q 4 to 6 h. Peds: 0.25 to 1 mg/kg PO/IM/PR q 4 to 6 h. Contraindicated if age younger than 2 yo; caution in older children. IV use common but not approved. [Generic only: Tabs/Suppository 12.5, 25, 50 mg. Syrup 6.25 mg/5 mL.] ▶LK ♀C ▷– $

SCOPOLAMINE (*Transderm-Scop, Scopace, ✦Transderm-V*) <u>Motion sickness:</u> Apply 1 disc (1.5 mg) behind ear 4 h prior to event; replace every 3 days. Tab: 0.4 to 0.8 mg PO 1 h before travel and q 8 h prn. [Trade only: Topical disc 1.5 mg/72 h, box of 4. Oral tablet 0.4 mg.] ▶L ♀C ▷+ $$

THIETHYLPERAZINE (*Torecan*) 10 mg PO/IM 1 to 3 times a day. [Trade only: Tabs 10 mg.] ▶L ♀? ▷? $

TRIMETHOBENZAMIDE (*Tigan*) 300 mg PO q 6 to 8 h, 200 mg IM q 6 to 8 h. [Generic/Trade: Cap 300 mg.] ▶LK ♀C ▷? $

Antiulcer—Antacids

ALKA-SELTZER (acetylsalicylic acid + citrate + bicarbonate) 2 regular-strength tabs in 4 oz water q 4 h PO prn (up to 8 tabs/day for age younger than 60 yo, up to 4 tabs/day for age 60 yo or greater) or 2 extra-strength tabs in 4 oz water q 6 h PO prn (up to 7 tabs/day for age less than 60 yo, up to 4 tabs/day for age 60 yo or greater). [OTC Trade only: Regular-strength, original: aspirin 325 mg + citric acid 1000 mg + sodium bicarbonate 1916 mg. Regular-strength lemon lime and cherry: 325 mg + 1000 mg + 1700 mg. Extra-strength: 500 mg + 1000 mg + 1985 mg. Not all forms of Alka Seltzer contain aspirin (eg, Alka Seltzer Heartburn Relief).] ▶LK ♀? (- 3rd trimester) ▷? $

ALUMINUM HYDROXIDE (*Alternagel, Amphojel, Alu-Tab, Alu-Cap, ✦Basalgel, Mucaine*) 5 to 10 mL or 300 to 600 mg PO up to 6 times per day. Constipating. [OTC Generic/Trade: Susp 320, 600 mg/ 5 mL.] ▶K ♀C ▷? $

CITROCARBONATE (bicarbonate + citrate)   1 to 2 teaspoons in cold water PO 15 min to 2 h after meals prn. [OTC Trade only: Sodium bicarbonate 0.78 g + sodium citrate anhydrous 1.82 g in each 1 teaspoonful dissolved in water 150, 300 g.]   ▶K ♀? ▶? \$

GAVISCON (aluminum hydroxide + magnesium carbonate)   2 to 4 tabs or 15 to 30 mL (regular strength) or 10 mL (extra strength) PO qid prn. [OTC Trade only: Tabs: Regular-strength (Al hydroxide 80 mg + Mg carbonate 20 mg), Extra-strength (Al hydroxide 160 mg + Mg carbonate 105 mg). Liquid: Regular-strength (Al hydroxide 95 mg + Mg carbonate 358 mg per 15 mL), Extra-strength (Al hydroxide 254 mg + Mg carbonate 237.5 mg per 30 mL).]   ▶K ♀? ▶? \$

MAALOX (aluminum hydroxide + magnesium hydroxide)   10 to 20 mL or 1 to 2 tabs PO prn. [OTC Generic/Trade: Regular-strength chewable tabs (Al hydroxide + Mg hydroxide 200/200 mg). Susp (225/200 mg per 5 mL). Other strengths available.]   ▶K ♀C ▶? \$

MAGALDRATE (*Riopan*)   5 to 10 mL PO prn. [OTC Trade only: Susp 540 mg/5 mL. Riopan Plus (with simethicone) available as susp 540/20 mg/5 mL, chewable tabs 540/20 mg.]   ▶K ♀C ▶? \$

MYLANTA (aluminum hydroxide + magnesium hydroxide + simethicone)   2 to 4 tabs or 10 to 20 mL PO prn. [OTC Generic/Trade: Liquid. Double-strength liquid. Tabs, Double-strength tabs. Trade only: Tabs sodium + sugar + dye-free.]   ▶K ♀C ▶? \$

ROLAIDS (calcium carbonate + magnesium hydroxide)   2 to 4 tabs PO q 1 h prn, max 12 tabs/day (regular strength) or 10 tabs/day (extra-strength). [OTC Trade only: Tabs regular-strength (Ca carbonate 550 mg, Mg hydroxide 110 mg), extra-strength (Ca carbonate 675 mg, Mg hydroxide 135 mg).]   ▶K ♀? ▶? \$

Antiulcer—H2 Antagonists

CIMETIDINE (*Tagamet, Tagamet HB*)   300 mg IV/IM/PO q 6 to 8 h, 400 mg PO bid, or 400 to 800 mg PO qhs. Erosive esophagitis: 800 mg PO bid or 400 mg PO qid. Continuous IV infusion 37.5 to 50 mg/h (900 to 1200 mg/day). [Tabs 200, 300, 400, 800 mg. Rx Generic only: Oral soln 300 mg/5 mL. OTC Generic/Trade: Tabs 200 mg.]   ▶LK ♀B ▶+ \$

FAMOTIDINE (*Pepcid, Pepcid AC, Maximum Strength Pepcid AC*)   20 mg IV q 12 h, 20 to 40 mg PO at bedtime, or 20 mg PO bid. [Generic/Trade: Tabs 10 mg (OTC, Pepcid AC Acid Controller), 20 mg (Rx and OTC, Maximum Strength Pepcid AC), 40 mg. Rx Generic/Trade: Susp 40 mg/5 mL.]   ▶LK ♀B ▶? \$

NIZATIDINE (*Axid, Axid AR*)   150 to 300 mg PO qhs, or 150 mg PO bid. [OTC Trade only (Axid AR): Tabs 75 mg. Rx Trade only: Oral soln 15 mg/mL (120, 480 mL). Rx Generic/Trade: Caps 150 mg. Generic: Caps 300 mg.]   ▶K ♀B ▶? \$\$\$\$

PEPCID COMPLETE (famotidine + calcium carbonate + magnesium hydroxide)   Treatment of heartburn: 1 tab PO prn. Max 2 tabs/day. [OTC trade/generic: Chewable tab, famotidine 10 mg with Ca carbonate 800 mg and Mg hydroxide 165 mg.]   ▶LK ♀B ▶? \$

RANITIDINE (*Zantac, Zantac Efferdose, Zantac 75, Zantac 150, Peptic Relief*) 150 mg PO bid or 300 mg PO at bedtime. 50 mg IV/IM q 8 h, or continuous infusion 6.25 mg/h (150 mg/day). [Generic/Trade: Tabs 75 (OTC: Zantac 75), 150 (OTC and Rx: Zantac 150), 300 mg. Syrup 75 mg/5 mL. Rx Trade only: Effervescent tabs 25, 150 mg. Rx Generic only: Caps 150, 300 mg.] ▶K ♀B ▶? $$$

Antiulcer—Helicobacter pylori Treatment

HELIDAC (bismuth subsalicylate + metronidazole + tetracycline) 1 dose PO qid for 2 weeks. To be given with an H2 antagonist. [Trade only: Each dose consists of bismuth subsalicylate 524 mg (2 × 262 mg) chewable tab + metronidazole 250 mg tab + tetracycline 500 mg cap.] ▶LK ♀D ▶– $$$$$
PREVPAC (lansoprazole + amoxicillin + clarithromycin) (*◆HP-Pac*) 1 dose PO bid for 10 to 14 days. [Trade only: Each does consists of lansoprazole 30 mg cap + amoxicillin 1 g (2 × 500 mg cap) + clarithromycin 500 mg tab.] ▶LK ♀C ▶? $$$$$
PYLERA (bismuth subcitrate potassium + metronidazole + tetracycline) 3 caps PO qid (after meals and at bedtime) for 10 days. Use with omeprazole 20 mg PO bid. [Trade only: Each cap contains biskalcitrate 140 mg + metronidazole 125 mg + tetracycline 125 mg.] ▶LK ♀D ▶– $$$$$

Antiulcer—Proton Pump Inhibitors

DEXLANSOPRAZOLE (*Dexilant*) <u>Erosive esophagitis:</u> 60 mg PO daily for up to 8 weeks. <u>Maintenance therapy after healing of erosive esophagitis:</u> 30 mg PO daily for up to 6 months. <u>GERD:</u> 30 mg PO daily for up to 4 weeks. [Trade only: Cap 30, 60 mg.] ▶L ♀B ▶? $$$$
ESOMEPRAZOLE (*Nexium*) <u>Erosive esophagitis:</u> 20 to 40 mg PO daily for 4 to 8 weeks. <u>Maintenance of erosive esophagitis:</u> 20 mg PO daily. <u>Zollinger-Ellison:</u> 40 mg PO bid for 4 to 8 weeks. <u>GERD:</u> 20 mg PO daily for 4 weeks. <u>GERD with esophagitis:</u> 20 to 40 mg IV daily for 10 days until taking PO. <u>Prevention of NSAID-associated gastric ulcer:</u> 20 to 40 mg PO daily for up to 6 months. <u>H. pylori eradication:</u> 40 mg PO daily with amoxicillin 1000 mg PO bid and clarithromycin 500 mg PO bid for 10 days. [Trade only: Cap delayed-release 20, 40 mg. Delayed-release granules for oral susp 10, 20, 40 mg per packet.] ▶L ♀B ▶? $$$$

HELICOBACTER PYLORI THERAPY

- Triple therapy PO for 10 to 14 days: clarithromycin 500 mg bid + amoxicillin 1 g bid (or metronidazole 500 mg bid) + PPI*
- Quadruple therapy PO for 14 days: bismuth subsalicylate 525 mg (or 30 mL) tid to qid plus metronidazole 500 mg tid to qid plus tetracycline 500 mg tid to qid plus a PPI* or a H2 blocker†
- PPI or H2 blocker may need to be continued past 14 days to heal the ulcer.

*PPIs include esomeprazole 40 mg qd, lansoprazole 30 mg bid, omeprazole 20 mg bid, pantoprazole 40 mg bid, rabeprazole 20 mg bid. †H₂ blockers include cimetidine 400 mg bid, famotidine 20 mg bid, nizatidine 150 mg bid, ranitidine 150 mg bid. Adapted from *Medical Letter Treatment Guidelines* 2008:55.

LANSOPRAZOLE (*Prevacid*) <u>Duodenal ulcer or maintenance therapy after healing of duodenal ulcer:</u> 15 mg PO daily for up to 12 months. <u>NSAID-induced Gastric ulcer:</u> 30 mg PO daily for 8 weeks (treatment), 15 mg PO daily for up to 12 weeks (prevention). <u>GERD:</u> 15 mg PO daily. <u>Gastric ulcer:</u> 30 mg PO daily. <u>Erosive esophagitis:</u> 30 mg PO daily for up to 8 weeks or 30 mg IV daily for 7 days or until taking PO. [OTC Trade only: Caps 15 mg. Rx Generic/Trade: 15, 30 mg. Rx Trade only: Susp 15, 30 mg packets. Orally disintegrating tab 15, 30 mg. Prevacid NapraPac: 7 lansoprazole 15 mg caps packaged with 14 naproxen tabs 375 mg or 500 mg.] ▶L ♀B ▶? $$$

OMEPRAZOLE (*Prilosec*, *◆Losec*) <u>GERD, duodenal ulcer, erosive esophagitis:</u> 20 mg PO daily. <u>Heartburn (OTC):</u> 20 mg PO daily for 14 days. <u>Gastric ulcer:</u> 40 mg PO daily. <u>Hypersecretory conditions:</u> 60 mg PO daily. [Rx Generic/Trade: Caps 10, 20, 40 mg. Trade only: Granules for oral susp 2.5 mg, 10 mg. OTC Trade only: Cap 20 mg.] ▶L ♀C ▶? OTC $, Rx $$$$

PANTOPRAZOLE (*Protonix*, *◆Pantoloc*) <u>GERD:</u> 40 mg PO daily. <u>Zollinger-Ellison syndrome:</u> 80 mg IV q 8 to 12 h for 7 days until taking PO. <u>GERD associated with a history of erosive esophagitis:</u> 40 mg IV daily for 7 to 10 days until taking PO. [Generic/Trade: Tabs 20, 40 mg. Trade only: Granules for susp 40 mg/packet.] ▶L ♀B ▶? $$$$

RABEPRAZOLE (*AcipHex*, *◆Pariet*) 20 mg PO daily. [Trade: Tabs 20 mg.] ▶L ♀B ▶? $$$$

ZEGERID (omeprazole + bicarbonate) <u>Duodenal ulcer, GERD, erosive esophagitis:</u> 20 mg PO daily for 4 to 8 weeks. <u>Gastric ulcer:</u> 40 mg PO once daily for 4 to 8 weeks. <u>Reduction of risk of upper GI bleed in critically ill (susp only):</u> 40 mg PO, then 40 mg 6 to 8 h later, then 40 mg once daily thereafter for up to 14 days. [OTC Trade only: Caps omeprazole/sodium bicarbonate 20 mg/1 g. Rx Trade only: 20 mg/1 g and 40 mg/1 g, powder packets for susp 20 mg/1g and 40 mg/1 g.] ▶L ♀C ▶? $$$$$

Antiulcer—Other

DICYCLOMINE (*Bentyl*, *◆Bentyol, Formulex, Protylol, Lomine*) 10 to 20 mg PO/IM qid up to 40 mg PO qid. [Generic/Trade: Tabs 20 mg. Caps 10 mg. Syrup 10 mg/5 mL. Generic only: Caps 20 mg.] ▶LK ♀B ▶– $

DONNATAL (phenobarbital + hyoscyamine + atropine + scopolamine) 1 to 2 tabs/caps or 5 to 10 mL PO tid to qid. 1 extended-release tab PO q 8 to 12 h. [Generic/trade: Phenobarbital 16.2 mg + hyoscyamine 0.1 mg + atropine 0.02 mg + scopolamine 6.5 mcg in each tab or 5 mL. Trade only: Extended-release tab 48.6 + 0.3111 + 0.0582 + 0.0195 mg.] ▶LK ♀C ▶– $$$

GI COCKTAIL (*green goddess*) <u>Acute GI upset:</u> Mixture of Maalox/Mylanta 30 mL + viscous lidocaine (2%) 10 mL + Donnatal 10 mL administered PO in a single dose. ▶L ♀See individual ▶See individual $

HYOSCINE (*◆Buscopan*) Canada: <u>GI or bladder spasm:</u> 10 to 20 mg PO/IV up to 60 mg daily (PO) or 100 mg daily (IV). [Canada Trade only: Tabs 10 mg.] ▶LK ♀C ▶? $$

HYOSCYAMINE (*Anaspaz, A-spaz, Cystospaz, ED Spaz, Hyosol, Hyospaz, Levbid, Levsin, Levsinex, Medispaz, NuLev, Spacol, Spasdel, Symax*) <u>Bladder spasm, control gastric secretion, GI hypermotility, irritable bowel syndrome:</u> 0.125 to 0.25 mg PO/SL q 4 h or prn. Extended-release: 0.375 to 0.75 mg PO q 12 h. Max 1.5 mg/day. [Generic/Trade: Tabs 0.125, 0.15 mg. Sublingual tabs 0.125 mg. Chewable tabs 0.125 mg. Extended-release tabs, caps 0.375 mg. Elixir 0.125 mg/5 mL. Gtts 0.125 mg/1 mL.] ▶LK ♀C ▶– $

MEPENZOLATE (*Cantil*) 25 to 50 mg PO qid, with meals and at bedtime. [Trade only: Tabs 25 mg.] ▶K + gut ♀B ▶? $$$$$

MISOPROSTOL (*PGE1, Cytotec*) <u>Prevention of NSAID-induced gastric ulcers:</u> Start 100 mcg PO bid, then titrate as tolerated up to 200 mcg PO qid. <u>Cervical ripening:</u> 25 mcg intravaginally q 3 to 6 h (or 50 mcg q 6 h). <u>First trimester pregnancy failure:</u> 800 mcg intravaginally, repeat on day 3 if expulsion incomplete. [Generic/Trade: Oral tabs 100, 200 mcg.] ▶LK ♀X ▶– $$$$

PROPANTHELINE (*Pro-Banthine, ✦Propanthel*) 7.5 to 15 mg PO 30 min after meals and 30 mg at bedtime. [Generic only: Tabs 15 mg.] ▶LK ♀C ▶– $$$

SIMETHICONE (*Mylicon, Gas-X, Phazyme, ✦Ovol*) 40 to 250 mg PO qid prn, max 500 mg/day. Infants: 20 mg PO qid prn. [OTC Generic/Trade: Chewable tabs 80, 125 mg. Gtts 40 mg/0.6 mL. Trade only: Softgels 166 mg (Gas-X) 180 mg (Phazyme). Strips, oral (Gas-X) 62.5 mg (adults), 40 mg (children).] ▶Not absorbed ♀C but + ▶? $

SUCRALFATE (*Carafate, ✦Sulcrate*) 1 g PO 1 h before meals (2 h before other medications) and at bedtime. [Generic/Trade: Tabs 1 g. Susp 1 g/10 mL.] ▶Not absorbed ♀B ▶? $$

Laxatives—Bulk-Forming

METHYLCELLULOSE (*Citrucel*) 1 heaping tablespoon in 8 oz. water PO daily (up to tid). [OTC Trade only: Regular and sugar-free packets and multiple-use canisters, Clear-mix soln, Caplets 500 mg.] ▶Not absorbed ♀+ ▶? $

POLYCARBOPHIL (*FiberCon, Konsyl Fiber, Equalactin, Psyllium*) <u>Laxative:</u> 1 g PO qid prn. <u>Diarrhea:</u> 1 g PO q 30 min. Max daily dose 6 g. [OTC Generic/Trade: Tabs/Caplets 625 mg. OTC Trade only: Chewable tabs 625 mg (Equalactin).] ▶Not absorbed ♀+ ▶? $

PSYLLIUM (*Metamucil, Fiberall, Konsyl, Hydrocil, ✦Prodium Plain*) 1 teaspoon in liquid, 1 packet in liquid, or 1 to 2 wafers with liquid PO daily (up to tid). [OTC Generic/Trade: Regular and sugar-free powder, Granules, Caps, Wafers, including various flavors and various amounts of psyllium.] ▶Not absorbed ♀+ ▶? $

Laxatives—Osmotic

GLYCERIN (*Fleet*) 1 adult or infant suppository PR prn. [OTC Generic/Trade: Suppository infant and adult, Soln (Fleet Babylax) 4 mL/applicator.] ▶Not absorbed ♀C ▶? $

LACTULOSE (*Enulose, Kristalose*) <u>Constipation:</u> 15 to 30 mL (syrup) or 10 to 20 g (powder for oral soln) PO daily. <u>Hepatic encephalopathy:</u> 30 to 45 mL (syrup) PO tid to qid, or 300 mL retention enema. [Generic/Trade: Syrup 10 g/15 mL. Trade only (Kristalose): 10, 20 g packets for oral soln.] ▶Not absorbed ♀B ▶? $$

MAGNESIUM CITRATE (*◆Citro-Mag*) 150 to 300 mL PO once or in divided doses. 2 to 4 mL/kg/day once or in divided doses for age younger than 6 yo. [OTC Generic only: Soln 300 mL/bottle. Low-sodium and sugar-free available.] ▶K ♀B ▶? $

MAGNESIUM HYDROXIDE (*Milk of Magnesia*) <u>Laxative:</u> 30 to 60 mL regular-strength liquid PO. <u>Antacid:</u> 5 to 15 mL regular-strength liquid or 622 to 1244 mg PO qid prn. [OTC Generic/Trade: Susp 400 mg/5 mL. Trade only: Chewable tabs 311, 400 mg. Generic only: Susp (concentrated) 1200 mg/5 mL, sugar-free 400 mg/5 mL.] ▶K ♀+ ▶? $

POLYETHYLENE GLYCOL (*MiraLax, GlycoLax*) 17 g (1 heaping tablespoon) in 4 to 8 oz water, juice, soda, coffee, or tea PO daily. [OTC Trade only: Powder for oral soln 17 g/scoop. Rx Generic/Trade: Powder for oral soln 17 g/scoop.] ▶Not absorbed ♀C ▶? $

POLYETHYLENE GLYCOL WITH ELECTROLYTES (*GoLytely, Colyte, TriLyte, NuLytely, Moviprep, HalfLytely and Bisacodyl Tablet Kit, ◆Klean-Prep, Electropeg, Peg-Lyte*) <u>Bowel prep:</u> 240 mL q 10 min PO or 20 to 30 mL/min per NG until 4 L is consumed. Moviprep: Follow specific instructions. [Generic/Trade: powder for oral solution in disposable jug 4 L or 2 L (Moviprep). Also, as a kit of 2 L bottle of polyethylene glycol with electrolytes and 2 or 4 bisacodyl tabs 5 mg (HalfLytely and Bisacodyl Tablet Kit). Trade only (GoLytely): packet for oral solution to make 3.785 L.] ▶Not absorbed ♀C ▶? $

SODIUM PHOSPHATE (*Fleet enema, Fleet Phospho-Soda, Fleet EZ-Prep, Accu-Prep, Osmoprep, Visicol, ◆Enemol, Phoslax*) 1 adult or pediatric enema PR or 20 to 30 mL of oral soln PO prn (max 45 mL/24 h). <u>Visicol:</u> <u>Evening before colonoscopy:</u> 3 tabs with 8 oz clear liquid q 15 min until 20 tabs are consumed. <u>Day of colonoscopy:</u> Starting 3 to 5 h before procedure, 3 tabs with 8 oz clear liquid q 15 min until 20 tabs are consumed. Osmoprep: 32 tabs (48 g of sodium phosphate) PO with total of 2 quarts clear liquids as follows: pm before procedure: 4 tabs PO with 8 oz of clear liquids q 15 min for a total of 20 tabs; day of procedure: 3 to 5 h before procedure, 4 tabs with 8 oz of clear liquids q 15 min for a total of 12 tabs. [OTC Generic/Trade: Adult enema, oral soln. OTC Trade only: Pediatric enema, bowel prep. Rx Trade only: Visicol, Osmoprep tab ($$$$) 1.5 g.] ▶Not absorbed ♀C ▶? $

SORBITOL 30 to 150 mL (of 70% soln) PO or 120 mL (of 25 to 30% soln) PR as a single dose. Cathartic: 4.3 mL/kg PO. [Generic only: Soln 70%.] ▶Not absorbed ♀C ▶? $

Laxatives—Stimulant

BISACODYL (*Correctol, Dulcolax, Feen-a-Mint, Fleet*) 10 to 15 mg PO prn, 10 mg PR prn, 5 to 10 mg PR prn if 2 to 11 yo. [OTC Generic/Trade: Tabs 5 mg. Suppository 10 mg. OTC Trade only (Fleet): Enema, 10 mg/30 mL.] ▶L ♀C ▶? $

CASCARA   325 mg PO at bedtime prn or 5 mL of aromatic fluid extract PO at bedtime prn. [OTC Generic only: Tabs 325 mg, liquid aromatic fluid extract.] ▶L ♀C ▶+ $

CASTOR OIL   Children: 5 to 15 mL/dose of castor oil PO or 7.5 to 30 mL emulsified castor oil PO once a day. Adult: 15 to 60 mL of castor oil or 30 to 60 mL emulsified castor oil PO once a day. [OTC Generic only: Oil 60, 120 mL.] ▶Not absorbed ♀− ▶? $

SENNA (*Senokot, SenokotXTRA, Ex-Lax, Fletcher's Castoria, ✦Glysennid*)   2 tabs or 1 teaspoon granules or 10 to 15 mL syrup PO. Max 8 tabs, 4 teaspoon granules, 30 mL syrup/day. Take granules with full glass of water. [OTC Generic/Trade (All dosing is based on sennosides content; 1 mg sennosides is equivalent to 21.7 mg standardized senna concentrate): Syrup 8.8 mg/5 mL. Liquid 3 mg/mL (Fletcher's Castoria). Tabs 8.6, 15, 17, 25 mg. Chewable tabs 15 mg.]   ▶L ♀C ▶+ $

Laxatives—Stool Softener

DOCUSATE (*Colace, Surfak, Kaopectate Stool Softener, Enemeez*)   Docusate calcium: 240 mg PO daily. Docusate sodium: 50 to 500 mg/day PO divided in 1 to 4 doses. Peds: Give 10 to 40 mg/day for age younger than 3 yo, give 20 to 60 mg/day for age 3 to 6 yo, give 40 to 150 mg/day for age 6 to 12 yo. In all cases doses are divided up to qid. <u>Cerumen impaction:</u> Instill 1 mL in affected ear. [Docusate calcium OTC Generic/Trade: Caps 240 mg. Docusate sodium OTC Generic/Trade: Caps 50, 100, 250 mg. Liquid 50 mg/5 mL. Syrup 20 mg/5 mL. Docusate sodium OTC Trade only (Enemeez): Enema, rectal 283 mg/5 mL.] ▶L ♀C ▶? $

Laxatives—Other or Combinations

LUBIPROSTONE (*Amitiza*)   <u>Chronic idiopathic constipation:</u> 24 mcg PO bid with food and water. <u>Irritable bowel syndrome with constipation in women age 18 yo or older:</u> 8 mcg PO bid. [Trade only: 8, 24 mcg caps.] ▶Gut ♀C ▶? $$$$$

MINERAL OIL (*Kondremul, Fleet Mineral Oil Enema, Liqui-Doss, ✦Lansoyl*)   15 to 45 mL PO. Peds: 5 to 15 mL/dose PO. Mineral oil enema: 60 to 150 mL PR. Peds 30 to 60 mL PR. [OTC Generic/Trade: Oil (30, 480 mL), Enema (Fleet). OTC Trade only: Oral liquid (Liqui-Doss) 13.5 mg/15 mL. Oral microemulsion (Kondremul) 2.5 mg/5 mL.] ▶Not absorbed ♀C ▶? $

PERI-COLACE (docusate + sennosides)   2 to 4 tabs PO once daily or in divided doses prn. [OTC Generic/Trade: Tabs 50 mg docusate + 8.6 mg sennosides.] ▶L ♀C ▶? $

SENOKOT-S (senna + docusate)   2 tabs PO daily. [OTC Generic/Trade: Tabs 8.6 mg senna concentrate/50 mg docusate.] ▶L ♀C ▶+ $

Ulcerative Colitis

BALSALAZIDE (*Colazal*)   2.25 g PO tid for 8 to 12 weeks. [Generic/Trade: Caps 750 mg.] ▶Minimal absorption ♀B ▶? $$$$$

MESALAMINE (*5-aminosalicylic acid, Apriso, 5-Aspirin, Asacol, Lialda, Pentasa, Canasa, Rowasa, ✦Mesasal, Salofalk*)   Apriso: 1.5 g (4 caps) PO qam. Asacol: 800 to 1600 mg PO tid. Pentasa: 1000 mg PO qid. Lialda: 2.4 to 4.8 g PO daily with a meal. Canasa: 500 mg PR bid to tid or 1000 mg PR at bedtime. [Trade only: delayed-release tab 400 mg (Asacol), 800 mg (Asacol HD). Controlled-release cap 250, 500 mg (Pentasa). Delayed-release tablet 1200 mg (Lialda). Rectal suppository 1000 mg (Canasa). Controlled-release cap 0.375 g (Apriso). Generic/Trade: Rectal susp 4 g/60 mL (Rowasa).] ▶Gut ♀C ▶? $$$$$

OLSALAZINE (*Dipentum*)   Ulcerative colitis: 500 mg PO bid with food. [Trade only: Caps 250 mg.] ▶L ♀C ▶– $$$$$

SULFASALAZINE (*Azulfidine, Azulfidine EN-tabs, ✦Salazopyrin En-tabs, S.A.S.*)   Colitis: 500 to 1000 mg PO qid. Peds: 30 to 60 mg/kg/day divided q 4 to 6 h. RA: 500 mg PO bid after meals up to 1 g PO bid. May turn body fluids, contact lenses, or skin orange-yellow. [Generic/Trade: Tabs 500 mg, scored. Enteric-coated, Delayed-release (EN-tabs) 500 mg.] ▶L ♀D ▶– $$

Other GI Agents

ALOSETRON (*Lotronex*)   Diarrhea-predominant irritable bowel syndrome in women who have failed conventional therapy: 0.5 mg PO bid for 4 weeks; discontinue in patients who become constipated. If well tolerated after 4 weeks, may increase to 1 mg PO bid. Discontinue if symptoms not controlled in 4 weeks on 1 mg PO bid. [Trade only: Tabs 0.5, 1 mg.] ▶L ♀B ▶? $$$$$

ALPHA-GALACTOSIDASE (*Beano*)   5 gtts or 1 tab per ½ cup gassy food, 3 tabs PO (chew, swallow, crumble) or 10 gtts per typical meal. [OTC Trade only: Oral gtts 150 IU/5 gtts, Tabs 150 IU.] ▶Minimal absorption ♀? ▶? $

ALVIMOPAN (*Entereg*)   Short-term (up to 15 doses) in hospitalized patients undergoing partial large or small bowel resection surgery with primary anastomosis: 12 mg PO 30 min to 5 h prior to surgery, then 12 mg PO bid starting the day after surgery for up to 7 days. [Trade only: Caps 12 mg.] ▶Intestinal flora ♀B ▶? ?

BUDESONIDE (*Entocort EC*)   9 mg PO daily for up to 8 weeks (remission induction) or 6 mg PO daily for 3 months (maintenance). [Trade only: Caps 3 mg.] ▶L ♀C ▶? $$$$$

CERTOLIZUMAB (*Cimzia*)   Crohn's: 400 mg SC at 0, 2, and 4 weeks. If response occurs, then 400 mg SC q 4 weeks. Rheumatoid arthritis: 400 mg SC at 0, 2, and 4 weeks. [Trade only: 400 mg kit.] ▶Plasma, K ♀B ▶? $$$$$

CHLORDIAZEPOXIDE-CLIDINIUM (*Librax*)   1 cap PO tid to qid. [Generic/Trade: Caps, chlordiazepoxide 5 mg + clidinium 2.5 mg.] ▶K ♀D ▶– $$$

GLYCOPYRROLATE (*Robinul, Robinul Forte*)   Peptic ulcer disease: 1 to 2 mg PO bid to tid. [Generic/Trade: Tabs 1, 2 mg.] ▶K ♀B ▶? $$$$

LACTASE (*Lactaid*)   Swallow or chew 3 caplets (Original strength), 2 caplets (Extra strength), 1 caplet (Ultra) with first bite of dairy foods. Adjust dose based on response. [OTC Generic/Trade: Caplets, Chewable tabs.] ▶Not absorbed ♀+ ▶+ $

METHYLNALTREXONE (Relistor) Less than 38 kg: 0.15 mg/kg SC every other day; 38 kg to 61 kg: 8 mg SC every other day; 62 kg to 114 kg: 12 mg SC every other day; 115 kg or greater: 0.15 mg/kg SC every other day. [Injectable soln 12 mg/0.6 mL.] ▶unchanged ♀B ▶? $$$$$

NEOMYCIN—ORAL (Neo-Fradin) Hepatic encephalopathy: 4 to 12 g/day PO divided q 4 to 6 h. Peds: 50 to 100 mg/kg/day PO divided q 6 to 8 h. [Generic only: Tabs 500 mg. Trade only: Soln 125 mg/5 mL.] ▶Minimally absorbed ♀D ▶? $$$

OCTREOTIDE (Sandostatin, Sandostatin LAR) Variceal bleeding: Bolus 25 to 50 mcg IV followed by infusion 25 to 50 mcg/h. AIDS diarrhea: 25 to 250 mcg SC tid. [Generic/Trade: Injection vials 0.05, 0.1, 0.2, 0.5, 1 mg. Trade only: Long-acting injectable susp (Sandostatin LAR) 10, 20, 30 mg.] ▶LK ♀B ▶? $$$$$

ORLISTAT (Alli, Xenical) Weight loss: 120 mg PO tid with meals. [OTC Trade only (Alli): Caps 60 mg. Rx Trade only (Xenical): Caps 120 mg.] ▶Gut ♀B ▶? $$$

PANCREATIN (Creon, Ku-Zyme, ✦Entozyme) 8,000 to 24,000 units lipase (1 to 2 tabs/caps) PO with meals and snacks. [Tabs, Caps with varying amounts of pancreatin, lipase, amylase, and protease.] ▶Gut ♀C ▶? $$$

PANCRELIPASE (Creon, Pancreaze, Viokase, Pancrease, Pancrecarb, Cotazym, Ku-Zyme HP, Zenpep) Varies by weight. Initial infant dose 2,000 to 4,000 lipase units per 120 mL formula or breast-feeding. 12 mo or older to younger than 4 yo: 1,000 lipase units/kg. 4 yo or older: 500 lipase units/kg per meal, max 2,500 lipase units/kg per meal. [Tabs, Caps, Powder with varying amounts of lipase, amylase, and protease.] ▶Gut ♀C ▶? $$$

PINAVERIUM (✦Dicetel) Canada only. 50 to 100 mg PO tid. [Trade only: tabs 50, 100 mg.] ▶? ♀C ▶- $$$

SECRETIN (SecreFlo, ChiRhoStim) Test dose 0.2 mcg IV. If tolerated, 0.2 to 0.4 mcg/kg IV over 1 min. ▶Serum ♀C ▶? $$$$$

URSODIOL (Actigall, URSO, URSO Forte) Gallstone dissolution (Actigall): 8 to 10 mg/kg/day PO divided bid to tid. Prevention of gallstones associated with rapid weight loss (Actigall): 300 mg PO bid. Primary biliary cirrhosis (URSO): 13 to 15 mg/kg/day PO divided in 2 to 4 doses. [Generic/Trade: Caps 300 mg, Tabs 250, 500 mg.] ▶Bile ♀B ▶? $$$$

HEMATOLOGY

Anticoagulants—LMW Heparins, & Fondaparinux

NOTE See cardiovascular section for antiplatelet drugs and thrombolytics.

DALTEPARIN (Fragmin) DVT prophylaxis, acute medical illness with restricted mobility: 5000 units SC daily. DVT prophylaxis, abdominal surgery: 2500 units SC 1 to 2 h pre-op and daily post-op. DVT prophylaxis, abdominal surgery in patients with malignancy: 5000 units SC evening before surgery and daily

(cont.)

post-op, or 2500 units 1 to 2 h pre-op and 12 h later, then 5000 units daily. <u>DVT prophylaxis, hip replacement:</u> Preop start (day of surgery): 2500 units SC given 2 h pre-op, 4 to 8 h post-op, then 5000 units daily starting at least 6 h after 2nd dose, or 5000 units 10 to 14 h pre-op, 4 to 8 h post-op, then daily (approximately 24 h between doses). Pre-op start (evening before surgery): 5000 units SC given evening before surgery then 5000 units daily starting at least 4 to 8 h post-op (approximately 24 h between doses). Post-op start: 2500 units 4 to 8 h post-op, then 5000 units daily starting at least 6 h after first dose. <u>Treatment of DVT/PE in cancer:</u> 200 units/kg SC daily for 1 month, then 150 units/kg SC daily for 5 months; max 18,000 units/day. <u>Unstable angina or non-Q-wave MI:</u> 120 units/kg up to 10,000 units SC q 12 h with aspirin (75 to 165 mg/day PO) until clinically stable. [Trade only: Single-dose syringes 2500, 5000 anti-Xa units/0.2 mL, 7500 anti-Xa/0.3 mL, 10,000 anti-Xa/1 mL, 12,500 anti-Xa/0.5 mL, 15,000 anti-Xa/0.6 mL, 18,000 anti-Xa units/0.72 mL; multidose vial 10,000 units/mL, 9.5 mL and 25,000 units/mL, 3.8 mL.] ▶KL ♀B ▶+ $$$$$

ENOXAPARIN (Lovenox) <u>DVT prophylaxis, acute medical illness with restricted mobility:</u> 40 mg SC daily (if CrCl < 30 mL/min: give 30 mg SC daily). <u>Hip/knee replacement:</u> 30 mg SC q 12 h starting 12 to 24 h post-op (if CrCl < 30 mL/min: give 30 mg SC daily). Alternative for hip replacement: 40 mg SC daily starting 12 h pre-op. <u>Abdominal surgery:</u> 40 mg SC daily starting 2 h pre-op (if CrCl < 30 mL/min: give 30 mg SC daily). <u>Outpatient treatment of DVT without pulmonary embolus:</u> 1 mg/kg SC q 12 h. Continue for at least 5 days and until therapeutic oral anticoagulation established. <u>Inpatient treatment of DVT with/without pulmonary embolus:</u> 1 mg/kg SC q 12 h or 1.5 mg/kg SC q 24 h (CrCl < 30 mL/min: 1 mg/kg SC daily). Continue for at least 5 days and until therapeutic oral anticoagulation established. <u>Unstable angina or non-Q-wave MI:</u> 1 mg/kg SC q 12 h with aspirin (100 to 325 mg PO daily) for at least 2 days and until clinically stable (if CrCl < 30 mL/min: give 1 mg/kg SC daily). <u>Acute ST-elevation MI:</u> For age 75 yo or younger: give 30 mg IV bolus, followed 15 min later by 1 mg/kg SC, then 1 mg/kg SC (max 100 mg/dose for the first two doses) q 12 h (if CrCl < 30 mL/min: give 30 mg IV bolus followed 15 min later by 1 mg/kg SC dose then 1 mg/kg SC daily); if older than 75 yo: 0.75 mg/kg SC q 12 h (max 75 mg/dose for the first two doses, no bolus) SC q 12 h (CrCl < 30 mL/min: 1 mg/kg SC daily, no bolus). [Trade only: Multidose vial 300 mg; Syringes 30, 40 mg; graduated syringes 60, 80, 100, 120, 150 mg. Concentration is 100 mg/mL except for 120, 150 mg, which are 150 mg/mL.] ▶KL ♀B ▶+ $$$$$

FONDAPARINUX (Arixtra) <u>DVT prophylaxis, hip/knee replacement or hip fracture surgery, abdominal surgery:</u> 2.5 mg SC daily starting 6 to 8 h post-op. <u>DVT/PE treatment</u> based on wt: 5 mg (if wt less than 50 kg), 7.5 mg (if 50 to 100 kg), 10 mg (if wt greater than 100 kg) SC daily for at least 5 day & therapeutic oral anticoagulation. [Trade only: Prefilled syringes 2.5 mg/0.5 mL, 5 mg/0.4 mL, 7.5 mg/0.6 mL, 10 mg/0.8 mL.] ▶K ♀B ▶? $$$$$

TINZAPARIN (Innohep) <u>DVT with/without pulmonary embolus:</u> 175 units/kg SC daily for at least 6 days and until adequate anticoagulation with warfarin. [Trade only: 20,000 anti-Xa units/mL, 2 mL multidose vial.] ▶K ♀B ▶+ $$$$$

WEIGHT-BASED HEPARIN DOSING FOR DVT/PE*

Initial dose: 80 units/kg IV bolus, then 18 units/kg/h. Check PTT in 6 h.

PTT less than 35 sec (less than 1.2 × control): 80 units/kg IV bolus, then increase infusion rate by 4 units/kg/h.

PTT 35–45 sec (1.2–1.5 × control): 40 units/kg IV bolus, then increase infusion rate by 2 units/kg/h.

PTT 46–70 sec (1.5–2.3 × control): No change.

PTT 71–90 sec (2.3–3 × control): decrease infusion rate by 2 units/kg/h.

PTT greater than 90 sec (greater than 3 × control): Hold infusion for 1 h, then decrease infusion rate by 3 units/kg/h.

*PTT = Activated partial thromboplastin time. Reagent-specific target PTT may differ; use institutional nomogram when available. Consider establishing a max bolus dose/max initial infusion rate or use an adjusted body wt in obesity. When PTT is stable within therapeutic range, monitor every morning. Therapeutic PTT range corresponds to anti-factor Xa activity of 0.3–0.7 units/mL. Recheck PTT 6 h after heparin initiation and 6 h after each dosage adjustment. Can begin warfarin on first day of heparin; continue heparin for ≥4 to 5 days of combined therapy. Adapted from *Ann Intern Med* 1993;119:874; *Chest* 2008:133:463S–464S, *Circulation* 2001; 103:2994.

Anticoagulants—Other

ARGATROBAN   HIT: Start 2 mcg/kg/min IV infusion. Get PTT at baseline and 2 h after starting infusion. Adjust dose (max dose: 10 mcg/kg/min) until PTT is 1.5 to 3X baseline (not > 100 sec). ACCP recommends starting at lower doses of 0.5 to 1.2 mcg/kg/min in patients with heart failure, multi-organ failure, anasarca, or post-cardiac surgery. ▶L ♀B ▶– $$$$$

BIVALIRUDIN (*Angiomax*)   Anticoagulation during PCI (patients with or at risk of HIT): 0.75 mg/kg IV bolus prior to intervention, then 1.75 mg/kg/h for duration of procedure (with provisional Gp IIb/IIIa inhibition). For CrCl < 30 mL/min, reduce infusion dose to 1 mg/kg/h after bolus. Use with aspirin 300 to 325 mg PO daily. Additional bolus of 0.3 mg/kg if activated clotting time > 225 sec. ▶proteolysis/K ♀B ▶? $$$$$

DABIGATRAN (*Pradaxa*)   Stroke prevention in atrial fibrillation: 150 mg PO BID (if CrCl 15–30 mL/min: 75 mg PO BID). [Trade only: caps 75, 150 mg.] ▶K ♀C ▶? $$$$$

DESIRUDIN (*Iprivask*)   DVT prophylaxis (hip replacement surgery): 15 mg SC q12 h (if CrCl 31 to 60 mL/min give 5 mg SC q12 h). ▶K ♀C ▶?

HEPARIN (+*Hepalean*)   Venous thrombosis/pulmonary embolus treatment: Load 80 units/kg IV, then initiate infusion at 18 units/kg/h. Adjust based on coagulation testing (PTT). Peds: Load 50 units/kg IV, then infuse 25 units/kg/h. DVT prophylaxis: 5000 units SC q 8 to 12 h. [Generic only: 1000, 5000, 10,000, 20,000 units/mL in various vial and syringe sizes.] ▶Reticuloendothelial system ♀C but + ▶+ $$

LEPIRUDIN (*Refludan*)   Anticoagulation in HIT and associated thromboembolic disease: Bolus 0.4 mg/kg up to 44 mg IV over 15 to 20 sec, then infuse 0.15 mg/kg up to 16.5 mg/h. Alternate initial dosing recommended by ACCP: Bolus 0.2 mg/kg IV (bolus only if life- or limb-threatening thrombosis) then infuse 0.05–0.1 mg/kg/h. Adjust dose to maintain APTT ratio of 1.5 to 2.5. ▶K ♀B ▶? $$$$$

WARFARIN (*Coumadin, Jantoven*)   Start 2 to 5 mg PO daily for 1 to 2 days, then adjust dose to maintain therapeutic PT/INR. [Generic/Trade: Tabs 1, 2, 2.5, 3, 4, 5, 6, 7.5, 10 mg.] ▶L ♀X ▶+ $

THERAPEUTIC GOALS FOR ANTICOAGULATION

INR Range*	Indication
2.0–3.0	Atrial fibrillation, deep venous thrombosis†, pulmonary embolism†, bio-prosthetic heart valve, mechanical prosthetic heart valve (aortic position, bileaflet or tilting disk with normal sinus rhythm and normal left atrium)
2.5–3.5	Mechanical prosthetic heart valve: (1) mitral position, (2) aortic position with atrial fibrillation, (3) caged ball or caged disk

*Aim for an INR in the middle of the INR range (eg, 2.5 for range of 2 to 3 and 3.0 for range of 2.5 to 3.5).
Adapted from: *Chest* 2008; 133: 456-7S, 459S, 547S, 594-5S; see this manuscript for additional information and other indications. †For first-event unprovoked DVT/PE, after 3 months of therapy at goal INR 2 to 3, may consider low-intensity therapy (INR range 1.5 to 2.0) in patients with strong preference for less frequent INR testing.

Colony Stimulating Factors

DARBEPOETIN (*Aranesp, NESP*)   <u>Anemia of chronic renal failure:</u> 0.45 mcg/kg IV/SC once a week, or 0.75 mcg/kg q 2 weeks in some nondialysis patients. <u>Cancer chemo anemia:</u> 2.25 mcg/kg SC weekly, or 500 mcg SC every 3 weeks. Adjust dose based on Hb. [Trade only: All forms are available with or without albumin. Single-dose vials: 25, 40, 60, 100, 200, 300, 500 mcg/1 mL, and 150 mcg/0.75 mL. Single-dose prefilled syringes or autoinjectors: 25 mcg/0.42 mL, 40 mcg/0.4 mL, 60 mcg/0.3 mL, 100 mcg/0.5 mL, 150 mcg/0.3 mL, 200 mcg/0.4 mL, 300 mcg/0.6 mL, 500 mcg/1 mL.] ▶cellular sialidases, L ♀C ▶? $$$$$

EPOETIN ALFA (*Epogen, Procrit, erythropoietin alpha, ✦Eprex*)   <u>Anemia:</u> 1 dose IV/SC 3 times a week. Initial dose if renal failure is 50 to 100 units/kg, Zidovudine-induced anemia is 100 units/kg, or chemo-associated anemia is 150 units/kg. <u>Alternate for chemo-associated anemia:</u> 40,000 units SC once a week. Adjust dose based on Hb. [Trade only: Single-dose 1 mL vials 2000, 3000, 4000, 10,000, 40,000 units/mL. Multidose vials 10,000 units/mL 2 mL, 20,000 units/mL 1 mL.] ▶L ♀C ▶? $$$$$

FILGRASTIM (*G-CSF, Neupogen*)   <u>Neutropenia:</u> 5 mcg/kg SC/IV daily. <u>Bone marrow transplant:</u> 10 mcg/kg/day SC/IV infusion. [Trade only: Single-dose vials: 300 mcg/1 mL, 480 mcg/1.6 mL. Single-dose syringes: 300 mcg/0.5 mL, 480 mcg/0.8 mL.] ▶L ♀C ▶? $$$$$

OPRELVEKIN (*Neumega*)   <u>Chemotherapy-induced thrombocytopenia in adults:</u> 50 mcg/kg SC daily. [Trade only: 5 mg single-dose vials with diluent.] ▶K ♀C ▶? $$$$$

PEGFILGRASTIM (*Neulasta*)   6 mg SC once each chemo cycle. [Trade only: Single-dose syringes 6 mg/0.6 mL.] ▶Plasma ♀C ▶? $$$$$

SARGRAMOSTIM (*GM-CSF, Leukine*)   Specialized dosing for <u>bone marrow transplant.</u> ▶L ♀C ▶? $$$$$

Other Hematological Agents

AMINOCAPROIC ACID (*Amicar*)   <u>Hemostasis:</u> 4 to 5 g PO/IV over 1 h, then 1 g/h prn. [Generic/Trade: Syrup 250 mg/mL, Tabs 500 mg. Trade only: Tabs 1000 mg.] ▶K ♀D ▶? $ IV $$$$$ Oral

DEFERASIROX (*Exjade*) Chronic iron overload: 20 mg/kg PO daily; adjust dose q 3 to 6 months based on ferritin trends. Max 40 mg/kg/day. [Trade only: Tabs for dissolving into oral susp 125, 250, 500 mg.] ▶L ♀B ▶? $$$$$

HYDROXYUREA (*Hydrea, Droxia*) Sickle cell anemia (Droxia): Start 15 mg/kg PO daily while monitoring CBC every 2 weeks. If no marrow depression, then increase dose every 12 weeks by 5 mg/kg/day (max 35 mg/kg/day). Give concomitant folic acid 1 mg/day. Chemotherapy: Doses vary by indication. [Generic/Trade: Caps 500 mg. Trade only: (Droxia) Caps 200, 300, 400 mg.] ▶LK ♀D ▶– $ varies by therapy

PROTAMINE Reversal of heparin: 1 mg antagonizes about 100 units heparin. Reversal of low-molecular-weight heparin: 1 mg protamine per 100 anti-Xa units of dalteparin or tinzaparin. 1 mg protamine per 1 mg enoxaparin. Give IV (max 50 mg) over 10 min. May cause allergy/anaphylaxis. ▶Plasma ♀C ▶? $

HERBAL & ALTERNATIVE THERAPIES

NOTE *In the United States, herbal and alternative therapy products are regulated as dietary supplements, not drugs. Premarketing evaluation and FDA approval are not required unless specific therapeutic claims are made. Because these products are not required to demonstrate efficacy, it is unclear whether many of them have health benefits. In addition, there may be considerable variability in content from lot to lot or between products. See www.tarascon.com/herbals for the evidence-based efficacy ratings used by Tarascon editorial staff.*

ALOE VERA (*acemannan, burn plant*) Topical: Efficacy unclear for seborrheic dermatitis, psoriasis, genital herpes, skin burns. Gel possibly effective for oral lichen planus. Do not apply to surgical incisions; impaired healing reported. Oral: Efficacy unclear for mild to moderate active ulcerative colitis, type 2 diabetes. OTC laxatives containing aloe were removed from US market due to possible increased risk of colon cancer. [Not by prescription.] ▶LK ♀oral– topical+? ▶oral– topical+? $

ARNICA (*Arnica montana, leopard's bane, wolf's bane*) Do not take by mouth or use on open wounds. Topical promoted for treatment of bruises, aches, and sprains; but insufficient data to assess efficacy. [Not by prescription.] ▶? ♀– ▶– $

ARTICHOKE LEAF EXTRACT (*Cynara scolymus*) May reduce total cholesterol, but clinical significance is unclear. Possibly effective for functional dyspepsia. [Not by prescription.] ▶? ♀? ▶? $

ASTRAGALUS (*Astragalus membranaceus, huang qi, Jin Fu Kang, vetch*) Used in combination with other herbs in traditional Chinese medicine for CAD, CHF, chronic liver disease, kidney disease, viral infections, and upper respiratory tract infection. Possibly effective for improving survival and performance status with platinum-based chemotherapy for non-small-cell lung cancer. However, astragalus-based herbal formula (Jin Fu Kang) did not affect survival or pharmacokinetics of docetaxel in phase II study of patients with non-small-cell lung cancer. [Not by prescription.] ▶? ♀? ▶? $

BILBERRY (*Vaccinium myrtillus, huckleberry, Tegens, VMA extract*) Insufficient data to evaluate efficacy for macular degeneration or prevention of cataracts. Does not appear to improve night vision. [Not by prescription.] ▶Bilke ♀– ▶– $

BITTER MELON (*Momordica charantia, ampalaya, karela*) Efficacy unclear for type 2 diabetes. Hypoglycemic coma reported in 2 children ingesting tea. Seeds can cause hemolytic anemia in G6PD deficiency. [Not by prescription.] ▶? ♀– ▶– $$

BUTTERBUR (*Petasites hybridus, Petadolex, Petaforce, Tesalin, ZE 339*) Migraine prophylaxis (possibly effective): Petadolex 50 to 75 mg PO bid. Allergic rhinitis prophylaxis (possibly effective): Petadolex 50 mg PO bid or Tesalin 1 tab PO qid or 2 tabs tid. Efficacy unclear for asthma. [Not by prescription. Standardized pyrrolizidine-free extracts: Petadolex (7.5 mg of petasin and isopetasin/50 mg tab). Tesalin (ZE 339; 8 mg petasin/tab).] ▶? ♀– ▶– $

CESIUM CHLORIDE Can cause life-threatening QT interval prolongation and torsades. Health Canada and FDA are taking action against Internet sellers promoting cesium chloride as alternative treatment of late-stage cancer. Evidence for benefit as cancer treatment is lacking. [Not by prescription.] ▶K♀– ▶– $$$

CHAMOMILE (*Matricaria recutita [German chamomile], Anthemis nobilis [Roman chamomile]*) Promoted as a sedative or anxiolytic, to relieve GI distress, for skin infections or inflammation, many other indications. Efficacy unclear for any indication. [Not by prescription.] ▶? ♀– ▶? $

CHASTEBERRY (*Vitex agnus castus fruit extract, Femaprin*) Premenstrual syndrome (possibly effective): 20 mg PO daily of extract ZE 440. [Not by prescription.] ▶? ♀– ▶– $

CHONDROITIN Does not appear effective for relief of OA pain overall. Chondroitin 400 mg PO tid + glucosamine may improve pain in subgroup of patients with moderate to severe knee OA. [Not by prescription.] ▶K ♀? ▶? $

COENZYME Q10 (*CoQ-10, ubiquinone*) Heart failure: 100 mg/day PO divided bid to tid (conflicting clinical trials; AHA does not recommend). Statin-induced myalgia: 100 to 200 mg PO daily (efficacy unclear; conflicting clinical trials). Parkinson's disease: 1200 mg/day PO divided qid ($$$$; efficacy unclear; might slow progression slightly, but the American Academy of Neurology does not recommend). Efficacy unclear for hypertension and improving athletic performance. Appears ineffective for diabetes. [Not by prescription.] ▶Bile ♀– ▶– $

CRANBERRY (*Cranactin, Vaccinium macrocarpon*) Prevention of UTI (possibly effective): 300 mL/day PO cranberry juice cocktail. Usual dose of cranberry juice extract caps/tabs is 300 to 400 mg PO bid. Insufficient data to assess efficacy for treatment of UTI. Potential increase in INR with warfarin. [Not by prescription.] ▶? ♀+ in food, – in supplements ▶+ in food, – in supplements $

CREATINE Promoted to enhance athletic performance. No benefit for endurance exercise; modest benefit for intense anaerobic tasks lasting less than 30 sec. Usual loading dose of 20 g/day PO for 5 days, then 2 to 5 g/day divided bid. [Not by prescription.] ▶LK ♀– ▶– $

DEHYDROEPIANDROSTERONE (*DHEA, Aslera, Fidelin, Prasterone*) Does not improve cognition, quality of life, or sexual function in elderly. Not recommended as androgen replacement in late-onset male hypogonadism. To improve well-being in women with adrenal insufficiency: 50 mg PO daily (possibly effective; conflicting clinical trials). [Not by prescription.] ▶Peripheral conversion to estrogens and androgens ♀–▶– $

DEVIL'S CLAW (*Harpagophytum procumbens, Phyto Joint, Doloteffin, Harpadol*) OA, acute exacerbation of chronic low-back pain (possibly effective): 2400 mg extract/day (50 to 100 mg harpagoside/day) PO divided bid to tid. [Not by prescription. Extracts standardized to harpagoside content.] ▶? ♀–▶– $

DONG QUAI (*Angelica sinensis*) Appears ineffective for postmenopausal symptoms; North American Menopause Society recommends against use. May increase bleeding risk with warfarin; avoid concurrent use. [Not by prescription.] ▶? ♀–▶– $

ELDERBERRY (*Sambucus nigra, Rubini, Sambucol, Sinupret*) Efficacy unclear for influenza, sinusitis, and bronchitis. [Not by prescription.] ▶? ♀–▶– $

EVENING PRIMROSE OIL (*Oenothera biennis*) Appears ineffective for premenstrual syndrome, postmenopausal symptoms, atopic dermatitis. Inadequate data to evaluate efficacy for cervical ripening. [Not by prescription.] ▶? ♀? ▶? $

FENUGREEK (*Trigonelle foenum-graecum*) Efficacy unclear for diabetes or hyperlipidemia. [Not by prescription.] ▶? ♀–▶? $$

FEVERFEW (*Chrysanthemum parthenium, MIG-99, Migra-Lief, MigraSpray, Tanacetum parthenium L.*) Prevention of migraine (possibly effective): 50 to 100 mg extract PO daily; 2 to 3 fresh leaves PO with or after meals daily; 50 to 125 mg freeze-dried leaf PO daily. May take 1 to 2 months to be effective. Inadequate data to evaluate efficacy for acute migraine. [Not by prescription.] ▶? ♀–▶– $

FLAVOCOXID (*Limbrel, UP446*) OA (efficacy unclear): 250 to 500 mg PO bid. [Caps 250, 500 mg. Marketed as medical food by prescription only (not all medical foods require a prescription). Medical foods are intended to be given under physician supervision to meet distinctive nutritional needs of a disease, but they do not undergo an approval process to establish safety and efficacy.] ▶L ♀–▶– $$$

GARCINIA (*Garcinia cambogia, Citri Lean*) Appears ineffective for wt loss. [Not by prescription.] ▶? ♀–▶– $

GARLIC SUPPLEMENTS (*Allium sativum, Kwai, Kyolic*) Ineffective for hyperlipidemia. Small reductions in BP, but efficacy in HTN unclear. Does not appear effective for diabetes. Significantly decreases saquinavir levels. May increase bleeding risk with warfarin with/without increase in INR. [Not by prescription.] ▶LK ♀–▶– $

GINGER (*Zingiber officinale*) Prevention of motion sickness (efficacy unclear): 500 to 1000 mg powdered rhizome PO single dose 1 h before exposure. Acute chemotherapy-induced nausea (possibly effective adjunct to standard antiemetics): 250 to 500 mg PO bid for 6 days, starting 3 days before chemo. Does not appear effective for post-op N/V. American College of Obstetrics and

(cont.)

Gynecology considers ginger 250 mg PO qid a nonpharmacologic option for N/V of pregnancy. Some experts advise pregnant women to limit dose to usual dietary amount (no more than 1 g/day). Some European countries advise pregnant women to avoid ginger supplements because it is cytotoxic in vitro. [Not by prescription.] ▶bile ♀? ▶? $

GINKGO BILOBA (*EGb 761, Ginkgold, Ginkoba*) Dementia (efficacy unclear): 40 mg PO tid of standardized extract containing 24% ginkgo flavone glycosides and 6% terpene lactones. The American Psychiatric Association and others find evidence too weak to recommend for Alzheimer's or other dementias. Does not prevent dementia in elderly or improve memory in people with normal cognitive function. Does not appear effective for intermittent claudication or prevention of acute altitude sickness. Possible risk of stroke. [Not by prescription.] ▶K ♀– ▶– $

GINSENG—AMERICAN (*Panax quinquefolius L., Cold-fX*) Reduction of postprandial glucose in type 2 diabetes (possibly effective): 3 g PO taken with or up to 2 h before meal. Cold-fX (1 cap PO bid) may modestly reduce the frequency of colds/flu; approved in Canada for adults and children 12 yo and older. [Not by prescription.] ▶K ♀– ▶– $

GINSENG—ASIAN (*Panax ginseng, Ginsana, G115, Korean red ginseng*) Promoted to improve vitality and well-being: 200 mg PO daily. Ginsana: 2 caps PO daily or 1 cap PO bid. Ginsana Sport: 1 cap PO daily. Preliminary evidence of efficacy for erectile dysfunction. Efficacy unclear for improving physical or psychomotor performance, diabetes, herpes simplex infections, cognitive, or immune function. American College of Obstetrics and Gynecologists and North American Menopause Society recommend against use for postmenopausal hot flashes. [Not by prescription.] ▶? ♀– ▶– $

GINSENG—SIBERIAN (*Eleutherococcus senticosus, Ci-wu-jia*) Does not appear effective for improving athletic endurance or chronic fatigue syndrome. May interfere with some digoxin assays. [Not by prescription.] ▶? ♀– ▶– $

GLUCOSAMINE (*Cosamin DS, Dona*) OA: Glucosamine HCl 500 mg PO tid or glucosamine sulfate (Dona $$) 1500 mg PO once daily. Appears ineffective overall for OA pain, but glucosamine plus chondroitin may improve pain in moderate to severe knee OA. [Not by prescription.] ▶L ♀– ▶– $

GOLDENSEAL (*Hydrastis canadensis*) Often used in attempts to achieve false-negative urine test for illicit drug use (efficacy unclear). Often combined with echinacea in cold remedies; but insufficient data to assess efficacy for common cold or URIs. [Not by prescription.] ▶? ♀– ▶– $

GRAPE SEED EXTRACT (*Vitis vinifera L., procyanidolic oligomers, PCO*) Small clinical trials suggest benefit in chronic venous insufficiency. No benefit in single study of seasonal allergic rhinitis. [Not by prescription.] ▶? ♀? ▶? $

GREEN TEA (*Camellia sinensis, Polyphenon E*) Efficacy unclear for cancer prevention, wt loss, hypercholesterolemia. Large doses may decrease INR with warfarin due to vitamin K content. Contains caffeine. [Not by prescription. Green tea extract available in caps standardized to polyphenol content.] ▶LK ♀+ in moderate amount in food, – in supplements ▶+ in moderate amount in food, – in supplements $

GUARANA (*Paullinia cupana*)   Marketed as a source of caffeine in wt-loss dietary supplements. [Not by prescription.] ▶? ♀+ in food, – in supplements ▶+ in food, – in supplements $

GUGGULIPID (*Commiphora mukul extract, guggul*)   Does not appear effective for hyperlipidemia. [Not by prescription.] ▶? ♀– ▶– $$

HAWTHORN (*Crataegus laevigata, monogyna, oxyacantha, standardized extract WS 1442—Crataegutt novo, HeartCare*)   Mild heart failure (possibly effective): 80 mg PO bid to 160 mg PO tid of standardized extract (19% oligomeric procyanidins; WS 1442; HeartCare 80 mg tabs). [Not by prescription.] ▶? ♀– ▶– $

HONEY (*Medihoney*)   Topical for burn/wound (including diabetic foot, stasis leg ulcers, pressure ulcers, 1st and 2nd degree partial thickness burns): Apply Medihoney for 12 to 24 h/day. Oral for nocturnal cough due to upper respiratory tract infection in children (efficacy unclear): Give PO within 30 min before sleep. Dose is ½ tsp for 2 to 5 yo, 1 tsp for 6 to 11 yo, 2 tsp for 12 to 18 yo. Do not feed honey to children younger than 1 yo due to risk of infant botulism. [Mostly not by prescription. Medihoney is FDA-approved.] ▶? ♀+ ▶+ $ for oral $$$ for Medihoney

HORSE CHESTNUT SEED EXTRACT (*Aesculus hippocastanum, buckeye, HCE50, Venastat*)   Chronic venous insufficiency (effective): 1 cap Venastat (16% aescin standardized extract) PO bid with water before meals. Am College of Cardiology found evidence insufficient to recommend for peripheral arterial disease. [Not by prescription.] ▶? ♀– ▶– $

LICORICE (*Cankermelt, Glycyrrhiza glabra, Glycyrrhiza uralensis*)   Insufficient data to assess efficacy for postmenopausal vasomotor symptoms. Chronic high doses can cause pseudo-primary aldosteronism (with HTN, edema, hypokalemia). Cancermelt (dissolving oral patch; efficacy unclear for aphthous ulcers): Apply patch to ulcer for 16 h/day until healed. [Not by prescription.] ▶Bile ♀– ▶– $

MELATONIN (*N-acetyl-5-methoxytryptamine*)   To reduce jet lag after flights over more than 5 time zones (effective): 0.5 to 5 mg PO at bedtime for 3 to 6 nights starting on day of arrival. [Not by prescription.] ▶L ♀– ▶– $

METHYLSULFONYLMETHANE (*MSM, dimethyl sulfone, crystalline DMSO2*)   Insufficient data to assess efficacy of oral and topical MSM for arthritis pain. [Not by prescription.] ▶? ♀– ▶– $

MILK THISTLE (*Silybum marianum, Legalon, silymarin, Thisylin*)   Hepatic cirrhosis (efficacy unclear): 100 to 200 mg PO tid of standardized extract with 70 to 80% silymarin. [Not by prescription.] ▶LK ♀– ▶– $

NETTLE ROOT (*stinging nettle, Urtica dioica radix*)   Efficacy unclear for treatment of BPH or OA. [Not by prescription.] ▶? ♀– ▶– $

NONI (*Morinda citrifolia*)   Promoted for many medical disorders; but insufficient data to assess efficacy. Potassium content comparable to orange juice; hyperkalemia reported in chronic renal failure. Case reports of hepatotoxicity. [Not by prescription.] ▶? ♀– ▶– $$$

PEPPERMINT OIL (*Mentha x piperita oil*)   Irritable bowel syndrome (possibly effective): 0.2 to 0.4 mL enteric-coated caps PO tid. Peds, 8 yo or older: 0.1 to 0.2 mL enteric-coated caps PO tid. Take before meals. [Not by prescription.] ▶LK ♀+ in food, ? in supplements ▶+ in food, ? in supplements $

POLICOSANOL (*CholeRx, Cholestin*) Ineffective for hyperlipidemia. [Not by prescription.] ▶? ♀– ▶– $

PROBIOTICS (*Acidophilus, Align, Bifantis, Bifidobacteria, Lactobacillus, Bacid, Culturelle, Florastor, IntestiFlora, Lactinex, LiveBac, Power-Dophilus, Primadophilus, Probiotica, Saccharomyces boulardii, VSL#3*) Prevention of antibiotic-associated diarrhea (effective): Forastor (Saccharomyces boulardii) 2 caps PO bid for adults; 1 cap PO bid for peds. Culturelle (Lactobacillus GG) 1 cap PO once daily or bid for peds. Give 2 h before/after antibiotic. IDSA recommends against probiotics to prevent C difficile associated diarrhea; safety and efficacy is unclear. Peds rotavirus gastroenteritis (effective): Lactobacillus GG at least 10 billion cells/day PO started early in illness. VSL#3 (approved as medical food) for ulcerative colitis or pouchitis: 1 to 8 packets/day or 4 to 32 caps/day for adults; peds dose based on wt and number of bowel movements. Irritable bowel syndrome: VSL#3 either ½ to 1 packet PO daily or 2 to 4 caps PO daily to relieve gas/bloating. Align: 1 cap PO once daily to relieve abdominal pain/bloating. [Not by prescription. Culturelle contains Lactobacillus GG 10 billion cells/cap. Florastor contains Saccharomyces boulardii 5 billion cells/250 mg cap. Probiotica contains Lactobacillus reuteri 100 million cells/chewable tab. VSL#3 contains 450 billion cells/packet, 225 billion cells/2 caps (Bifidobacterium breve, longum, infantis; Lactobacillus acidophilus, plantarum, casei, bulgaricus; Streptococcus thermophilus). Align contains Bifidobacterium infantis 35624, 1 billion cells/cap. VSL#3 is marketed as nonprescription medical food. Medical foods are intended to be given under physician supervision to meet distinctive nutritional needs of a disease, but they do not undergo an approval process to establish safety and efficacy.] ▶? ♀+ ▶+ $

PYCNOGENOL (*French maritime pine tree bark*) Promoted for many medical disorders; but efficacy unclear for chronic venous insufficiency, HTN, sperm dysfunction, melasma, OA, diabetes, and ADHD. [Not by prescription.] ▶L ♀? ▶? $

PYGEUM AFRICANUM (*African plum tree*) BPH (may have modest efficacy): 50 to 100 mg PO bid or 100 mg PO daily of standardized extract containing 14% triterpenes. [Not by prescription.] ▶? ♀– ▶– $

RED CLOVER (*red clover isoflavone extract, Trifolium pratense, trefoil, Promensil, Rimostil, Trinovin*) Postmenopausal vasomotor symptoms (conflicting evidence; does not appear effective overall, but may have modest benefit for severe symptoms): Promensil 1 tab PO daily to bid with meals. [Not by prescription. Isoflavone content (genistein, daidzein, biochanin, formononetin) is 40 mg/tab in Promensil and Trinovin, 57 mg/tab in Rimostil.] ▶Gut, L, K ♀– ▶– $$

RED YEAST RICE (*Monascus purpureus, Xuezhikang, Zhibituo, Hypocol, Lipolysar*) Hyperlipidemia: Usual dose is 1200 mg PO bid. Efficacy depends on whether formulation contains lovastatin or other statins. In the US, red yeast rice should not contain more than trace amounts of statins, but some products contain up to 10 mg lovastatin per cap. Some clinicians consider red

(cont.)

yeast rice an alternative for patients who develop myalgia with prescription statins. Can cause myopathy. Some formulations may contain citrinin, a potential nephrotoxin. [Not by prescription.] Xuezhikang marketed in Asia, Norway (HypoCol), Italy (Lipolysar).] ▶L ♀– ▶– $$

S-ADENOSYLMETHIONINE (*SAM-e, sammy*) Mild to moderate depression (effective): 800 to 1600 mg/day PO in divided doses with meals. Efficacy unclear for OA. [Not by prescription.] ▶L ♀? ▶? $$$

SAINT JOHN'S WORT (*Hypericum perforatum, Kira, Movana, LI-160*) Mild to moderate depression (effective): 300 mg PO tid of standardized extract (0.3% hypericin). Does not appear effective for ADHD. May decrease efficacy of other drugs (eg, ritonavir, oral contraceptives) by inducing liver metabolism. May cause serotonin syndrome with SSRIs, MAOIs. [Not by prescription.] ▶L ♀– ▶– $

SAW PALMETTO (*Serenoa repens*) BPH (does not appear effective): 160 mg PO bid or 320 mg PO daily of standardized liposterolic extract. Take with food. [Not by prescription.] ▶? ♀– ▶– $

SHARK CARTILAGE (*BeneFin, Cartilade*) Appears ineffective for palliative care of advanced cancer. [Not by prescription.] ▶? ♀– ▶– $$$$$

SOY (*Genisoy, Healthy Woman, Novasoy, Phytosoya, Supro*) Cardiovascular risk reduction: at least 25 g/day soy protein (50 mg/day isoflavones) PO. Hypercholesterolemia: about 50 g/day soy protein PO reduces LDL cholesterol by about 3%; no apparent benefit for isoflavone supplements. Postmenopausal vasomotor symptoms (modest benefit if any): 20 to 60 g/day soy protein PO (40 to 80 mg/day isoflavones). Conflicting clinical trials for postmenopausal bone loss. [Not by prescription.] ▶Gut, L, K ♀+ for food, ? for supplements ▶+ for food, ? for supplements $

STEVIA (*Stevia rebaudiana*) Leaves traditionally used as sweetener. Rebaudioside A (a component of stevia) is FDA approved as a general purpose sweetener. Unrefined stevia is available as dietary supplement in US, but not FDA approved as a sweetener. [Not by prescription. Rebaudioside A available as Rebiana, Truvia, PureVia.] ▶L ♀– ▶? $

TEA TREE OIL (*melaleuca oil, Melaleuca alternifolia*) Not for oral use; CNS toxicity reported. Efficacy unclear for topical treatment of onychomycosis, tinea pedis, acne vulgaris, dandruff, pediculosis. [Not by prescription.] ▶? ♀– ▶– $

VALERIAN (*Valeriana officinalis, Alluna*) Insomnia (possibly modestly effective; conflicting clinical trials): 400 to 900 mg of standardized extract PO 30 min before bedtime. Alluna: 2 tabs PO 1 h before bedtime. [Not by prescription.] ▶? ♀– ▶– $

WILD YAM (*Dioscorea villosa*) Ineffective as topical "natural progestin." Was used historically to synthesize progestins, cortisone, and androgens; it is not converted to them or dehydroepiandrosterone (DHEA) in the body. [Not by prescription.] ▶L ♀? ▶? $

WILLOW BARK EXTRACT (*Salix alba, Salicis cortex, Assalix, salicin*) OA, low-back pain (possibly effective): 60 to 240 mg/day salicin PO divided bid to tid. [Not by prescription. Some products standardized to 15% salicin content.] ▶K ♀– ▶– $

YOHIMBE (*Corynanthe yohimbe, Pausinystalia yohimbe*)   Non-prescription yohimbe promoted for impotence and as aphrodisiac, but some products contain little yohimbine. FDA considers yohimbe bark in herbal remedies an unsafe herb. [Yohimbine is the primary alkaloid in the bark of the yohimbe tree. Yohimbine HCl is a prescription drug in the United States; yohimbe bark is available without prescription. Yohimbe bark (not by prescription) and prescription yohimbine HCl are not interchangeable.] ▶L ♀– ▶– $

IMMUNOLOGY

Immunizations

NOTE *For vaccine info see CDC website (www.cdc.gov).*

AVIAN INFLUENZA VACCINE H5N1—INACTIVATED INJECTION   1 mL IM for 2 doses, separated by 21 to 35 days.   ♀C ▶? ?

BCG VACCINE (*Tice BCG, ✦Oncotice, Immucyst*)   0.2 to 0.3 mL percutaneously.   ♀C ▶? $$$$

COMVAX (haemophilus B vaccine + hepatitis B vaccine)   Infants born of HBsAg (negative) mothers: 0.5 mL IM for 3 doses, given at 2, 4, and 12 to 15 months.   ♀C ▶? $$$

DIPHTHERIA, TETANUS, AND ACELLULAR PERTUSSIS VACCINE (*DTaP, Tdap, Tripedia, Infanrix, Daptacel, Boostrix, Adacel, ✦Tripacel*)   0.5 mL IM. Do not use Boostrix or Adacel for primary childhood vaccination series.   ♀C ▶– $$

DIPHTHERIA-TETANUS TOXOID (*Td, DT, ✦D2T5*)   0.5 mL IM. [Injection DT (pediatric: 6 weeks to 6 yo). Td (adult and children at least 7 yo).]   ♀C ▶? $

HAEMOPHILUS B VACCINE (*ActHIB, HibTITER, PedvaxHIB*)   0.5 mL IM. Dosing schedule varies depending on formulation used and age of child at first dose.   ♀C ▶? $$

HEPATITIS A VACCINE (*Havrix, Vaqta, ✦Avaxim, Epaxal*)   Adult formulation 1 mL IM, repeat in 6 to 12 months. Peds: 0.5 mL IM for age 1 yo or older, repeat 6 to 18 months later. [Single-dose vial (specify pediatric or adult).]   ♀C ▶+ $$$

HEPATITIS B VACCINE (*Engerix-B, Recombivax HB*)   Adults: 1 mL IM, repeat in 1 and 6 months later. Separate pediatric formulations and dosing.   ♀C ▶+ $$$

HUMAN PAPILLOMAVIRUS RECOMBINANT VACCINE (*Gardasil*)   0.5 mL IM, then repeat in 2 and 6 months later.   ♀B ▶? $$$$$

INFLUENZA VACCINE—INACTIVATED INJECTION (*Agriflu, Afluria, Fluarix, FluLaval, Fluzone, Fluvirin, ✦Fluviral, Influvac, Intanza, Vaxigrip*)   0.5 mL IM. Fluarix and FluLaval not indicated for age younger than 18 yo, Fluvirin not indicated if age younger than 4 yo.   ♀C ▶+ $

INFLUENZA VACCINE—LIVE INTRANASAL (*FluMist*)   1 dose (0.2 mL) intranasally. Use only if 2 to 49 yo.   ♀C ▶+ $

JAPANESE ENCEPHALITIS VACCINE (*JE-Vax*)   1 mL SC for 3 doses on day 0, 7, and 30.   ♀C ▶? $$$$

MEASLES, MUMPS, AND RUBELLA VACCINE (*M-M-R II*, ✦*Priorix*)   0.5 mL (1 vial) SC.   ♀C ▶+ $$$

MENINGOCOCCAL VACCINE (*Menomune-A/C/Y/W-135, Menactra,* ✦*Menjugate*)   0.5 mL SC (Menomune) or IM (Menactra).   ♀C ▶? $$$$

PEDIARIX (diphtheria tetanus and acellular pertussis vaccine + hepatitis B vaccine + polio vaccine)   0.5 mL IM at 2, 4, 6 mo.   ♀C ▶? $$$

PLAGUE VACCINE   1 mL IM first dose, then 0.2 mL IM 1 to 3 months after the first injection, then 0.2 mL IM 5 to 6 months later for age 18 to 61 yo.   ♀C ▶+ $

PNEUMOCOCCAL 23-VALENT VACCINE (*Pneumovax,* ✦*Pneumo 23*)   0.5 mL IM or SC.   ♀C ▶+ $$

PNEUMOCOCCAL 7-VALENT CONJUGATE VACCINE (*Prevnar*)   0.5 mL IM for 3 doses 6 to 8 weeks apart starting at age 2 to 6 mo, followed by a 4th dose at 12 to 15 mo.   ♀C ▶? $$$$

POLIO VACCINE (*IPOL*)   0.5 mL IM or SC.   ♀C ▶? $$

PROQUAD (measles mumps & rubella vaccine + varicella vaccine, MMRV)   0.5 mL (1 vial) SC for age 12 mo to 12 yo.   ♀C ▶? $$$$

RABIES VACCINE (*RabAvert, Imovax Rabies, BioRab, Rabies Vaccine Adsorbed*)   1 mL IM in deltoid region on day 0, 3, 7, 14, 28.   ♀C ▶? $$$$$

ROTAVIRUS VACCINE (*RotaTeq, Rotarix*)   RotaTeq: Give the first dose (2 mL PO) between 6 to 12 weeks of age, and then 2nd and 3rd doses at 4 to 10 week intervals thereafter (last dose no later than 32 weeks). Rotarix: Give first dose (1 mL) at 6 weeks of age, and 2nd dose (1 mL) at least 4 weeks later, and last dose prior to 24 weeks of age. [Trade only: Oral susp 2 mL (RotaTeq), 1 mL (Rotarix).]   ▶? $$$$$

TETANUS TOXOID   0.5 mL IM or SC.   ♀C ▶+ $$

TRIHIBIT (haemophilus B vaccine + diphtheria tetanus and acellular pertussis vaccine)   Use for 4th dose only, age 15 to 18 mo: 0.5 mL IM.   ♀C ▶– $$$

TWINRIX (hepatitis A vaccine + hepatitis B vaccine)   Adults: 1 mL IM in deltoid, repeat at 1 and 6 months later. Accelerated dosing schedule: 0, 7, 21 to 30 days and booster dose at 12 months.   ♀C ▶? $$$$

TYPHOID VACCINE—INACTIVATED INJECTION (*Typhim Vi,* ✦*Typherix*)   0.5 mL IM single dose. May revaccinate q 2 to 5 years if high risk.   ♀C ▶? $$

TYPHOID VACCINE—LIVE ORAL (*Vivotif Berna*)   1 cap every other day for 4 doses. May revaccinate q 2 to 5 years if high risk. [Trade only: Caps.]   ♀C ▶? $$

VARICELLA VACCINE (*Varivax,* ✦*Varilrix*)   Children 1 to 12 yo: 0.5 mL SC. Repeat dose at ages 4 to 6 yo. Age 13 yo or older: 0.5 mL SC, repeat 4 to 8 weeks later.   ♀C ▶? $$$$

YELLOW FEVER VACCINE (*YF-Vax*)   0.5 mL SC.   ♀C ▶+ $$$

ZOSTER VACCINE—LIVE (*Zostavax*)   0.65 mL SC single dose for age 60 yo or older.   ♀C ▶? $$$$

Immunoglobulins

ANTIVENIN—CROTALIDAE IMMUNE FAB OVINE POLYVALENT (*CroFab*)   Rattlesnake envenomation: Give 4 to 6 vials IV infusion over 60 min, within 6 h of bite if possible. Administer 4 to 6 additional vials if no initial control of envenomation syndrome, then 2 vials q 6 h for up to 18 h (3 doses) after initial control has been established.   ▶? ♀C ▶? $$$$$

BOTULISM IMMUNE GLOBULIN (*BabyBIG*) <u>Infant botulism:</u> give 1 mL/kg (50 mg/kg) IV for age younger than 1 yo. ▶L ♀? ▶? $$$$$

HEPATITIS B IMMUNE GLOBULIN (*H-BIG, HyperHep B, HepaGam B, NABI-HB*) 0.06 mL/kg IM within 24 h of <u>needlestick, ocular, or mucosal exposure,</u> repeat in 1 month. ▶L ♀C ▶? $$$

IMMUNE GLOBULIN—INTRAMUSCULAR (*Baygam, ✦Gamastan*) <u>Hepatitis A prophylaxis:</u> 0.02 to 0.06 mL/kg IM depending on length of travel to endemic area. <u>Measles</u> (within 6 days postexposure): 0.2 to 0.25 mL/kg IM. ▶L ♀C ▶? $$$$

IMMUNE GLOBULIN—INTRAVENOUS (*Carimune, Flebogamma, Gammagard, Gammaplex, Gamunex, Octagam, Privigen*) IV dosage varies by indication and product. ▶L ♀C ▶? $$$$$

IMMUNE GLOBULIN—SUBCUTANEOUS (*Vivaglobulin, Hizentra*) 100 to 200 mg/kg SC weekly. ▶L ♀C ▶? $$$$$

LYMPHOCYTE IMMUNE GLOBULIN (*Atgam*) Specialized dosing. ▶L ♀C ▶? $$$$$

RABIES IMMUNE GLOBULIN HUMAN (*Imogam Rabies-HT, HyperRAB S/D*) 20 units/kg, as much as possible infiltrated around bite, the rest IM. ▶L ♀C ▶? $$$$$

CHILDHOOD IMMUNIZATION SCHEDULE*

				Months						Years	
Age	Birth	1	2	4	6	12	15	18	2	4–6	11–12
Hepatitis B	HB	HB				HB					
Rotavirus			Rota	Rota	Rota@						
DTP			DTaP	DTaP	DTaP		DTaP			DTaP	DTaP***
H influenza b			Hib	Hib	Hib	Hib					
Pneumococci**			PCV	PCV	PCV	PCV					
Polio			IPV	IPV		IPV				IPV#	
Influenza†						Influenza (yearly)†					
MMR						MMR				MMR	
Varicella						Varicella				Vari	
Hepatitis A¶						Hep A × 2¶					
Papillomavirus§											HPV × 3§
Meningococcal^											MCV^

*2010 schedule from the CDC, ACIP, AAP, & AAFP, see CDC website (www.cdc.gov/vaccines/recs/schedules/default.htm).

**Administer 1 dose to all healthy children 24–59 months having an incomplete schedule.

***When immunizing adolescents 10 yo or older, consider DTaP if patient has never received a pertussis booster (*Boostrix* if 10–18 yo, *Adacel* if 11–64 yo).

@If using *Rotarix* at 2 and 4 months, dose at 6 months is not indicated.

Give IPV on or after 4th birthday, and at least 6 months since last dose. If 4 doses given before 4th birthday, give 5th dose at ages 4 to 6 yo.

†For healthy patients age 2 yo or greater can use intranasal form. If age less than 9 yo and receiving for first time, administer 2 doses 4 or more weeks apart for injected form and 6 or more weeks apart for intranasal form.

¶Two doses at least 6 months apart. §Second and third doses 2 and 6 months after first dose. Also approved for males 9–18 yo to reduce risk of genital warts. ^For children 2–10 yo at high risk for meningococcal disease, vaccinate with meningococcal polysaccharide vaccine (*Menactra*). Revaccinate after 3 years (if first dose was at 2–6 yo) for children who remain at high risk after 5 years (if first dose was a 7 yo or older).

RSV IMMUNE GLOBULIN (*RespiGam*) IV infusion for <u>RSV</u>. ▶Plasma ♀C ▶? $$$$$

TETANUS IMMUNE GLOBULIN (*BayTet*, ✚*Hypertet*) Prophylaxis: 250 units IM. ▶L ♀C ▶? $$$$

VARICELLA-ZOSTER IMMUNE GLOBULIN (*VariZIG, VZIG*) Specialized dosing. ▶L ♀C ▶? $$$$$

Immunosuppression

BASILIXIMAB (*Simulect*) Specialized dosing for organ transplantation. ▶Plasma ♀B ▶? $$$$$

CYCLOSPORINE (*Sandimmune, Neoral, Gengraf*) Specialized dosing for <u>organ transplantation, RA, and psoriasis.</u> [Generic/Trade: Microemulsion Caps 25, 100 mg. Generic/Trade: Caps (Sandimmune) 25, 100 mg. Soln (Sandimmune) 100 mg/mL. Microemulsion soln (Neoral, Gengraf) 100 mg/mL.] ▶L ♀C ▶– $$$$$

DACLIZUMAB (*Zenapax*) Specialized dosing for <u>organ transplantation.</u> ▶L ♀C ▶? $$$$$

MYCOPHENOLATE MOFETIL (*Cellcept, Myfortic*) Specialized dosing for <u>organ transplantation.</u> [Generic/Trade: Caps 250 mg. Tabs 500 mg. Trade only (CellCept): Susp 200 mg/mL. Trade only (Myfortic): Tabs Extended-release: 180, 360 mg.] ▶? ♀D ▶? $$$$$

SIROLIMUS (*Rapamune*) Specialized dosing for <u>organ transplantation.</u> [Trade only: Soln 1 mg/mL (60 mL). Tabs 1, 2 mg.] ▶L ♀C ▶– $$$$$

TACROLIMUS (*Prograf, FK506*) Specialized dosing for <u>organ transplantation</u>. [Generic/Trade: Caps 0.5, 1, 5 mg.] ▶L ♀C ▶– $$$$$

Other

HYMENOPTERA VENOM Specialized <u>desensitization</u> dosing protocol. ▶Serum ♀C ▶? $$$$

TUBERCULIN PPD (*Aplisol, Tubersol, Mantoux, PPD*) 5 tuberculin units (0.1 mL) intradermally, read 48 to 72 h later. ▶L ♀C ▶+ $

TETANUS WOUND CARE (www.cdc.gov)		
	Unknown or less than 3 prior tetanus immunizations	3 or more prior tetanus immunizations
Non-tetanus prone wound (e.g., clean and minor)	Td (DT age younger than 7 yo)	Td if more than 10 years since last dose
Tetanus prone wound (eg, dirt, contamination, punctures, crush components)	Td (DT age younger than 7 yo), tetanus immune globulin 250 units IM at site other than Td	Td if more than 5 years since last dose

If patient age 10 yo or older has never received a pertussis booster consider DTaP (*Boostrix* if 10–18 yo, *Adacel* if 11–64 yo).

NEUROLOGY

Alzheimer's Disease—Cholinesterase Inhibitors

DONEPEZIL (*Aricept*)   Start 5 mg PO at bedtime. May increase to 10 mg PO at bedtime in 4 to 6 weeks for mild to moderate disease. For moderate to severe disease (MMSE 10 or less), may increase after 3 months to 23 mg/day. [Generic/Trade: Tabs 5, 10 mg. Trade only: Tab 23 mg. Orally disintegrating tabs 5, 10 mg.]   ▶LK ♀C ▶? $$$$

GALANTAMINE (*Razadyne, Razadyne ER, ✦Reminyl*)   Extended-release: Start 8 mg PO daily; increase to 16 mg after 4 weeks. May increase to 24 mg after another 4 weeks. Immediate-release: Start 4 mg PO bid with food; increase to 8 mg bid after 4 weeks. May increase to 12 mg bid after another 4 weeks. [Generic/Trade: Tabs (Razadyne) 4, 8, 12 mg. Extended-release caps (Razadyne ER) 8, 16, 24 mg. Oral soln 4 mg/mL. Prior to April 2005 was called Reminyl.]   ▶LK ♀B ▶? $$$$

RIVASTIGMINE (*Exelon, Exelon Patch*)   Alzheimer's disease: Start 1.5 mg PO bid with food. Increase to 3 mg bid after 2 weeks. Max 12 mg/day. Patch: Start 4.6 mg/24 h once daily; may increase after 1 month or more to max 9.5 mg/24 h. Dementia associated with Parkinson's disease: Start 1.5 mg PO bid with food. Increase by 3 mg/day at intervals greater than 4 weeks to max 12 mg/day. Patch: Start 4.6 mg/24 h once daily; may increase after 1 month or more to max 9.5 mg/24 h. [Trade only: Caps 1.5, 3, 4.5, 6 mg. Oral soln 2 mg/mL (120 mL). Transdermal patch: 4.6 mg/24 h (9 mg/patch), 9.5 mg/24 h (18 mg/patch).]   ▶K ♀B ▶? $$$$$

Alzheimer's Disease—NMDA Receptor Antagonists

MEMANTINE (*Namenda, Namenda XR, ✦Ebixa*)   Start 5 mg PO daily. Increase by 5 mg/day at weekly intervals to max 20 mg/day. Doses greater than 5 mg/day should be divided. Extended-release: start 7 mg once daily. Increase at weekly intervals to target dose of 28 mg/day. Reduce to 14 mg/day with renal impairment. [Trade only: Tabs 5, 10 mg. Oral soln 2 mg/mL. Extended-release caps 7, 14, 21, 28 mg.]   ▶LK ♀B ▶? $$$$

Anticonvulsants

CARBAMAZEPINE (*Tegretol, Tegretol XR, Carbatrol, Epitol, Equetro*)   Epilepsy: 200 to 400 mg PO bid to qid. Extended-release: 200 mg PO bid. Age younger than 6 yo: 10 to 20 mg/kg/day PO divided bid to qid. Age 6 to 12 yo: 100 mg PO bid or 50 mg PO qid; increase by 100 mg/day at weekly intervals divided tid to qid (regular-release), bid (extended-release), or qid (susp). Bipolar disorder, acute manic/mixed episodes (Equetro): Start 200 mg PO bid; increase by 200 mg/day to max 1600 mg/day. Aplastic anemia, agranulocytosis, many drug interactions. [Generic/Trade: Tabs 200 mg, Chewable tabs 100 mg, Susp 100 mg/5 mL. Extended-release tabs (Tegretol XR) 100, 200, 400 mg. Generic only: Tabs 100, 300, 400 mg, Chewable tabs 200 mg. Trade only: Extended-release caps (Carbatrol and Equetro): 100, 200, 300 mg.]   ▶LK ♀D ▶+ $$

CLOBAZAM (*★Frisium*) Canada only. Adults: Start 5 to 15 mg PO daily. Increase prn to max 80 mg/day. Children younger than 2 yo: 0.5 to 1 mg/kg PO daily. Children age 2 to 16 yo: Start 5 mg PO daily. May increase prn to max 40 mg/day. [Generic/Trade: Tabs 10 mg.] ▶L ♀X (first trimester) D (second/third trimesters) ▶– $

ETHOSUXIMIDE (*Zarontin*) <u>Absence seizures</u>, age 3 to 6 yo: Start 250 mg PO daily (or divided bid). Age older than 6 yo: Start 500 mg PO daily or bid. Max 1.5 g/day. [Generic/Trade: Caps 250 mg. Syrup 250 mg/5 mL.] ▶LK ♀C ▶+ $$$$

FELBAMATE (*Felbatol*) Start 400 mg PO tid. Max 3600 mg/day. Peds: Start 15 mg/kg/day PO divided tid to qid. Max 45 mg/kg/day. Aplastic anemia, hepatotoxicity. Not first line. Requires written informed consent. [Trade only: Tabs 400, 600 mg. Susp 600 mg/5 mL.] ▶KL ♀C ▶– $$$$$

FOSPHENYTOIN (*Cerebyx*) Load: 15 to 20 mg "phenytoin equivalents" (PE) per kg IM/IV no faster than 150 PE/min. Maintenance: 4 to 6 PE/kg/day. ▶L ♀D ▶+ $$$$$

GABAPENTIN (*Neurontin*) <u>Partial seizures, adjunctive therapy:</u> Start 300 mg PO at bedtime. Increase gradually to 300 to 600 mg PO tid. Max 3600 mg/day. <u>Postherpetic neuralgia:</u> Start 300 mg PO on day 1; increase to 300 mg bid on day 2, and to 300 mg tid on day 3. Max 1800 mg/day. <u>Partial seizures, initial monotherapy:</u> Titrate as above. Usual effective dose is 900 to 1800 mg/day. [Generic only: Tabs 100, 300, 400 mg. Generic/Trade: Caps 100, 300, 400 mg. Tabs scored 600, 800 mg. Soln 50 mg/mL.] ▶K ♀C ▶? $$$$

LACOSAMIDE (*Vimpat*) <u>Partial onset seizures, adjunctive</u> (17 yo and older): Start 50 mg PO/IV bid. Increase by 50 mg bid to recommended dose of 100 to 200 mg bid. Max 600 mg/day or 300 mg/day in mild/mod hepatic or severe renal impairment. [Trade only: Tabs 50, 100, 150, 200 mg.] ▶KL ♀C ▶? $$$$$

LAMOTRIGINE (*Lamictal, Lamictal CD, Lamictal ODT*) <u>Partial seizures, Lennox-Gastaut syndrome, or generalized tonic-clonic seizures adjunctive therapy with a single enzyme-inducing anticonvulsant.</u> Age 2 to 12 yo: dosing is based on wt and concomitant meds (see package insert). Age older than 12 yo: 50 mg PO daily for 2 weeks, then 50 mg bid for 2 weeks, then gradually increase to 150 to 250 mg bid. Also approved for conversion to monotherapy (age 16 yo or older): See package insert. Drug interaction with valproate (see package insert for adjusted dosing guidelines). Potentially life-threatening rashes reported in 0.3% of adults and 0.8% of children; discontinue at first sign of rash. [Generic/Trade: Chewable dispersible tabs (Lamictal CD) 2, 5, 25 mg. Tabs, 25, 100, 150, 200 mg. Trade only: Orally disintegrating tabs (Lamictal ODT) 25, 50, 100, 200 mg. Chewable dispersible tabs (Lamictal CD) 2 mg may not be available in all pharmacies; obtain through manufacturer representative, or by calling 888-825-5249.] ▶LK ♀C (see notes) ▶– $$$$

LEVETIRACETAM (*Keppra, Keppra XR*) <u>Partial seizures, juvenile myoclonic epilepsy (JME), or primary generalized tonic-clonic seizures (GTC), adjunctive:</u> Start 500 mg PO/IV bid or 1000 mg/day (Keppra XR, partial seizures only);

(cont.)

increase by 1000 mg/day q 2 weeks prn to max 3000 mg/day (partial seizures) or to target dose of 3000 mg/day (JME or GTC). IV route not approved for GTC or if age less than 16 yo. [Generic/Trade: Tabs 250, 500, 750, 1000 mg, Oral soln 100 mg/mL. Trade only: Tabs extended-release 500, 750 mg.] ▶K ♀C ▶? $$$$$

OXCARBAZEPINE (*Trileptal*) Start 300 mg PO bid. Titrate to 1200 mg/day (adjunctive) or 1200 to 2400 mg/day (monotherapy). Peds 2 to 16 yo: Start 8 to 10 mg/kg/day divided bid. Life-threatening rashes and hypersensitivity reactions. [Generic/Trade: Tabs (scored) 150, 300, 600 mg. Trade only: Oral susp 300 mg/5 mL.] ▶LK ♀C ▶– $$$$$

PHENOBARBITAL (*Luminal*) Load: 20 mg/kg IV at rate no faster than 60 mg/min. Maintenance: 100 to 300 mg/day PO given once daily or divided bid. Peds 3 to 5 mg/kg/day PO divided bid to tid. Many drug interactions. [Generic only: Tabs 15, 16.2, 30, 32.4, 60, 100 mg. Elixir 20 mg/5 mL.] ▶L ♀D –©IV $

PHENYTOIN (*Dilantin, Phenytek*) <u>Status epilepticus:</u> Load 15-20 mg/kg IV no faster than 50 mg/min, then 100 mg IV/PO q 6 to 8 h. <u>Epilepsy:</u> Oral load: 400 mg PO initially, then 300 mg in 2 h and 4 h. Maintenance: 5 mg/kg (or 300 mg PO) given once daily (extended-release) or divided tid (standard-release) and titrated to a therapeutic level. [Generic/Trade: Extended-release caps 30, 100 mg (Dilantin). Susp 125 mg/5 mL. Trade only: Extended-release caps 200, 300 mg (Phenytek). Chewable tabs 50 mg (Dilantin Infatabs). Generic only: Extended-release caps 200, 300 mg.] ▶L ♀D ▶+ $$

PREGABALIN (*Lyrica*) <u>Painful diabetic peripheral neuropathy:</u> Start 50 mg PO tid; may increase within 1 week to max 100 mg PO tid. <u>Postherpetic neuralgia:</u> Start 150 mg/day PO divided bid to tid. May increase within 1 week to max 300 mg/day divided bid to tid; max 600 mg/day. <u>Partial seizures</u> (adjunctive): Start 150 mg/day PO divided bid to tid; increase prn to max 600 mg/day divided bid to tid. <u>Fibromyalgia:</u> Start 75 mg PO bid; may increase to 150 mg bid within 1 week; max 225 mg bid. [Trade only: Caps 25, 50, 75, 100, 150, 200, 225, 300 mg. Oral solution 20 mg/mL (480 mL).] ▶K ♀C ▶? –©V $$$$$

PRIMIDONE (*Mysoline*) Start 100 to 125 mg PO at bedtime. Increase over 10 days to 250 mg tid to qid. Max 2 g/day. Metabolized to phenobarbital. [Generic/Trade: Tabs 50, 250 mg.] ▶LK ♀D ▶– $$$$

RUFINAMIDE (*Banzel*) Start 400 to 800 mg/day PO divided bid. Increase by 400 to 800 mg/day q 2 day to max 3200 mg/day. [Trade only: Tabs 200, 400 mg.] ▶K ♀C ▶? $$$$$

TIAGABINE (*Gabitril*) Start 4 mg PO daily. Increase by 4 to 8 mg/day at weekly intervals prn to max 32 mg/day for age 12 to 18 yo or max 56 mg/day for age older than 18 yo divided bid to qid. Avoid off-label use. [Trade only: Tabs 2, 4, 12, 16 mg.] ▶L ♀C ▶? $$$$$

TOPIRAMATE (*Topamax*) <u>Partial seizures or primary generalized tonic-clonic seizures, monotherapy</u> for age older than 10 yo: Start 25 mg PO bid (week 1), 50 mg bid (week 2), 75 mg bid (week 3), 100 mg bid (week 4), 150 mg bid (week 5), then 200 mg bid as tolerated. <u>Partial seizures, primary generalized tonic-clonic seizures, or Lennox-Gastaut syndrome,</u>

(cont.)

adjunctive therapy: Start 25 to 50 mg PO at bedtime. Increase weekly by 25 to 50 mg/day to usual effective dose of 200 mg PO bid. Doses greater than 400 mg/day not shown to be more effective. Migraine prophylaxis: Titrate to 50 mg PO bid over 4 weeks. [Trade: Tabs 25, 50, 100, 200 mg. Sprinkle Caps 15, 25 mg.] ▶K ♀C ▶? $$$$$

VALPROIC ACID (*Depakene, Depakote, Depakote ER, Depacon, Stavzor, divalproex, sodium valproate, ✦Epival, Deproic*) Epilepsy: 10 to 15 mg/kg/day PO/IV divided bid to qid (standard-release, delayed-release, or IV) or given once daily (Depakote ER). Titrate to max 60 mg/kg/day. Use rate no faster than 20 mg/min when given IV. Migraine prophylaxis: Start 250 mg PO bid (Depakote or Stavzor) or 500 mg PO daily (Depakote ER) for 1 week, then increase to max 1000 mg/day PO divided bid (Depakote or Stavzor) or given once daily (Depakote ER). Hepatotoxicity, drug interactions, reduce dose in elderly. [Generic/Trade: Immediate-release caps 250 mg (Depakene), syrup (Depakene, valproic acid) 250 mg/5 mL. Delayed-release tabs (Depakote) 125, 250, 500 mg, Extended-release tabs (Depakote ER) 250, 500 mg, Delayed-release sprinkle caps (Depakote) 125 mg. Trade only (Stavzor): Delayed-release caps 125, 250, 500 mg.] ▶L ♀D ▶+ $$$$

ZONISAMIDE (*Zonegran*) Start 100 mg PO daily. Titrate every 2 weeks to 200 to 400 mg/day given once daily or divided bid. Max 600 mg/day. Drug interactions. Contraindicated in sulfa allergy. [Generic/Trade: Caps 25, 50, 100 mg.] ▶LK ♀C ▶? $$$$

Migraine Therapy—Triptans (5-HT1 Receptor Agonists)

NOTE *May cause vasospasm. Avoid in ischemic or vasospastic heart disease, cerebrovascular syndromes, peripheral arterial disease, uncontrolled HTN, and hemiplegic or basilar migraine. Do not use within 24 h of ergots or other triptans. Risk of serotonin syndrome if used with SSRIs or MAOIs.*

ALMOTRIPTAN (*Axert*) 6.25 to 12.5 mg PO. May repeat in 2 h prn. Max 25 mg/day. Avoid MAOIs. [Trade only: Tabs 6.25, 12.5 mg.] ▶LK ♀C ▶? $$

ELETRIPTAN (*Relpax*) 20 to 40 mg PO. May repeat in 2 h prn. Max 40 mg/dose or 80 mg/24 h. Drug interactions. Avoid MAOIs. [Trade only: Tabs 20, 40 mg.] ▶LK ♀C ▶? $$$

FROVATRIPTAN (*Frova*) 2.5 mg PO. May repeat in 2 h prn. Max 7.5 mg/24 h. [Trade only: Tabs 2.5 mg.] ▶LK ♀C ▶? $

NARATRIPTAN (*Amerge*) 1 to 2.5 mg PO. May repeat in 4 h prn. Max 5 mg/24 h. [Generic/Trade: Tabs 1, 2.5 mg.] ▶KL ♀C ▶? $$$

RIZATRIPTAN (*Maxalt, Maxalt MLT*) 5 to 10 mg PO. May repeat in 2 h prn. Max 30 mg/24 h. MLT form dissolves on tongue without liquids. Avoid MAOIs. [Trade only: Tabs 5, 10 mg. Orally disintegrating tabs (MLT) 5, 10 mg.] ▶LK ♀C ▶? $$

SUMATRIPTAN (*Imitrex, Alsuma*) 4 to 6 mg SC. May repeat in 1 h prn. Max 12 mg/24 h. Tabs: 25 to 100 mg PO (50 mg most common). May repeat q 2 h prn with 25 to 100 mg doses. Max 200 mg/24 h. Intranasal spray: 5 to 20 mg q 2 h. Max 40 mg/24 h. Avoid MAOIs. [Injection (STATdose System) 4, 6 mg prefilled cartridges.] ▶LK ♀C ▶+ $$$

TREXIMET (sumatriptan + naproxen) 1 tab PO at onset; may repeat in 2 h. Max 2 tabs/24 h. [Trade only: Tabs 85 mg sumatriptan + 500 mg naproxen sodium.] ▶LK ♀C ▶– $$

ZOLMITRIPTAN (*Zomig, Zomig ZMT*) 1.25 to 2.5 mg PO q 2 h. Max 10 mg/ 24 h. Orally disintegrating tabs (ZMT) 2.5 mg PO. May repeat in 2 h prn. Max 10 mg/24 h. Nasal spray: 5 mg (1 spray) in 1 nostril. May repeat in 2 h. Max 10 mg/24 h. [Trade only: Tabs 2.5, 5 mg. Orally disintegrating tabs (ZMT) 2.5, 5 mg. Nasal spray 5 mg/spray.] ▶L ♀C ▶? $$

Migraine Therapy—Other

CAFERGOT (ergotamine + caffeine) 2 tabs PO at onset, then 1 tab q 30 min prn. Max 6 tabs/attack or 10/week. Drug interactions. Fibrotic complications. [Trade only: Tabs 1/100 mg ergotamine/caffeine.] ▶L ♀X ▶– $

DIHYDROERGOTAMINE (*D.H.E. 45, Migranal*) Soln (DHE 45) 1 mg IV/ IM/SC. May repeat in 1 h prn. Max 2 mg (IV) or 3 mg (IM/SC) per d. Nasal spray (Migranal): 1 spray in each nostril. May repeat in 15 min prn. Max 6 sprays/24 h or 8 sprays/week. Drug interactions. Fibrotic complications. [Trade only: Nasal spray 0.5 mg/spray (Migranal). Self-injecting soln (D.H.E 45): 1 mg/mL.] ▶L ♀X ▶– $$

FLUNARIZINE (*◆Sibelium*) Canada only. 10 mg PO at bedtime. [Generic/ Trade: Caps 5 mg.] ▶L ♀C ▶– $$

MIDRIN (isometheptene + dichloralphenazone + acetaminophen, Amidrine, Durdrin, Migquin, Migratine, Migrazone, Va-Zone) <u>Tension and vascular headache treatment:</u> 1 to 2 caps PO q 4 h. Max 8 caps/day. <u>Migraine treatment:</u> 2 caps PO single dose, then 1 cap q 1 h prn to max 5 caps within 12 h. [Generic only: Caps (isometheptene/dichloralphenazone/acetaminophen) 65/100/325 mg.] ▶L ♀? ▶? ©IV $

Multiple Sclerosis

DALFAMPRIDINE (*Ampyra*) 10 mg PO bid [Trade: Extended-release tabs 10 mg.] ▶K– ♀C ▶?

GLATIRAMER (*Copaxone*) <u>Multiple sclerosis:</u> 20 mg SC daily. [Trade only: Injection 20 mg single-dose vial.] ▶Serum ♀B ▶? $$$$$

INTERFERON BETA-1A (*Avonex, Rebif*) <u>Multiple sclerosis:</u> Avonex 30 mcg (6 million units) IM q week. Rebif start 8.8 mcg SC 3 times a week; titrate over 4 weeks to maintenance dose of 44 mcg 3 times a week. Suicidality, hepatotoxicity, blood dyscrasias. Follow LFTs and CBC. [Trade only (Avonex): Injection 30 mcg single-dose vial with or without albumin. Prefilled syringe 30 mcg. Trade only (Rebif): Starter kit 20 mcg prefilled syringe. Prefilled syringe 22, 44 mcg.] ▶L ♀C ▶? $$$$$

INTERFERON BETA-1B (*Betaseron*) <u>Multiple sclerosis:</u> Start 0.0625 mg SC every other day; titrate over 6 weeks to 0.25 mg (8 million units) SC every other day. Suicidality, hepatotoxicity. Follow LFTs. [Trade only: Injection 0.3 mg (9.6 million units) single-dose vial.] ▶L ♀C ▶? $$$$$

Dermatomes

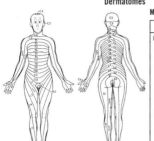

MOTOR FUNCTION BY NERVE ROOTS

Level	Motor Function
C3/C4/C5	Diaphragm
C5/C6	Deltoid/biceps
C7/C8	Triceps
C8/T1	Finger flexion/intrinsics
T1–T12	Intercostal/abd muscles
L2/L3	Hip flexion
L2/L3/L4	Hip adduction/quads
L4/L5	Ankle dorsiflexion
S1/S2	Ankle plantarflexion
S2/S3/S4	Rectal tone

LUMBOSACRAL NERVE ROOT COMPRESSION	Root	Motor	Sensory	Reflex
	L4	quadriceps	medial foot	knee-jerk
	L5	dorsiflexors	dorsum of foot	medial hamstring
	S1	plantarflexors	lateral foot	ankle-jerk

GLASGOW COMA SCALE		
Eye Opening	Verbal Activity	Motor Activity
4. Spontaneous	5. Oriented	6. Obeys commands
3. To command	4. Confused	5. Localizes pain
2. To pain	3. Inappropriate	4. Withdraws to pain
1. None	2. Incomprehensible	3. Flexion to pain
	1. None	2. Extension to pain
		1. None

Myasthenia Gravis

EDROPHONIUM (*Tensilon, Enlon*) Evaluation for myasthenia gravis: 2 mg IV over 15 to 30 sec (test dose) while on cardiac monitor, then 8 mg IV after 45 sec. Atropine should be readily available in case of cholinergic reaction. Duration of effect is 5 to 10 min. [10 mg/mL MDV vial.] ▶Plasma ♀C ▶? $

NEOSTIGMINE (*Prostigmin*) 15 to 375 mg/day PO in divided doses, or 0.5 mg IM/SC. [Trade only: Tabs 15 mg.] ▶L ♀C ▶? $$$$

PYRIDOSTIGMINE (*Mestinon, Mestinon Timespan, Regonal*) Myasthenia gravis: 60 to 200 mg PO tid (standard-release) or 180 mg PO daily or divided bid (extended-release). [Generic/Trade: Tabs 60 mg. Trade only: Extended-release tabs 180 mg. Syrup 60 mg/ 5 mL.] ▶Plasma, K ♀C ▶+ $$

Parkinsonian Agents—Anticholinergics

BENZTROPINE MESYLATE (*Cogentin*) <u>Parkinsonism:</u> 0.5 to 2 mg IM/PO/IV given once daily or divided bid. <u>Drug-induced extrapyramidal disorders:</u> 1 to 4 mg PO/IM/IV given once daily or divided bid. [Generic only: Tabs 0.5, 1, 2 mg.] ▶LK ♀C ▶? $

BIPERIDEN (*Akineton*) 2 mg PO tid to qid, max 16 mg/day. [Trade only: Tabs 2 mg.] ▶LK ♀C ▶? $$$

TRIHEXYPHENIDYL (*Artane*) Start 1 mg PO daily. Gradually increase to 6 to 10 mg/day divided tid. Max 15 mg/day. [Generic only: Tabs 2, 5 mg. Elixir 2 mg/5 mL.] ▶LK ♀C ▶? $

Parkinsonian Agents—COMT Inhibitors

ENTACAPONE (*Comtan*) Start 200 mg PO with each dose of carbidopa/levodopa. Max 8 tabs (1600 mg)/day. [Trade only: Tabs 200 mg.] ▶L ♀C ▶? $$$$$

Parkinsonian Agents—Dopaminergic Agents & Combinations

APOMORPHINE (*Apokyn*) Start 0.2 mL SC prn. May increase in 0.1 mL increments every few day. Monitor for orthostatic hypotension after initial dose and with dose escalation. Max 0.6 mL/dose or 2 mL/d. Potent emetic, pretreat with trimethobenzamide 300 mg PO tid starting 3 days prior to use and continue for age 2 mo or older. Contains sulfites. [Trade only: Cartridges (for injector pen, 10 mg/mL) 3 mL. Ampules (10 mg/mL) 2 mL.] ▶L ♀C ▶? $$$$$

CARBIDOPA-LEVODOPA (*Sinemet, Sinemet CR, Parcopa*) Start 1 tab (25/100 mg) PO tid. Increase q 1 to 4 days prn. Sustained-release: Start 1 tab (50/200 mg) PO bid; increase q 3 days prn. [Generic/Trade: Tabs (carbidopa/levodopa) 10/100, 25/100, 25/250 mg. sustained-release (Sinemet CR, carbidopa-levodopa ER) 25/100, 50/200 mg. Trade only: Orally disintegrating tablet (Parcopa) 10/100, 25/100, 25/250.] ▶L ♀C ▶– $$$$

PRAMIPEXOLE (*Mirapex, Mirapex ER*) Parkinson's disease: Start 0.125 mg PO tid. Gradually increase to 0.5 to 1.5 mg PO tid. Extended release: start 0.375 mg PO daily. May increase q 5 to 7 days first to 0.75 mg daily, then by 0.75 mg/d increments to max 4.5 mg/d. Restless leg syndrome: Start 0.125 mg PO 2 to 3 h prior to hs. May increase q 4 to 7 days to max 0.5 mg/dose. [Generic/Trade: Tabs 0.125, 0.25, 0.5, 1, 1.5 mg. Trade only: Tabs 0.75 mg, Tabs extended release 0.375, 0.75, 1.5, 3, 4.5 mg.] ▶K ♀C ▶? $$$$$

ROPINIROLE (*Requip, Requip XL*) Parkinson's disease: Start 0.25 mg PO tid, then gradually increase to 1 mg PO tid. Extended-release: Start 2 mg PO daily, then gradually titrate dose at weekly intervals. Max 24 mg/day. Restless legs syndrome: Start 0.25 mg PO 1 to 3 h before sleep for 2 d, then increase to 0.5 mg/day on day 3 to 7. Increase by 0.5 mg at weekly intervals per to max 4 mg/day given 1 to 3 h before sleep. [Generic/Trade: Tabs, immediate-release 0.25, 0.5, 1, 2, 3, 4, 5 mg. Trade only: Tabs extended-release 2, 3, 4, 6, 8 mg.] ▶L ♀C ▶? $$$$$

STALEVO (carbidopa + levodopa + entacapone) <u>Parkinson's disease</u> (converting from prior treatment using carbidopa-levodopa with or without entacapone): Start Stalevo tab that contains the same amount of carbidopa-levodopa as the patient was previously taking and titrate to desired response. May need to reduce levodopa dose if not already taking entacapone. [Trade only: Tabs (carbidopa/levodopa/entacapone): Stalevo 50 (12.5/50/200 mg), Stalevo 75 (18.75/75/200), Stalevo 100 (25/100/200 mg), Stalevo 125 (31.25/125/200), Stalevo 150 (37.5/150/200 mg), Stalevo 200 (50/200/200 mg).] ▶L ♀C ▶– $$$$$

Parkinsonian Agents—Monoamine Oxidase Inhibitors (MAOIs)

RASAGILINE (Azilect) <u>Parkinson's disease, monotherapy:</u> 1 mg PO every morning. <u>Parkinson's disease, adjunctive:</u> 0.5 mg PO every morning. Max 1 mg/day. Requires an MAOI diet. [Trade only: Tabs 0.5, 1 mg.] ▶L ♀C ▶? $$$$$

SELEGILINE (Eldepryl, Zelapar) 5 mg PO every morning and at noon, max 10 mg/day. Zelapar ODT: 1.25 to 2.5 mg every morning, max 2.5 mg/day. [Generic/Trade: Caps 5 mg. Tabs 5 mg. Trade only: Oral disintegrating tabs (Zelapar ODT) 1.25 mg.] ▶LK ♀C ▶? $$$$

Other Agents

BOTULINUM TOXIN TYPE A (Botox, Botox Cosmetic) Dose varies based on indication. [Trade only: 100 unit single-use vials.] ▶Not absorbed ♀C ▶? $$$$$

MANNITOL (Osmitrol, Resectisol) <u>Intracranial HTN:</u> 0.25 to 2 g/kg IV over 30 to 60 min. ▶K ♀C ▶? $$

MILNACIPRAN (Savella) Day 1: 12.5 mg PO once. Days 2 to 3: 12.5 mg BID. Days 4 to 7: 25 mg bid, then 50 mg bid thereafter. Max 200 mg/day. [Trade only: Tabs 12.5, 25, 50, 100 mg.] ▶LK ♀C ▶? $$$$

NIMODIPINE (Nimotop) <u>Subarachnoid hemorrhage:</u> 60 mg PO q 4 h for 21 days. [Generic only: Caps 30 mg.] ▶L ♀C ▶– $$$$$

OXYBATE (Xyrem, GHB, gamma hydroxybutyrate) <u>Narcolepsy-associated cataplexy or excessive daytime sleepiness:</u> 2.25 g PO at bedtime. Repeat in 2.5 to 4 h. May increase by 1.5 g/day at 2 week intervals to max 9 g/day. From a centralized pharmacy. [Trade only: Soln 180 mL (500 mg/mL) supplied with measuring device and child-proof dosing cups.] ▶L ♀B ▶? ©III $$$$$

RILUZOLE (Rilutek) <u>ALS:</u> 50 mg PO q 12 h. Monitor LFTs. [Trade only: Tabs 50 mg.] ▶LK ♀C ▶– $$$$$

TETRABENAZINE (Xenazine, ✦Nitoman) Start 12.5 mg PO every morning. Increase after 1 week to 12.5 mg PO bid. May increase by 12.5 mg/day weekly. For doses greater than 37.5 to 50 mg/day divide doses tid. For doses greater than 50 mg/day genotype for CYP2D6 and titrate by 12.5 mg/day weekly and divide tid to max 100 mg/day and 37.5 mg/dose (extensive/intermediate metabolizers) or 50 mg/day and 25 mg/dose (poor metabolizers). [Trade only: Tabs 12.5, 25 mg.] ▶L ♀C ▶? ? $$$$$

OB/GYN

Contraceptives—Oral Monophasic

OGESTREL (ethinyl estradiol + norgestrel) 1 subdermal implant q 3 years. [Trade only: Tabs: 50 mcg ethinyl estradiol/0.5 mg norgestrel.] ▶L ♀X ▶– $$

Contraceptives—Other

LEVONORGESTREL (Plan B) <u>Emergency contraception:</u> 1 tab PO ASAP but within 72 h of intercourse. 2nd tab 12 h later. [OTC Trade only: Kit contains 2 tabs 0.75 mg.] ▶L ♀X ▶– $$
LEVONORGESTREL 1S (Plan B One-Step) <u>Emergency contraception:</u> 1 tab PO ASAP but within 72 h of intercourse. [OTC Trade only: Tabs 1.5 mg.] ▶L ♀X ▶– $$
NUVARING (ethinyl estradiol vaginal ring + etonogestrel) 1 ring intravaginally for 3 weeks each month. [Trade only: Flexible intravaginal ring, 15 mcg ethinyl estradiol/0.120 mg etonogestrel/day in 1, 3 rings/box.] ▶L ♀X ▶– $$$
ORTHO EVRA (norelgestromin + ethinyl estradiol transdermal) (✚Evra) <u>Contraception:</u> 1 patch q week for 3 weeks, then 1 week patch-free. [Trade only: Transdermal patch: 150 mcg norelgestromin/20 mcg ethinyl estradiol/day in 1, 3 patches/box.] ▶L ♀X ▶– $$$

Estrogens

NOTE See also Hormone Combinations.

ESTERIFIED ESTROGENS (Menest) 0.3 to 1.25 mg PO daily. [Trade only: Tabs 0.3, 0.625, 1.25, 2.5 mg.] ▶L ♀X ▶– $$
ESTRADIOL (Estrace, Gynodiol) 1 to 2 mg PO daily. [Generic/Trade: Tabs, micronized 0.5, 1, 2 mg, scored. Trade only: 1.5 mg (Gynodiol).] ▶L ♀X ▶– $
ESTRADIOL ACETATE (Femtrace) 0.45 to 1.8 mg PO daily. [Trade only: Tabs, 0.45, 0.9, 1.8 mg.] ▶L ♀X ▶– $$
ESTRADIOL ACETATE VAGINAL RING (Femring) Insert and replace after 90 days. [Trade only: 0.05 mg/day and 0.1 mg/day.] ▶L ♀X ▶– $$$
ESTRADIOL CYPIONATE (Depo-Estradiol) 1 to 5 mg IM q 3 to 4 weeks. ▶L ♀X ▶– $
ESTRADIOL GEL (Divigel, Estrogel, Elestrin) Thinly apply contents of 1 complete pump depression to one entire arm (Estrogel) or upper arm (Elestrin) or contents of 1 foil packet (Divigel) to one upper thigh. [Trade only: Gel 0.06% in nonaerosol, metered-dose pump with #64 or #32 1.25 g doses (Estrogel), #100 0.87 g doses (Elestrin). Gel 0.1% in single-dose foil packets of 0.25, 0.5, 1.0 g, carton of 30 (Divigel).] ▶L ♀X ▶– $$$
ESTRADIOL TOPICAL EMULSION (Estrasorb) Rub in contents of 1 pouch each to left and right legs (spread over thighs and calves) qam. Daily dose is equivalent to two 1.74 g pouches. [Trade only: Topical emulsion, 56 pouches/carton.] ▶L ♀X ▶– $$

ESTRADIOL TRANSDERMAL PATCH (Alora, Climara, Esclim, Estraderm, FemPatch, Menostar, Vivelle, Vivelle Dot, ✦Estradot, Oesclim) Apply 1 patch weekly (Climara, FemPatch, Estradiol, Menostar) or twice a week (Esclim, Estraderm, Vivelle, Vivelle Dot, Alora). [Generic/Trade: Transdermal patches doses in mg/day: Climara (once a week) 0.025, 0.0375, 0.05, 0.075, 0.1. Trade only: FemPatch (once a week) 0.025. Esclim (twice per week) 0.025, 0.0375, 0.05, 0.075, 0.1. Vivelle, Vivelle Dot (twice per week) 0.025, 0.0375, 0.05, 0.075, 0.1. Estraderm (twice per week) 0.05, 0.1. Alora (twice per week) 0.025, 0.05, 0.075, 0.1.] ▶L ♀X ▶– $$

ESTRADIOL TRANSDERMAL SPRAY (Evamist) 1 to 3 sprays daily to forearm. [Trade only: Spray: 1.53 mg estradiol per 90 mcL spray, 56 sprays per metered-dose pump.] ▶L ♀X ▶– $$$

ESTRADIOL VAGINAL RING (Estring) Insert and replace after 90 days. [Trade only: 2 mg ring single pack.] ▶L ♀X ▶– $$$

ESTRADIOL VAGINAL TAB (Vagifem) 1 tab vaginally daily for 2 weeks, then 1 tab vaginally twice a week. [Trade only: Vaginal tab: 25 mcg in disposable single-use applicators, 8, 18/pack.] ▶L ♀X ▶– $$$

ESTRADIOL VALERATE (Delestrogen) 10 to 20 mg IM q 4 weeks. ▶L ♀X ▶– $$

ESTROGEN VAGINAL CREAM (Premarin, Estrace) Menopausal atrophic vaginitis: Premarin: 0.5 to 2 g daily. Estrace: 2 to 4 g daily for 2 weeks, then reduce. Moderate to severe menopausal dyspareunia: Premarin: 0.5 g daily, then reduce to twice a week. [Trade only: Vaginal cream (Premarin) 0.625 mg conjugated estrogens/g in 42.5 g with or without calibrated applicator. Estrace: 0.1 mg estradiol/g in 42.5 g with calibrated applicator. Generic only: Cream 0.625 mg synthetic conjugated estrogens/g in 30 g with calibrated applicator.] ▶L ♀X ▶? $$$$

ESTROGENS CONJUGATED (Premarin, C.E.S., Congest) 0.3 to 1.25 mg PO daily. Abnormal uterine bleeding: 25 mg IV/IM. Repeat in 6 to 12 h if needed. [Trade only: Tabs 0.3, 0.45, 0.625, 0.9, 1.25 mg.] ▶L ♀X ▶– $$$

ESTROGENS SYNTHETIC CONJUGATED A (Cenestin) 0.3 to 1.25 mg PO daily. [Trade only: Tabs 0.3, 0.45, 0.625, 0.9, 1.25 mg.] ▶L ♀X ▶– $$$

ESTROGENS SYNTHETIC CONJUGATED B (Enjuvia) 0.3 to 1.25 mg PO daily. [Trade only: Tabs 0.3, 0.45, 0.625, 0.9, 1.25 mg.] ▶L ♀X ▶– $$

ESTROPIPATE (Ogen, Ortho-Est) 0.75 to 6 mg PO daily. [Generic/Trade: Tabs 0.75, 1.5, 3, 6 mg of estropipate.] ▶L ♀X ▶– $

Hormone Combinations

NOTE See also Estrogens.

ACTIVELLA (estradiol + norethindrone) 1 tab PO daily. [Trade only: Tabs 1/0.5 and 0.5/0.1 mg estradiol/norethindrone acetate in calendar dial pack dispenser.] ▶L ♀X ▶– $$$

ANGELIQ (estradiol + drospirenone) 1 tab PO daily. [Trade only: Tabs 1 mg estradiol/0.5 mg drospirenone.] ▶L ♀X ▶– $$$

CLIMARA PRO (estradiol + levonorgestrel) 1 patch weekly. [Trade only: Transdermal 0.045/0.015 estradiol/levonorgestrel in mg/day, 4 patches/box.] ▶L ♀X ▶– $$$

EMERGENCY CONTRACEPTION Emergency contraception within 72 h of unprotected sex. Progestin-only methods (causes less nausea & may be more effective): *Plan B One-Step* (levonorgestrel 1.5 mg tab, OTC for age at least 17 yo): take one pill. *Plan B* (levonorgestrel 0.75 mg, OTC for age at least 18 yo): take one tab ASAP and 2nd dose 12 h later. Progestin and estrogen method: Dose is defined as 2 pills of *Ovral* or *Ogestrel*, 4 pills of *Cryselle, Levlen, Levora, Lo/Ovral, Nordette, Tri-Levlen*, Triphasil*, Trivora**, or *Low Ogestrel*, or 5 pills of *Alesse, Aviane, Lessina*, or *Levlit*: Take first dose ASAP and 2nd dose 12 h later. If vomiting occurs within 1 h of taking dose, consider repeating that dose with an antiemetic 1 h prior. More info at: www.not-2-late.com.

*Use 0.125 mg levonorgestrel/30 mcg ethinyl estradiol tabs.

COMBIPATCH (estradiol + norethindrone) (✦*Estalis*) 1 patch twice a week. [Trade only: Transdermal patch 0.05 estradiol/0.14 norethindrone and 0.05 estradiol/0.25 norethindrone in mg/day, 8 patches/box.] ▶L ♀X ▶– $$$

ESTRATEST (esterified estrogens + methyltestosterone) 1 tab PO daily. [Trade only: Tabs 1.25 mg esterified estrogens/2.5 mg methyltestosterone.] ▶L ♀X ▶– $$$$

ESTRATEST H.S. (esterified estrogens + methyltestosterone) 1 tab PO daily. [Trade only: Tabs 0.625 mg esterified estrogens/1.25 mg methyltestosterone.] ▶L ♀X ▶– $$$

FEMHRT (ethinyl estradiol + norethindrone) 1 tab PO daily. [Trade only: Tabs 5/1, 2.5/0.5 mcg ethinyl estradiol/mg norethindrone, 28/blister card.] ▶L ♀X ▶– $$$

PREFEST (estradiol + norgestimate) 1 pink tab PO daily for 3 days followed by 1 white tab PO daily for 3 days, sequentially throughout the month. [Trade only: Tabs in 30 days blister packs 1 mg estradiol (15 pink), 1 mg estradiol/0.09 mg norgestimate (15 white).] ▶L ♀X ▶– $$$

PREMPHASE (estrogens conjugated + medroxyprogesterone) 1 tab PO daily. [Trade only: Tabs in 28 days EZ-Dial dispensers: 0.625 mg conjugated estrogens (14), 0.625 mg/5 mg conjugated estrogens/medroxyprogesterone (14).] ▶L ♀X ▶– $$$

PREMPRO (estrogens conjugated + medroxyprogesterone) (✦*Premplus*) 1 tab PO daily. [Trade only: Tabs in 28-day EZ-Dial dispensers: 0.625 mg/5 mg, 0.625 mg/2.5 mg, 0.45 mg/1.5 mg (Prempro low dose), and 0.3 mg/1.5 mg conjugated estrogens/medroxyprogesterone.] ▶L ♀X ▶– $$$

SYNTEST D.S. (esterified estrogens + methyltestosterone) 1 tab PO daily. [Generic only: Tabs 1.25 mg esterified estrogens/2.5 mg methyltestosterone.] ▶L ♀X ▶– $$$

SYNTEST H.S. (esterified estrogens + methyltestosterone) 1 tab PO daily. [Generic only: Tabs 0.625 mg esterified estrogens/1.25 mg methyltestosterone.] ▶L ♀X ▶– $$$

Labor Induction/Cervical Ripening

DINOPROSTONE (*PGE2, Prepidil, Cervidil, Prostin E2*) Cervical ripening: 1 syringe of gel placed directly into the cervical os for cervical ripening or 1 insert in the posterior fornix of the vagina. [Trade only: Gel (Prepidil) 0.5 mg/3 g syringe. Vaginal insert (Cervidil) 10 mg. Vaginal supps (Prostin E2) 20 mg.] ▶Lung ♀C ▶? $$$$$

ORAL CONTRACEPTIVES* ▶L ♀X Monophasic	Estrogen (mcg)	Progestin (mg)
Norinyl 1+50, Ortho-Novum 1/50, Necon 1/50	50 mestranol	1 norethindrone
Ovcon-50		
Demulen 1/50, Zovia 1/50E	50 ethinyl estradiol	1 ethynodiol
Ovral, Ogestrel		0.5 norgestrel
Norinyl 1+35, Ortho-Novum 1/35, Necon 1/35, Nortrel 1/35		1 norethindrone
Brevicon, Modicon, Necon 0.5/35, Nortrel 0.5/35		0.5 norethindrone
Ovcon-35, Femcon Fe, Balziva	35 ethinyl estradiol	0.4 norethindrone
Previfem		0.18 norgestimate
Ortho-Cyclen, MonoNessa, Sprintec-28		0.25 norgestimate
Demulen 1/35, Zovia 1/35E, Kelnor 1/35		1 ethynodiol
Loestrin 21 1.5/30, Loestrin Fe 1.5/30, Junel 1.5/30, Junel 1.5/30 Fe, Microgestin Fe 1.5/30		1.5 norethindrone
Cryselle, Lo/Ovral, Low-Ogestrel		0.3 norgestrel
Apri, Desogen, Ortho-Cept, Reclipsen	30 ethinyl estradiol	0.15 desogestrel
Levlen, Levora, Nordette, Portia, Solia		0.15 levonorgestrel
Yasmin, Ocella		3 drospirenone
Loestrin 21 1/20, Loestrin Fe 1/20, Loestrin 24 Fe, Junel 1/20, Junel Fe 1/20, Microgestin 1/20		1 norethindrone
Alesse, Aviane, Lessina, Levlite, Lutera, Sronyx	20 ethinyl estradiol	0.1 levonorgestrel
Lybrel†		0.09 levonorgestrel
Yaz		3 drospirenone
Kariva, Mircette	20/10 eth estrad	0.15 desogestrel
Progestin-only		
Micronor, Nor-Q.D., Camila, Errin, Jolivette, Nora-BE	none	0.35 norethindrone
Biphasic (estrogen & progestin contents vary)		
Ortho Novum 10/11, Necon 10/11	35 eth estradiol	0.5/1 norethindrone
Triphasic (estrogen & progestin contents vary)		
Cyclessa, Velivet, Cesia	25 ethinyl estradiol	0.100/0.125/0.150 desogestrel
Ortho-Novum 7/7/7, Necon 7/7/7, Nortrel 7/7/7	35 ethinyl estradiol	0.5/0.75/1 norethindr
Tri-Norinyl, Leena, Aranelle		0.5/1/0.5 norethindrone
Enpresse, Tri-Levlen, Triphasil, Trivora-28	30/40/30 ethinyl estradiol	0.5/0.75/0.125 levonorgestrel
Ortho Tri-Cyclen, Trinessa, Tri-Sprintec, Tri-Previfem	35 eth estradiol	00.18/0.215/0.25 norgestimate
Ortho Tri-Cyclen Lo	25 eth estradiol	
Estrostep Fe, Tri-Legest, Tri-Legest Fe, Tilia Fe	20/30/35 eth estr	1 norethindrone
Extended Cycle††		
Seasonale, Quasense, Jolessa	30 ethinyl estradiol	0.15 levonorgestrel
Seasonique	30/10 eth estrad	0.15 levonorgestrel
LoSeasonique	20 ethinyl estradiol	0.1 levonorgestrel

*All: Not recommended in smokers. Increase risk of thromboembolism, CVA, MI, hepatic neoplasia, & gallbladder disease. Nausea, breast tenderness, & breakthrough bleeding are common transient side effects. Effectiveness reduced by hepatic enzyme-inducing drugs such as certain anticonvulsants and barbiturates, rifampin, rifabutin, griseofulvin, & protease inhibitors. Coadministration with St. John's wort may decrease efficacy. Vomiting or diarrhea may also increase the risk of contraceptive failure. Consider an additional form of birth control in above circumstances. See product insert for instructions on missing doses. Most available in 21 and 28 day packs. **Progestin only:** Must be taken at the same time every day. Because much of the literature regarding OC adverse effects pertains mainly to estrogen/progestin combinations, the extent to which progestin-only contraceptives cause these effects is unclear. No significant interaction has been found with broad-spectrum antibiotics. The effect of St. John's wort is unclear. Start new pack immediately after finishing current one. Available in 28 day packs. Readers may find the following website useful: www.managingcontraception.com. † Approved for continuous use without a "pill-free" period. †† 84 active pills and 7 placebo pills.

MISOPROSTOL- OB (*PGE1, Cytotec*) Cervical ripening: 25 mcg intravaginally q 3 to 6 h (or 50 mcg q 6 h). First trimester pregnancy failure: 800 mcg intravaginally, repeat on day 3 if expulsion incomplete. [Generic/Trade: Oral tabs 100, 200 mcg.] ▶LK ♀X ▶– $$$$

OXYTOCIN (*Pitocin*) Labor induction: 10 units in 1000 mL NS (10 milliunits/mL), start at 6 to 12 mL/h (1 to 2 milliunits/min). Postpartum bleeding: 10 units IM or 10 to 40 units in 1000 mL NS IV, infuse 20 to 40 milliunits/min. ▶LK ♀? ▶– $

Ovulation Stimulants

CLOMIPHENE (*Clomid, Serophene*) Specialized dosing for ovulation induction. [Generic/Trade: Tabs 50 mg, scored.] ▶L ♀D ▶? $$$$$

Progestins

HYDROXYPROGESTERONE CAPROATE Amenorrhea, dysfunctional uterine bleeding, metrorrhagia: 375 mg IM. Production of secretory endometrium and desquamation: 125 to 250 mg IM on 10th day of the cycle, repeat q 7 days until suppression no longer desired. ▶L ♀X ▶?

MEDROXYPROGESTERONE (*Provera*) 10 mg PO daily for last 10 to 12 days of month, or 2.5 to 5 mg PO daily. Secondary amenorrhea, abnormal uterine bleeding: 5 to 10 mg PO daily for 5 to 10 days. Endometrial hyperplasia: 10 to 30 mg PO daily. [Generic/Trade: Tabs 2.5, 5, 10, scored.] ▶L ♀X ▶+ $

MEDROXYPROGESTERONE—INJECTABLE (*Depo-Provera, depo-subQ provera 104*) Contraception/Endometriosis: 150 mg IM in deltoid or gluteus maximus or 104 mg SC in anterior thigh or abdomen q 13 weeks. ▶L ♀X ▶+ $

MEGESTROL (*Megace, Megace ES*) Endometrial hyperplasia: 40 to 160 mg PO daily for 3 to 4 months. AIDS anorexia: 800 mg (20 mL) susp PO daily or 625 mg (5 mL) ES daily. [Generic/Trade: Tabs 20, 40 mg. Susp 40 mg/mL in 240 mL. Trade only: Megace ES susp 125 mg/mL (150 mL).] ▶L ♀D ▶? $$$$$

NORETHINDRONE (*Aygestin, Micronor, Nor-Q.D., Camila, Errin, Jolivette, Nora-BE*) Amenorrhea, abnormal uterine bleeding: 2.5 to 10 mg PO daily for 5 to 10 days during the 2nd half of the menstrual cycle. Endometriosis: 5 mg PO daily for 2 weeks. Increase by 2.5 mg every 2 weeks to 15 mg. [Generic/Trade: Tabs scored 5 mg. Trade only: 0.35 mg tabs.] ▶L ♀D/X ▶See notes $

PROGESTERONE GEL (*Crinone, Prochieve*) Secondary amenorrhea: 45 mg (4%) intravaginally every other day up to 6 doses. If no response, use 90 mg (8%) every other day up to 6 doses. Infertility: Special dosing. [Trade only: 4%, 8% single-use, prefilled applicators.] ▶Plasma ♀– ▶? $$$

PROGESTERONE MICRONIZED (*Prometrium*) 200 mg PO at bedtime 10 to 12 days per month or 100 mg at bedtime daily. Secondary amenorrhea: 400 mg PO at bedtime for 10 days. Contraindicated in peanut allergy. [Trade only: Caps 100, 200 mg.] ▶L ♀B ▶+ $$

PROGESTERONE VAGINAL INSERT (*Endometrin*) Infertility: Special dosing. [Trade only: 100 mg vaginal insert.] ▶Plasma ♀– ▶? $$$$

Selective Estrogen Receptor Modulators

RALOXIFENE (*Evista*) <u>Osteoporosis</u> prevention/treatment, <u>breast cancer prevention:</u> 60 mg PO daily. [Trade only: Tabs 60 mg.] ▶L ♀X ▶− $$$$

TAMOXIFEN (*Nolvadex, Soltamox, Tamone, ✦Tamofen*) <u>Breast cancer prevention:</u> 20 mg PO daily for 5 years. <u>Breast cancer:</u> 10 to 20 mg PO bid. [Generic/Trade: Tabs 10, 20 mg. Trade only (Soltamox): Sugar-free soln 10 mg/5 mL (150 mL).] ▶L ♀D ▶− $$

Uterotonics

CARBOPROST (*Hemabate, 15-methyl-prostaglandin F2 alpha*) <u>Refractory postpartum uterine bleeding:</u> 250 mcg deep IM. ▶LK ♀C ▶? $$$

METHYLERGONOVINE (*Methergine*) <u>Refractory postpartum uterine bleeding:</u> 0.2 mg IM/PO tid–qid prn. [Trade only: Tabs 0.2 mg.] ▶LK ♀C ▶? $$

Vaginitis Preparations

NOTE See also STD/vaginitis table in antimicrobial section.

BORIC ACID <u>Resistant vulvovaginal candidiasis:</u> 1 vaginal suppository qhs for 2 weeks. [No commercial preparation; must be compounded by pharmacist. Vaginal supps 600 mg in gelatin caps.] ▶Not absorbed ♀? ▶− $

BUTOCONAZOLE (*Gynazole, Mycelex-3*) <u>Vulvovaginal candidiasis:</u> Mycelex 3: 1 applicatorful qhs for 3 to 6 days. Gynazole-1: 1 applicatorful intravaginally once qhs. [OTC Trade only (Mycelex 3): 2% vaginal cream in 5 g prefilled applicators (3s), 20 g tube with applicators. Rx: Trade only (Gynazole-1): 2% vaginal cream in 5 g prefilled applicator.] ▶LK ♀C ▶? $(OTC), $$$(Rx)

CLINDAMYCIN—VAGINAL (*Cleocin, Clindesse, ✦Dalacin*) <u>Bacterial vaginosis:</u> Cleocin: 1 applicatorful cream qhs for 7 days or 1 vaginal suppository qhs for 3 days. Clindesse: 1 applicatorful once. [Generic/Trade: 2% vaginal cream in 40 g tube with 7 disposable applicators (Cleocin). Vaginal suppository (Cleocin Ovules) 100 mg (3) with applicator. 2% vaginal cream in a single-dose prefilled applicator (Clindesse).] ▶L ♀− ▶+ $$

DRUGS GENERALLY ACCEPTED AS SAFE IN PREGNANCY (selected)

<u>Analgesics:</u> acetaminophen, codeine*, meperidine*, methadone*. <u>Antimicrobials:</u> penicillins, cephalosporins, erythromycins (not estolate), azithromycin, nystatin, clotrimazole, metronidazole, nitrofurantoin***, *Nix.* <u>Antivirals:</u> acyclovir, valacyclovir, famciclovir. <u>CV:</u> labetalol, methyldopa, hydralazine, nifedipine. <u>Derm:</u> erythromycin, clindamycin, benzoyl peroxide. <u>Endo:</u> insulin, liothyronine, levothyroxine. <u>ENT:</u> chlorpheniramine, diphenhydramine, dimenhydrinate, dextromethorphan, guaifenesin, nasal steroids, nasal cromolyn. <u>GI:</u> trimethobenzamide, antacids*, simethicone, cimetidine, famotidine, ranitidine, nizatidine, psyllium, metoclopramide, bisacodyl, docusate, doxylamine, meclizine. <u>Heme:</u> Heparin, low molecular wt heparins. <u>Psych:</u> desipramine, doxepin. <u>Pulmonary:</u> short-acting inhaled beta-2 agonists, cromolyn, nedocromil, beclomethasone, budesonide, theophylline, prednisone**.   *Except if used long-term or in high dose at term. **Except 1st trimester.   ***Contraindicated at term and during labor and delivery.

CLOTRIMAZOLE—VAGINAL (*Mycelex 7, Gyne-Lotrimin, ✦Canesten, Clotrimaderm*) <u>Vulvovaginal candidiasis:</u> 1 applicatorful 1% cream qhs for 7 days. 1 applicatorful 2% cream qhs for 3 days. 1 vaginal suppository 100 mg qhs for 7 days. 200 mg suppository qhs for 3 days. [OTC Generic/ Trade: 1% vaginal cream with applicator (some prefilled). 2% vaginal cream with applicator and 1% topical cream in some combination packs. OTC Trade only (Gyne-Lotrimin): Vaginal suppository 100 mg (7), 200 mg (3) with applicators.] ▶LK ♀B ▶? $

METRONIDAZOLE—VAGINAL (*MetroGel-Vaginal, Vandazole*) <u>Bacterial vaginosis:</u> 1 applicatorful qhs or bid for 5 days. [Generic/Trade: 0.75% gel in 70 g tube with applicator.] ▶LK ♀B ▶? $$

MICONAZOLE (*Monistat, Femizol-M, M-Zole, Micozole, Monazole*) <u>Vulvovaginal candidiasis:</u> 1 applicatorful qhs for 3 (4%) or 7 (2%) days. 100 mg vaginal suppository qhs for 7 days. 400 mg vaginal suppository qhs for 3 days. 1200 mg vaginal suppository once. [OTC Generic/Trade: 2% vaginal cream in 45 g with 1 applicator or 7 disposable applicators. Vaginal suppository 100 mg (7) OTC Trade only: 400 mg (3), 1200 mg (1) with applicator. Generic/Trade: 4% vaginal cream in 25 g tubes or 3 prefilled applicators. Some in combination packs with 2% miconazole cream for external use.] ▶LK ♀+ ▶? $

NYSTATIN—VAGINAL (*Mycostatin, ✦Nilstat, Nyaderm*) <u>Vulvovaginal candidiasis:</u> 1 vaginal tab qhs for 14 days. [Generic only: Vaginal tabs 100,000 units in 15s with applicator.] ▶Not metabolized ♀A ▶? $$

TERCONAZOLE (*Terazol*) <u>Vulvovaginal candidiasis:</u> 1 applicatorful of 0.4% cream qhs for 7 days, or 1 applicatorful of 0.8% cream qhs for 3 days, or 80 mg vaginal suppository qhs for 3 days. [All forms supplied with applicators: Generic/Trade: Vaginal cream 0.4% (Terazol 7) in 45 g tube, 0.8% (Terazol 3) in 20 g tube. Vaginal suppository (Terazol 3) 80 mg (#3).] ▶LK ♀C ▶– $$

TIOCONAZOLE (*Monistat 1-Day, Vagistat-1*) <u>Vulvovaginal candidiasis:</u> 1 applicatorful of 6.5% ointment intravaginally qhs single-dose. [OTC Trade only: Vaginal ointment: 6.5% (300 mg) in 4.6 g prefilled single-dose applicator.] ▶Not absorbed ♀C ▶– $

Other OB/GYN Agents

DANAZOL (*Danocrine, ✦Cyclomen*) <u>Endometriosis:</u> Start 400 mg PO bid, then titrate downward to maintain amenorrhea for 3 to 6 months. <u>Fibrocystic breast disease:</u> 100 to 200 mg PO bid for 4 to 6 months. [Generic only: Caps 50, 100, 200 mg.] ▶L ♀X ▶– $$$$$

MIFEPRISTONE (*Mifeprex, RU-486*) 600 mg PO 1 followed by 400 mcg misoprostol on day 3, if abortion not confirmed. [Trade only: Tabs 200 mg.] ▶L ♀X ▶? $$$$$

PREMESIS-RX (pyridoxine + folic acid + cyanocobalamin + calcium carbonate) <u>Pregnancy-induced nausea:</u> 1 tab PO daily. [Trade only: Tabs 75 mg vitamin B6 (pyridoxine), sustained-release, 12 mcg vitamin B12 (cyanocobalamin), 1 mg folic acid, and 200 mg calcium carbonate.] ▶L ♀A ▶+ $$

RHO IMMUNE GLOBULIN (*HyperRHO S/D, MICRhoGAM, RhoGAM, Rhophylac, WinRho SDF*) 300 mcg vial IM to mother at 28 weeks gestation followed by a second dose within 72 h of delivery (if mother Rh− and baby is or might be Rh+). Microdose (50 mcg, MICRhoGAM) is appropriate if spontaneous abortion less than 12 weeks gestation. ▶L ♀C ▶? $$$$$

ONCOLOGY

ALKYLATING AGENTS altretamine (*Hexalen*), bendamustine (*Treanda*), busulfan (*Myleran, Busulfex*), carmustine (*BCNU, BiCNU, Gliadel*), chlorambucil (*Leukeran*), cyclophosphamide (*Cytoxan, Neosar*), dacarbazine (*DTIC-Dome*), ifosfamide (*Ifex*), lomustine (*CeeNu, CCNU, CCNU*), mechlorethamine (*Mustargen*), melphalan (*Alkeran*), procarbazine (*Matulane*), streptozocin (*Zanosar*), temozolomide (*Temodar*, ✦*Temodal*), thiotepa (*Thioplex*). **ANTIBIOTICS:** bleomycin (*Blenoxane*), dactinomycin (*Cosmegen*), daunorubicin (*Cerubidine*), doxorubicin liposomal (*Doxil*, ✦*Caelyx, Myocet*), doxorubicin non-liposomal (*Adriamycin, Rubex*), epirubicin (*Ellence*, ✦*Pharmorubicin*), idarubicin (*Idamycin*), mitomycin (*Mutamycin, Mitomycin-C*), mitoxantrone (*Novantrone*), valrubicin (*Valstar*, ✦*Valtaxin*). **ANTIMETABOLITES:** azacitidine (*Vidaza*), capecitabine (*Xeloda*), cladribine (*Leustatin, chlorodeoxyadenosine*), clofarabine (*Clolar*), cytarabine (*Cytosar, AraC*), cytarabine liposomal (*Depo-Cyt*), decitabine (*Dacogen*), floxuridine (*FUDR*), fludarabine (*Fludara*), fluorouracil (*Adrucil, 5-FU*), gemcitabine (*Gemzar*), hydroxyurea (*Hydrea, Droxia*), mercaptopurine (*6-MP, Purinethol*), methotrexate, nelarabine (*Arranon*), pemetrexed (*Alimta*), pentostatin (*Nipent*), pralatrexate (*Folotyn*), thioguanine (*Tabloid*, ✦*Lanvis*). **CYTOPROTECTIVE AGENTS:** amifostine (*Ethyol*), dexrazoxane (*Zinecard, Totect*), mesna (*Mesnex*, ✦*Uromitexan*), palifermin (*Kepivance*). **HORMONES:** anastrozole (*Arimidex*), bicalutamide (*Casodex*), cyproterone, (✦*Androcur, Androcur Depot*), degarelix (*Firmagon*), estramustine (*Emcyt*), exemestane (*Aromasin*), flutamide (*Eulexin*, ✦*Euflex*), fulvestrant (*Faslodex*), goserelin (*Zoladex*), histrelin (*Vantas, Supprelin LA*), letrozole (*Femara*), leuprolide (*Eligard, Lupron, Lupron Depot, Lupron Depot-Ped*), nilutamide (*Nilandron*),raloxifene (*Evista*), toremifene (*Fareston*), triptorelin (*Trelstar Depot*). **IMMUNOMODULATORS:** aldesleukin (*Proleukin, interleukin-2*), alemtuzumab (*Campath*, ✦*MabCampath*), BCG (*Bacillus of Calmette & Guerin, Pacis, TheraCys, Tice BCG*, ✦*Oncotice*, ✦*Immucyst*), bevacizumab (*Avastin*), cetuximab (*Erbitux*), denileukin (*Ontak*), everolimus (*Afinitor*), ibritumomab (*Zevalin*), interferon alfa-2b (*Intron-A*), lenalidomide (*Revlimid*), ofatumumab (*Arzerra*), panitumumab (*Vectibix*), rituximab (*Rituxan*), temsirolimus (*Torisel*), thalidomide (*Thalomid*) tositumomab (*Bexxar*), trastuzumab (*Herceptin*). **MITOTIC INHIBITORS:** cabazitaxel (*Jevtana*), docetaxel (*Taxotere*), ixabepilone (*Ixempra*), paclitaxel (*Taxol, Abraxane, Onxol*), vinblastine (*Velban, VLB*), vincristine (*Oncovin*,

(cont.)

Vincasar, VCR), vinorelbine (*Navelbine*). **PLATINUM-CONTAINING AGENTS:** carboplatin (*Paraplatin*), cisplatin (*Platinol-AQ*), oxaliplatin (*Eloxatin*). **RADIOPHARMACEUTICALS:** samarium 153 (*Quadramet*), strontium-89 (*Metastron*). **TOPOISOMERASE INHIBITORS:** etoposide (*VP-16, Etopophos, Toposar, VePesid*), irinotecan (*Camptosar*), teniposide (*Vumon, VM-26*), topotecan (*Hycamtin*) **MISCELLANEOUS:** arsenic trioxide (*Trisenox*), asparaginase (*Elspar, ✦Kidrolase*), bexarotene (*Targretin*), bortezomib (*Velcade*), dasatinib (*Sprycel*), erlotinib (*Tarceva*) gefitinib (*Iressa*), imatinib (*Gleevec*), lapatinib (*Tykerb*), leucovorin (*folinic acid*), levoleucovorin (*Fusilev*), mitotane (*Lysodren*), nilotinib (*Tasigna*), pazopanib (*Votrient*), pegaspargase (*Oncaspar*), porfimer (*Photofrin*), rasburicase (*Elitek*), romidepsin (*Istodax*), sorafenib (*Nexavar*), sunitinib (*Sutent*), tretinoin (*Vesanoid*), vorinostat (*Zolinza*).

OPHTHALMOLOGY

NOTE *Most eye medications can be administered 1 gtt at a time despite common manufacturer recommendations of 1 to 2 gtts concurrently. Even a single gtt is typically more than the eye can hold, and thus a second gtt is wasteful and increases the possibility of systemic toxicity. If 2 gtts of the medication are desired, separate single gtt by at least 5 min.*

Antiallergy—Decongestants & Combinations

NAPHAZOLINE (*Albalon, All Clear, AK-Con, Naphcon, Clear Eyes*) 1 to 2 gtts in each affected eye qid for up to 3 days. [OTC Generic/Trade: Soln 0.012, 0.025% (15, 30 mL). Rx Generic/Trade: 0.1% (15 mL).] ▶? ♀C ▶? \$
NAPHCON-A (naphazoline + pheniramine, *Visine-A*) 1 gtt in each affected eye qid prn for up to 3 days. [OTC Trade only: Soln 0.025% + 0.3% (15 mL).] ▶L ♀C ▶? \$
VASOCON-A (naphazoline + antazoline) 1 gtt in each affected eye qid prn for up to 3 days. [OTC Trade only: Soln 0.05% + 0.5% (15 mL).] ▶L ♀C ▶? \$

Antiallergy—Dual Antihistamine & Mast Cell Stabilizer

AZELASTINE—OPHTHALMIC (*Optivar*) 1 gtt in each affected eye bid. [Trade only: Soln 0.05% (6 mL).] ▶L ♀C ▶? \$\$\$
EPINASTINE (*Elestat*) 1 gtt in each affected eye bid. [Trade only: Soln 0.05% (5 mL).] ▶K ♀C ▶? \$\$\$\$
KETOTIFEN—OPHTHALMIC (*Alaway, Zaditor*) 1 gtt in each affected eye q 8 to 12 h. [OTC Generic/Trade: Soln 0.025% (5 mL).] ▶Minimal absorption ♀C ▶? \$
OLOPATADINE (*Pataday, Patanol*) 1 gtt of 0.1% soln in each affected eye bid (Patanol) or 1 gtt of 0.2% soln in each affected eye daily (Pataday). [Trade only: Soln 0.1% (5 mL, Patanol), 0.2% (2.5 mL, Pataday).] ▶K ♀C ▶? \$\$\$\$

Antiallergy—Pure Antihistamines

BEPOTASTINE (*Bepreve*) 1 gtt in each affected eye(s) bid [Trade only: Soln 1.5% (2.5, 5, 10 mL)] ▶L (but minimal absorption) - ♀C ▶? $$$

EMEDASTINE (*Emadine*) 1 gtt in each affected eye daily to qid. [Trade only: Soln 0.05% (5 mL).] ▶L ♀B ▶? $$$

LEVOCABASTINE—OPHTHALMIC (*Livostin*) 1 gtt in each affected eye daily to qid for 2 weeks. [Trade only: Susp 0.05% (5, 10 mL).] ▶Minimal absorption ♀C ▶? $$$

Antiallergy—Pure Mast Cell Stabilizers

CROMOLYN—OPHTHALMIC (*Crolom, Opticrom*) 1 to 2 gtts in each affected eye 4 to 6 times a day. [Generic/Trade: Soln 4% (10 mL).] ▶LK ♀B ▶? $$

LODOXAMIDE (*Alomide*) 1 to 2 gtts in each affected eye qid. [Trade only: Soln 0.1% (10 mL).] ▶K ♀B ▶? $$$

NEDOCROMIL—OPHTHALMIC (*Alocril*) 1 to 2 gtts in each affected eye bid. [Trade only: Soln 2% (5 mL).] ▶L ♀B ▶? $$$

PEMIROLAST (*Alamast*) 1 to 2 gtts in each affected eye qid. [Trade only: Soln 0.1% (10 mL).] ▶? ♀C ▶? $$$

Antibacterials—Aminoglycosides

GENTAMICIN—OPHTHALMIC (*Garamycin, Genoptic, Gentak, ✦Diogent*) 1 to 2 gtts in each affected eye q 2 to 4 h; ½ inch ribbon of ointment bid to tid. [Generic/Trade: Soln 0.3% (5, 15 mL), Ointment 0.3% (3.5 g tube).] ▶K ♀C ▶? $

TOBRAMYCIN—OPHTHALMIC (*Tobrex*) 1 to 2 gtts in each affected eye q 1 to 4 h or ½ inch ribbon of ointment q 3 to 4 h or bid to tid. [Generic/Trade: Soln 0.3% (5 mL). Trade only: Ointment 0.3% (3.5 g tube).] ▶K ♀B ▶− $

Antibacterials—Fluoroquinolones

BESIFLOXACIN (*Besivance*) 1 gtt in each affected eye tid for 7 days. [Trade: solution 0.6% (5 mL).] ▶LK ♀C ▶? ?

CIPROFLOXACIN—OPHTHALMIC (*Ciloxan*) 1 to 2 gtts in each affected eye q 1 to 6 h or ½ inch ribbon ointment bid to tid. [Generic/Trade: Soln 0.3% (2.5, 5, 10 mL). Trade only: Ointment 0.3% (3.5 g tube).] ▶LK ♀C ▶? $$

GATIFLOXACIN—OPHTHALMIC (*Zymaxid*) 1 to 2 gtts in each affected eye q 2 h while awake (up to 8 times per day) on day 1 and 2, then 1 to 2 gtts q 4 h (up to qid) on days 3 to 7. [Trade only: Soln 0.3% (5 mL).] ▶K ♀C ▶? $$$

LEVOFLOXACIN—OPHTHALMIC (*Iquix, Quixin*) Quixin: 1 to 2 gtts in each affected eye q 2 h while awake (up to 8 times per day) on days 1 and 2, then 1 to 2 gtts q 4 h (up to qid) on days 3 to 7. Iquix: 1 to 2 gtts q 30 min to 2 h while awake and q 4 to 6 h overnight on days 1 to 3, then 1 to 2 gtts q 1 to 4 h while awake on day 4 to completion of therapy. [Trade only: Soln 0.5% (Quixin, 5 mL), 1.5% (Iquix, 5 mL).] ▶KL ♀C ▶? $$$

MOXIFLOXACIN—OPHTHALMIC (*Vigamox*) 1 gtt in each affected eye tid for 7 days. [Trade only: Soln 0.5% (3 mL).] ▶LK ♀C ▶? $$$

OFLOXACIN—OPHTHALMIC (*Ocuflox*) 1 to 2 gtts in each affected eye q 1 to 6 h for 7 to 10 days. [Generic/Trade: Soln 0.3% (5, 10 mL).] ▶LK ♀C ▶? $$

Antibacterials—Other

AZITHROMYCIN—OPHTHALMIC (*Azasite*) 1 gtt in each affected eye bid for 2 days, then 1 gtt once daily for 5 more days. [Trade only: Soln 1% (2.5 mL).] ▶L ♀B ▶? $$$

BACITRACIN—OPHTHALMIC (*AK Tracin*) Apply ¼ to ½ inch ribbon of ointment in each affected eye q 3 to 4 h or bid to qid for 7 to 10 days. [Generic/Trade: Ointment 500 units/g (3.5 g tube).] ▶L ♀C ▶? $

ERYTHROMYCIN—OPHTHALMIC (*Ilotycin, AK-Mycin*) ½ inch ribbon of ointment in each affected eye q 3 to 4 h or 2 to 6 times per day. [Generic only: Ointment 0.5% (1, 3.5 g tube).] ▶L ♀B ▶+ $

NEOSPORIN OINTMENT—OPHTHALMIC (neomycin + bacitracin + polymyxin) ½ inch ribbon of ointment in each affected eye q 3 to 4 h for 7 to 10 days or ½ inch ribbon 2 to 3 times per day for mild to moderate infection. [Generic only: Ointment. (3.5 g tube).] ▶K ♀C ▶? $

NEOSPORIN SOLUTION—OPHTHALMIC (neomycin + polymyxin + gramicidin) 1 to 2 gtts in each affected eye q 4 to 6 h for 7 to 10 days. [Generic/Trade: Soln (10 mL).] ▶KL ♀C ▶? $$

POLYSPORIN—OPHTHALMIC (polymyxin + bacitracin) ½ inch ribbon of ointment in each affected eye q 3 to 4 h for 7 to 10 days or ½ inch ribbon bid to tid for mild to moderate infection. [Generic only: Ointment (3.5 g tube).] ▶K ♀C ▶? $$

POLYTRIM—OPHTHALMIC (polymyxin + trimethoprim) 1 to 2 gtts in each affected eye q 4 to 6 h (up to 6 gtts/day) for 7 to 10 days. [Generic/Trade: Soln (10 mL).] ▶KL ♀C ▶? $$

SULFACETAMIDE—OPHTHALMIC (*Bleph-10, Sulf-10*) 1 to 2 gtts in each affected eye q 2 to 6 h for 7 to 10 days or ½ inch ribbon of ointment q 3 to 8 h for 7 to 10 days. [Generic/Trade: Soln 10% (15 mL), Ointment 10% (3.5 g tube). Generic only: Soln 30% (15 mL).] ▶K ♀C ▶– $

Antiviral Agents

GANCICLOVIR (*Zirgan*) <u>Herpetic keratitis:</u> 1 gtt 5 times per day (approximately q3h) until ulcer heals, then 1 gtt 3 times/day for 7 days. [Trade only: Gel 0.15% (5g).] ▶Minimal absorption ♀C ▶? $$$$

TRIFLURIDINE (*Viroptic*) <u>Herpes:</u> 1 gtt q 2 to 4 h for 7 to 14 days, max 9 gtts per day and max of 21 days of therapy. [Generic/Trade Soln 1% (7.5 mL).] ▶Minimal absorption ♀C ▶– $$$

Corticosteroid & Antibacterial Combinations

NOTE *Recommend that only ophthalmologists or optometrists prescribe due to infection, cataract, corneal/scleral perforation, and glaucoma risk from prolonged use. Monitor intraocular pressure.*

BLEPHAMIDE **(prednisolone—ophthalmic + sulfacetamide)** 1 to 2 gtts in each affected eye q 1 to 8 h or ½ inch ribbon to lower conjunctival sac 3 to 4 times per day and 1 to 2 times at bedtime. [Generic/Trade: Soln/Susp (5, 10 mL). Trade only: Ointment (3.5 g tube).] ▶KL ♀C ▶? $

CORTISPORIN—OPHTHALMIC **(neomycin + polymyxin + hydrocortisone - ophthalmic)** 1 to 2 gtts or ½ inch ribbon of ointment in each affected eye q 3 to 4 h or more frequently prn. [Generic only: Susp (7.5 mL). Ointment (3.5 g tube).] ▶LK ♀C ▶? $

FML-S LIQUIFILM **(prednisolone - ophthalmic + sulfacetamide)** 1 to 2 gtts in each affected eye q 1 to 8 h or ½ inch ribbon of ointment daily to qid. [Trade only: Susp (10 mL).] ▶KL ♀C ▶? $$

MAXITROL **(dexamethasone—ophthalmic + neomycin + polymyxin)** Ointment: Small amount (about ½ inch) in affected eye 3 to 4 times per day or at bedtime as an adjunct with gtts. Susp: 1 to 2 gtts into affected eye q 3 to 4 h; in severe disease, gtts may be used hourly and tapered to discontinuation. [Generic/Trade: Susp (5 mL), Ointment (3.5 g tube).] ▶L ♀C ▶? $

PRED G **(prednisolone—ophthalmic + gentamicin)** 1 to 2 gtts in each affected eye q 1 to 8 h daily to qid or ½ inch ribbon of ointment bid to qid. [Trade only: Susp (2, 5, 10 mL). Ointment (3.5 g tube).] ▶KL ♀C ▶? $$

TOBRADEX **(tobramycin + dexamethasone—ophthalmic)** 1 to 2 gtts in each affected eye q 2 to 6 h or ½ inch ribbon of ointment bid to qid. [Trade only (tobramycin 0.3%/dexamethasone 0.1%): Susp (2.5, 5, 10 mL), Ointment (3.5 g tube).] ▶L ♀C ▶? $$$

TOBRADEX ST **(tobramycin + dexamethasone—ophthalmic)** 1 gtt in each affected eye q 2 to 6 h. [Trade only: Susp (tobramycin 0.3%/dexamethasone 0.05%: Susp (2.5, 5, 10 mL).] ▶L ♀C ▶? $$$

VASOCIDIN **(prednisolone—ophthalmic + sulfacetamide)** 1 to 2 gtts in each affected eye q 1 to 8 h or ½ inch ribbon of ointment daily to qid. [Generic only: Soln (5, 10 mL).] ▶KL ♀C ▶? $

ZYLET **(loteprednol + tobramycin)** 1 to 2 gtts in each affected eye q 1 to 2 h for 1 to 2 days then 1 to 2 gtts q 4 to 6 h. [Trade only: Susp 0.5% loteprednol + 0.3% tobramycin (2.5, 5, 10 mL).] ▶LK ♀C ▶? $$$

Corticosteroids

NOTE *Recommend that only ophthalmologists or optometrists prescribe due to infection, cataract, corneal/scleral perforation, and glaucoma risk from prolonged use. Monitor intraocular pressure.*

DIFLUPREDNATE (***Durezol***) 1 gtt into affected eye qid, beginning 24 h after surgery for 2 weeks, then 1 gtt into affected eye bid for 1 week, then taper based on response. [Trade only: Ophthalmic emulsion 0.05% (2.5, 5 mL).] ▶Not absorbed ♀C ▶? $$$$

FLUOROMETHOLONE (***FML, FML Forte, Flarex***) 1 to 2 gtts in each affected eye q 1 to 12 h or ½ inch ribbon of ointment q 4 to 24 h. [Trade only: Susp (5, 10, 15 mL), 0.25% (2, 5, 10, 15 mL); Ointment 0.1% (3.5 g tube).] ▶L ♀C ▶? $$

LOTEPREDNOL (*Alrex, Lotemax*) 1 to 2 gtts in each affected eye qid. [Trade only: Susp 0.2% (Alrex 5, 10 mL), 0.5% (Lotemax 2.5, 5, 10, 15 mL).] ▶L ♀C ▶? $$$

PREDNISOLONE—OPHTHALMIC (*Pred Forte, Pred Mild, Inflamase Forte, Econopred Plus, ✦AK Tate, Diopred*) Soln: 1 to 2 gtts in each affected eye (up to q 1 h during day and q 2 h at night); when response observed, then 1 gtt in each affected eye q 4 h, then 1 gtt tid to qid. Susp: 1 to 2 gtts in each affected eye bid to qid. [Generic/Trade: Soln, Susp 1% (5, 10, 15 mL). Trade only (Pred Mild): Susp 0.12% (5, 10 mL). Susp (Pred Forte) 1% (1 mL).] ▶L ♀C ▶? $$

RIMEXOLONE (*Vexol*) 1 to 2 gtts in each affected eye q 1 to 6 h. [Trade only: Susp 1% (5, 10 mL).] ▶L ♀C ▶? $$

Glaucoma Agents—Beta-Blockers

NOTE *Use caution in cardiac conditions and asthma.*

BETAXOLOL—OPHTHALMIC (*Betoptic, Betoptic S*) 1 to 2 gtts in each affected eye bid. [Trade only: Susp 0.25% (5, 10, 15 mL). Generic only: Soln 0.5% (5, 10, 15 mL).] ▶LK ♀C ▶? $

CARTEOLOL—OPHTHALMIC (*Ocupress*) 1 gtt in each affected eye bid. [Generic only: Soln 1% (5, 10, 15 mL).] ▶LK ♀C ▶? $

LEVOBUNOLOL (*Betagan*) 1 to 2 gtts in each affected eye daily to bid. [Generic/Trade: Soln 0.25% (5, 10 mL), 0.5% (5, 10, 15 mL. Trade only: Soln 0.25% 2 mL).] ▶? ♀C ▶– $$

METIPRANOLOL (*Optipranolol*) 1 gtt in each affected eye bid. [Generic/Trade: Soln 0.3% (5, 10 mL).] ▶? ♀C ▶? $

TIMOLOL—OPHTHALMIC (*Betimol, Timoptic, Timoptic XE, Istalol, Timoptic Ocudose*) 1 gtt in each affected eye bid. Timoptic XE, Istalol: 1 gtt in each affected eye daily. [Generic/Trade: Soln 0.25, 0.5% (5, 10, 15 mL). Preservative-free soln (Timoptic Ocudose) 0.25% (0.2 mL). Gel-forming soln (Timoptic XE) 0.25, 0.5% (2.5, 5 mL).] ▶LK ♀C ▶+ $$

Glaucoma Agents—Carbonic Anhydrase Inhibitors

NOTE *Sulfonamide derivatives; verify absence of sulfa allergy before prescribing.*

BRINZOLAMIDE (*Azopt*) 1 gtt in each affected eye tid. [Trade only: Susp 1% (5, 10, 15 mL).] ▶LK ♀C ▶? $$$

DORZOLAMIDE (*Trusopt*) 1 gtt in each affected eye tid. [Generic/Trade: Soln 2% (5, 10 mL).] ▶KL ♀C ▶– $$$

METHAZOLAMIDE (*Neptazane*) 25 to 50 mg PO daily (up to tid). [Generic only: Tabs 25, 50 mg.] ▶LK ♀C ▶? $$

Glaucoma Agents—Miotics

PILOCARPINE—OPHTHALMIC (*Pilopine HS, Isopto Carpine, ✦Diocarpine, Akarpine*) 1 gtt in each affected eye up to qid or ½ inch ribbon of gel bedtime.

(cont.)

[Generic only: Soln 0.5% (15 mL), 1% (2 mL), 2% (2 mL), 3% (15 mL), 4% (2 mL), 6% (15 mL). Trade only (Pilopine HS): Gel 4% (4 g tube).] ▶Plasma ♀C ▶? $

Glaucoma Agents—Prostaglandin Analogs

BIMATOPROST (*Lumigan, Latisse*) 1 gtt to eyelashes at bedtime. [Trade only: Soln 0.03% (Lumigan, 2.5, 5, 7.5 mL), (Latisse, 3 mL with 60 sterile, disposable applicators).] ▶LK ♀C ▶? $$$

LATANOPROST (*Xalatan*) 1 gtt in each affected eye at bedtime. [Trade only: Soln 0.005% (2.5 mL).] ▶LK ♀C ▶? $$$

TRAVOPROST (*Travatan, Travatan Z*) 1 gtt in each affected eye at bedtime. [Trade only: Soln (Travatan), benzalkonium chloride-free (Travatan Z) 0.004% (2.5, 5 mL).] ▶L ♀C ▶? $$$

Glaucoma Agents—Sympathomimetics

BRIMONIDINE (*Alphagan P, ◆Alphagan*) 1 gtt in each affected eye tid. [Trade only: Soln 0.1% (5, 10, 15 mL). Generic/Trade: Soln 0.15% (5, 10, 15 mL). Generic only: Soln 0.2% (5, 10, 15 mL).] ▶L ♀B ▶? $$

Glaucoma Agents—Combinations and Other

COMBIGAN (brimonidine + timolol) 1 gtt in each affected eye q 12 h. [Trade only: Soln brimonidine 0.2% + timolol 0.5% (5, 10 mL).] ▶LK ♀C ▶– $$$

COSOPT (dorzolamide + timolol) 1 gtt in each affected eye bid. [Generic/Trade: Soln dorzolamide 2% + timolol 0.5% (5, 10 mL).] ▶LK ♀D ▶– $$$

Mydriatics & Cycloplegics

ATROPINE—OPHTHALMIC (*Isopto Atropine, Atropine Care*) 1 to 2 gtts in each affected eye before procedure or daily to qid or ⅛ to ¼ inch ointment before procedure or daily to tid. Cycloplegia may last up to 5 to 10 days and mydriasis may last up to 7 to 14 days. [Generic/Trade: Soln 1% (2, 5, 15 mL) Generic only: Ointment 1% (3.5 g tube).] ▶L ♀C ▶+ $

CYCLOPENTOLATE (*AK-Pentolate, Cyclogyl, Pentolair*) 1 to 2 gtts in each affected eye for 1 to 2 doses before procedure. Cycloplegia may last 6 to 24 h; mydriasis may last 1 day. [Generic/Trade: Soln 1% (2, 15 mL). Trade only (Cyclogyl): 0.5% (15 mL), 1% (5 mL) and 2% (2, 5, 15 mL).] ▶? ♀C ▶? $

HOMATROPINE (*Isopto Homatropine*) 1 to 2 gtts in each affected eye before procedure or bid to tid. Cycloplegia and mydriasis lasts 1 to 3 days. [Trade only: Soln 2% (5 mL), 5% (15 mL). Generic/Trade: Soln 5% (5 mL).] ▶? ♀C ▶? $

PHENYLEPHRINE—OPHTHALMIC (*AK-Dilate, Altafrin, Mydfrin, Refresh*) 1 to 2 gtts in each affected eye before procedure or tid to qid. No cycloplegia; mydriasis may last up to 5 h. [Rx Generic/Trade: Soln 2.5% (2, 3, 5, 15 mL), 10% (5 mL). OTC Trade only (Altafrin and Refresh): Soln 0.12% (15 mL).] ▶Plasma, L ♀C ▶? $

TROPICAMIDE (*Mydriacyl, Tropicacyl*) 1 to 2 gtts in each affected eye before procedure. Mydriasis may last 6 h. [Generic/Trade: Soln 0.5% (15 mL), 1% (3, 15 mL). Generic only: Soln 1% (2 mL).] ▶? ♀? ▶? $

Non-Steroidal Anti-Inflammatories

BROMFENAC—OPHTHALMIC (*Xibrom*) 1 gtt in each affected eye bid for 2 weeks. [Trade only: Soln 0.09% (2.5, 5 mL).] ▶Minimal absorption ♀C, D (3rd trimester) ▶? $$$$$
DICLOFENAC—OPHTHALMIC (*Voltaren, ✦Voltaren Ophtha*) 1 gtt in each affected eye daily to qid. [Generic/Trade: Soln 0.1% (2.5, 5 mL).] ▶L ♀B, D (3rd trimester) ▶? $$$
KETOROLAC—OPHTHALMIC (*Acular, Acular LS*) 1 gtt in each affected eye qid. [Generic/Trade: Soln (Acular LS) 0.4% (5 mL). Trade only: Acular 0.5% (3, 5, 10 mL), preservative-free Acular 0.5% unit dose (0.4 mL).] ▶L ♀C ▶? $$$$
NEPAFENAC (*Nevanac*) 1 gtt in each affected eye tid for 2 weeks. [Trade only: Susp 0.1% (3 mL).] ▶Minimal absorption ♀C ▶? $$$

Other Ophthalmologic Agents

ARTIFICIAL TEARS (*Tears Naturale, Hypotears, Refresh Tears, GenTeal, Systane*) 1 to 2 gtts in each eye tid to qid prn. [OTC Generic/Trade: Soln (15, 30 mL, among others.)] ▶Minimal absorption ♀A ▶+ $
CYCLOSPORINE—OPHTHALMIC (*Restasis*) 1 gtt in each eye q 12 h. [Trade only: Emulsion 0.05% (0.4 mL single-use vials).] ▶Minimal absorption ♀C ▶? $$$$
HYDROXYPROPYL CELLULOSE (*Lacrisert*) <u>Moderate–severe dry eyes:</u> 1 insert in each eye daily. Some patients may require bid use. [Trade only: Ocular insert 5 mg.] ▶Minimal absorption ♀+ ▶+ $$$
LIDOCAINE—OPHTHALMIC (*Akten*) Do not prescribe for unsupervised or prolonged use. Corneal toxicity and ocular infections may occur with repeated use. 2 gtts before procedure, repeat prn. [Generic only: Gel 3.5% (5 mL).] ▶L ♀B ▶? ?
PETROLATUM (*Lacrilube, Dry Eyes, Refresh PM, ✦Duolube*) Apply ¼ to ½ inch ointment to inside of lower lid prn. [OTC Trade only: Ointment (3.5, 7 g) tube.] ▶Minimal absorption ♀A ▶+ $
PROPARACAINE (*Ophthaine, Ophthetic, ✦Alcaine*) Do not prescribe for unsupervised or prolonged use. Corneal toxicity and ocular infections may occur with repeated use. 1 to 2 gtts into affected eye before procedure. [Generic/Trade: Soln 0.5% (15 mL).] ▶L ♀C ▶? $
TETRACAINE—OPHTHALMIC (*Pontocaine*) Do not prescribe for unsupervised or prolonged use. Corneal toxicity and ocular infections may occur with repeated use. 1 to 2 gtts or ½ to 1 inch ribbon of ointment in each affected eye before procedure. [Generic only: Soln 0.5% (15 mL), unit-dose vials (0.7, 2 mL).] ▶Plasma ♀C ▶? $

PSYCHIATRY

Antidepressants—Heterocyclic Compounds

AMITRIPTYLINE (*Elavil*) Start 25 to 100 mg PO at bedtime; gradually increase to usual effective dose of 50 to 300 mg/day. Primarily inhibits serotonin reuptake. Demethylated to nortriptyline, which primarily inhibits norepinephrine reuptake. [Generic: Tabs 10, 25, 50, 75, 100, 150 mg. Elavil brand name no longer available; has been retained in this entry for name recognition purposes only.] ▶L ♀D ▶– $$

CLOMIPRAMINE (*Anafranil*) Start 25 mg PO at bedtime; gradually increase to usual effective dose of 150 to 250 mg/day. Max 250 mg/day. Primarily inhibits serotonin reuptake. [Generic/Trade: Caps 25, 50, 75 mg.] ▶L ♀C ▶+ $$$

DESIPRAMINE (*Norpramin*) Start 25 to 100 mg PO given once daily or in divided doses. Gradually increase to usual effective dose of 100 to 200 mg/day, max 300 mg/day. Primarily inhibits norepinephrine reuptake. [Generic/Trade: Tabs 10, 25, 50, 75, 100, 150 mg.] ▶L ♀C ▶+ $$

DOXEPIN (*Sinequan, Silenor*) Start 75 mg PO at bedtime. Gradually increase to usual effective dose of 75 to 150 mg/day, max 300 mg/day. Primarily inhibits norepinephrine reuptake. Insomnia (Silenor): 6 mg PO 30 min before bedtime, 3 mg in age 65 yo or older [Generic/Trade: Caps 10, 25, 50, 75, 100, 150 mg. Oral concentrate 10 mg/mL.] ▶L ♀C ▶– $$

IMIPRAMINE (*Tofranil, Tofranil PM*) <u>Depression:</u> Start 75 to 100 mg PO at bedtime or in divided doses; gradually increase to max 300 mg/day. <u>Enuresis:</u> 25 to 75 mg PO at bedtime. [Generic/Trade: Tabs 10, 25, 50 mg. Caps 75, 100, 125, 150 mg (as pamoate salt).] ▶L ♀D ▶– $$$

NORTRIPTYLINE (*Aventyl, Pamelor*) Start 25 mg PO given once daily or divided bid to qid. Usual effective dose is 75 to 100 mg/day, max 150 mg/day. Primarily inhibits norepinephrine reuptake. [Generic/Trade: Caps 10, 25, 50, 75 mg. Oral soln 10 mg/5 mL.] ▶L ♀D ▶+ $$$

PROTRIPTYLINE (*Vivactil*) <u>Depression:</u> 15 to 40 mg/day PO divided tid to qid. Max 60 mg/day. [Trade only: Tabs 5, 10 mg.] ▶L ♀C ▶+ $$$$

Antidepressants—Monoamine Oxidase Inhibitors (MAOIs)

NOTE *Must be on tyramine-free diet throughout treatment and for 2 weeks after discontinuation. Numerous drug interactions; risk of hypertensive crisis and serotonin syndrome with many medications, including OTC. Allow ≥ 2 weeks wash-out when converting from an MAOI to an SSRI (6 weeks after fluoxetine), TCA, or other antidepressant.*

ISOCARBOXAZID (*Marplan*) Start 10 mg PO bid; increase by 10 mg q 2 to 4 days. Usual effective dose is 20 to 40 mg/day. MAOI diet. [Trade only: Tabs 10 mg.] ▶L ♀C ▶? $$$

PHENELZINE (*Nardil*) Start 15 mg PO tid. Usual effective dose is 60 to 90 mg/day in divided doses. MAOI diet. [Trade only: Tabs 15 mg.] ▶L ♀C ▶? $$$

SELEGILINE—TRANSDERMAL (*Emsam*) <u>Depression:</u> Start 6 mg/24 h patch, change daily. Max 12 mg/24 h. MAOI diet for doses 9 mg/day or higher. [Trade only: Transdermal patch 6 mg/day, 9 mg/24 h, 12 mg/24 h.] ▶L ♀C ▶? $$$$$

TRANYLCYPROMINE (*Parnate*) Start 10 mg PO every morning; increase by 10 mg/day at 1 to 3 week intervals to usual effective dose of 10 to 40 mg/day divided bid. MAOI diet. [Generic/Trade: Tabs 10 mg.] ▶L ♀C ▶– $$

Antidepressants—Selective Serotonin Reuptake Inhibitors (SSRIs)

CITALOPRAM (*Celexa*) <u>Depression:</u> Start 20 mg PO daily; usual effective dose is 20 to 40 mg/day, max 60 mg/day. Suicidality. [Generic/Trade: Tabs 10, 20, 40 mg. Oral soln 10 mg/5 mL. Generic only: Oral disintegrating tab 10, 20, 40 mg.] ▶LK ♀C but - in third trimester ▶– $$$

ESCITALOPRAM (*Lexapro*, ✦*Cipralex*) <u>Depression-generalized anxiety disorder,</u> adults and age 12 yo or older: Start 10 mg PO daily; max 20 mg/day. Suicidality. [Generic/Trade: Tabs 5, 10, 20 mg. Trade only: Oral soln 1 mg/mL.] ▶LK ♀C but - in 3rd trimester ▶– $$$

FLUOXETINE (*Prozac, Prozac Weekly, Sarafem*) <u>Depression, OCD:</u> Start 20 mg PO every morning; usual effective dose is 20 to 40 mg/day, max 80 mg/day. <u>Depression,</u> maintenance: 20 to 40 mg/day (standard-release) or 90 mg PO once a week (Prozac Weekly) starting 7 days after last standard-release dose. <u>Bulimia:</u> 60 mg PO daily; may need to titrate slowly, over several days. <u>Panic disorder:</u> Start 10 mg PO every morning; titrate to 20 mg/day after 1 week, max 60 mg/day. <u>Premenstrual Dysphoric Disorder</u> (Sarafem): 20 mg PO daily, given either throughout the menstrual cycle or for 14 days prior to menses; max 80 mg/day. Doses greater than 20 mg/day can be divided bid (in morning and at noon). <u>Bipolar Depression, olanzapine + fluoxetine:</u> Start 5 mg olanzapine + 20 mg fluoxetine daily in the evening. Increase to usual range of 5 to 12.5 mg olanzapine plus 20 to 50 mg fluoxetine as tolerated. <u>Treatment-resistant Depression, olanzapine + fluoxetine:</u> Start 5 mg olanzapine + 20 mg fluoxetine daily in the evening. Increase to usual range of 5 to 20 mg olanzapine plus 20 to 50 mg fluoxetine as tolerated. Suicidality, many drug interactions. [Generic/Trade: Tabs 10 mg. Caps 10, 20, 40 mg. Oral soln 20 mg/5 mL. Caps (Sarafem): 10, 20 mg. Trade only: Tabs (Sarafem) 10, 15, 20 mg. Caps delayed-release (Prozac Weekly) 90 mg. Generic only: Tabs 20, 40 mg.] ▶L ♀C but - in 3rd trimester ▶– $$$

FLUVOXAMINE (*Luvox, Luvox CR*) <u>OCD:</u> Start 50 mg PO at bedtime; usual effective dose is 100 to 300 mg/day divided bid, max 300 mg/day. <u>OCD and Social Anxiety Disorder (CR):</u> Start 100 mg PO at bedtime; increase by 50 mg/day q week prn to max 300 mg/day. <u>OCD (children age 8 yo or older):</u> Start 25 mg PO at bedtime; usual effective dose is 50 to 200 mg/day divided bid, max 200 mg/day. Don't use with thioridazine, pimozide, alosetron, cisapride, tizanidine, tryptophan, or MAOIs; use caution with benzodiazepines, TCAs, theophylline, and warfarin. Suicidality. [Generic/Trade: Tabs 25, 50, 100 mg. Trade only: Caps extended-release 100, 150 mg.] ▶L ♀C but - in third trimester ▶– $$$$

PAROXETINE (*Paxil, Paxil CR, Pexeva*) <u>Depression:</u> Start 20 mg PO every morning, max 50 mg/day. Depression, controlled-release: Start 25 mg PO every morning, max 62.5 mg/day. <u>OCD:</u> Start 10 to 20 mg PO every morning, max 60 mg/day. <u>Social anxiety disorder:</u> Start 10 to 20 mg PO every morning, max 60 mg/day. <u>Social anxiety disorder, controlled-release:</u> Start 12.5 mg PO every morning, max 37.5 mg/day. <u>Generalized anxiety disorder:</u> Start 20 mg PO every morning, max 50 mg/day. <u>Panic disorder:</u> Start 10 mg PO every morning, increase by 10 mg/day at intervals of 1 week or more to usual effective dose of 10 to 60 mg/day; max 60 mg/day. <u>Panic disorder, controlled-release:</u> Start 12.5 mg PO every morning, max 75 mg/day. <u>Post-traumatic stress disorder:</u> Start 20 mg PO every morning, max 50 mg/day. <u>Premenstrual dysphoric disorder (PMDD), continuous dosing:</u> Start 12.5 mg PO every morning (controlled-release); may increase dose after 1 week to max 25 mg every morning. PMDD, intermittent dosing (given for 2 weeks prior to menses): 12.5 mg PO every morning (controlled-release), max 25 mg/day. Suicidality, many drug interactions. [Generic/Trade: Tabs 10, 20, 30, 40 mg. Oral susp 10 mg/5 mL. Controlled-release tabs 12.5, 25 mg. Trade only: (Paxil CR) 37.5 mg.] ▶LK ♀D ▶? $$$

SERTRALINE (*Zoloft*) <u>Depression, OCD:</u> Start 50 mg PO daily; usual effective dose is 50 to 200 mg/day, max 200 mg/day. <u>Panic disorder, post-traumatic stress disorder, social anxiety disorder:</u> Start 25 mg PO daily, max 200 mg/day. <u>Premenstrual dysphoric disorder (PMDD), continuous dosing:</u> Start 50 mg PO daily, max 150 mg/day. PMDD, intermittent dosing (given for 14 days prior to menses): Start 50 mg PO daily for 3 days, then increase to 100 mg/day. Suicidality. [Generic/Trade: Tabs 25, 50, 100 mg. Oral concentrate 20 mg/mL (60 mL).] ▶LK ♀C but - in third trimester ▶+ $$$

Antidepressants—Serotonin-Norepinephrine Reuptake Inhibitors (SNRIs)

DESVENLAFAXINE (*Pristiq*) 50 mg PO daily. Max 400 mg/day. [Trade only: Tabs extended-release 50, 100 mg.] ▶LK ♀C ▶? $$$$

DULOXETINE (*Cymbalta*) <u>Depression:</u> 20 mg PO bid; max 60 mg/day given once daily or divided bid. <u>Generalized anxiety disorder:</u> Start 30 to 60 mg PO daily, max 120 mg/day. <u>Diabetic peripheral neuropathic pain:</u> 60 mg PO daily. <u>Fibromyalgia:</u> Start 30 to 60 mg PO daily, max 60 mg/day. Suicidality, hepatotoxicity, many drug interactions. [Trade only: Caps 20, 30, 60 mg.] ▶L ♀C ▶? $$$$

VENLAFAXINE (*Effexor, Effexor XR*) <u>Depression/anxiety:</u> Start 37.5 to 75 mg PO daily (Effexor XR) or 75 mg/day divided bid to tid (Effexor). Usual effective dose is 150 to 225 mg/day, max 225 mg/day (Effexor XR) or 375 mg/day (Effexor). <u>Generalized anxiety disorder:</u> Start 37.5 to 75 mg PO daily (Effexor XR), max 225 mg/day. <u>Social anxiety disorder:</u> 75 mg PO daily (Effexor XR). <u>Panic disorder:</u> Start 37.5 mg PO daily (Effexor XR), may titrate by 75 mg/day at weekly intervals to max 225 mg/day. Suicidality, seizures, HTN. [Generic/Trade: Caps extended-release 37.5, 75, 150 mg. Tabs 25, 37.5, 50, 75, 100 mg. Generic only: Tabs extended-release 37.5, 75, 150, 225 mg.] ▶LK ♀C but - in 3rd trimester ▶? $$$$

Antidepressants—Other

BUPROPION (*Wellbutrin, Wellbutrin SR, Wellbutrin XL, Aplenzin, Zyban, Buproban*) Depression: Start 100 mg PO bid (immediate-release tabs); can increase to 100 mg tid after 4 to 7 days. Usual effective dose is 300 to 450 mg/day, max 150 mg/dose and 450 mg/day. Sustained-release: Start 150 mg PO every morning; may increase to 150 mg bid after 4 to 7 days, max 400 mg/day. Give last dose no later than 5 pm. Extended-release: Start 150 mg PO every morning; may increase to 300 mg every morning after 4 days, max 450 mg every morning. Extended-release (Aplenzin): Start 174 mg PO every morning; increase to target dose of 348 mg/day after 4 days or more. May increase to max dose of 522 mg/day after 4 weeks or more. Seasonal affective disorder: Start 150 mg of extended-release PO every morning in autumn; can increase to 300 mg every morning after 1 week, max 300 mg/day. In the spring, decrease to 150 mg/day for 2 weeks and then discontinue. Smoking cessation (Zyban, Buproban): Start 150 mg PO every morning for 3 days, then increase to 150 mg PO bid for 7 to 12 weeks. Max 150 mg PO bid. Give last dose no later than 5 pm. Seizures, suicidality. [Generic/Trade (for depression, bupropion HCl): Tabs 75, 100 mg. Sustained-release tabs 100, 150, 200 mg. Extended-release tabs 150, 300 mg (Wellbutrin XL). Generic/Trade (Smoking cessation): Sustained-release tabs 150 mg (Zyban, Buproban). Trade only: Extended-release (Aplenzin, bupropion hydrobromide) tabs 174, 348, 522 mg.] ▶LK ♀C ▶− $$$$

MIRTAZAPINE (*Remeron, Remeron SolTab*) Start 15 mg PO at bedtime. Usual effective dose is 15 to 45 mg/day. Agranulocytosis in 0.1% of patients. Suicidality. [Generic/Trade: Tabs 15, 30, 45 mg. Tabs orally disintegrating (SolTab) 15, 30, 45 mg. Generic only: Tabs 7.5 mg.] ▶LK ♀C ▶? $$

TRAZODONE (*Desyrel, Oleptro*) Depression: Start 50 to 150 mg/day PO in divided doses; usual effective dose is 400 to 600 mg/day. Extended release: Start 150 mg PO at bedtime. May increase by 75 mg/day every 3 days to max 375 mg/day. Insomnia: 50 to 150 mg PO at bedtime. [Trade only: Extended release tabs (Oleptro) 150, 300 mg. Generic only: Tabs 50, 100, 150, 300 mg.] ▶L ♀C ▶− $

Antimanic (Bipolar) Agents

LAMOTRIGINE (*Lamictal, Lamictal CD, Lamictal ODT, Lamictal XR*) Adults with bipolar disorder (maintenance): Start 25 mg PO daily, 50 mg PO daily if on enzyme-inducing drugs, or 25 mg PO every other day if on valproate; titrate to 200 mg/day, 400 mg/day divided bid if on enzyme-inducing drugs, or 100 mg/day if on valproate. Potentially life-threatening rashes in 0.3% of adults and 0.8% of children; discontinue at first sign of rash. Drug interaction with valproic acid; see product information for adjusted dosing guidelines. [Generic/Trade: Chewable dispersible tabs (Lamictal CD) 5, 25 mg. Tabs 25, 100, 150, 200 mg. Trade only: Orally disintegrating tabs (ODT) 25, 50, 100, 200 mg. Extended-release tabs (XR) 25, 50, 100, 200 mg.] ▶LK ♀C (see notes) ▶− $$$$

LITHIUM (*Eskalith, Eskalith CR, Lithobid, ✦Lithane*)   <u>Acute mania:</u> Start 300 to 600 mg/day PO bid to tid; usual effective dose is 900 to 1800 mg/day. Steady state is achieved in 5 days. <u>Bipolar maintenance</u> usually 900 to 1200 mg/day titrated to therapeutic trough level of 0.6 to 1.2 mEq/L. [Generic/Trade: Caps 300, Extended-release caps 300, 450 mg. Generic only: Caps 150, 600 mg, Tabs 300 mg, Syrup 300/5 mL.] ▶K ♀D ▬ $

TOPIRAMATE (*Topamax*)   <u>Bipolar disorder (unapproved):</u> Start 25 to 50 mg/day PO. Titrate prn to max 400 mg/day divided bid. [Generic/Trade: Tabs 25, 50, 100, 200 mg. Sprinkle caps 15, 25 mg.] ▶K ♀C ? $$$$$

VALPROIC ACID (*Depakote, Depakote ER, Stavzor, divalproex, ✦Epiject, Epival, Deproic*)   <u>Mania:</u> 250 mg PO tid (Depakote) or 25 mg/kg once daily (Depakote ER); max 60 mg/kg/day. Hepatotoxicity, drug interactions, reduce dose in the elderly. [Generic only: Syrup (Valproic acid) 250 mg/5 mL. Generic/Trade: Delayed-release tabs (Depakote) 125, 250, 500 mg. Extended-release tabs (Depakote ER) 250, 500 mg. Delayed-release sprinkle caps (Depakote) 125 mg. Trade only (Stavzor): Delayed-release caps 125, 250, 500 mg.] ▶L ♀D ▶+ $$$$

Antipsychotics—1st Generation (Typical)

CHLORPROMAZINE (*Thorazine*)   Start 10 to 50 mg PO/IM bid to tid, usual dose 300 to 800 mg/day. [Generic only: Tabs 10, 25, 50, 100, 200 mg. Generic/Trade: Oral concentrate 30 mg/mL, 100 mg/mL. Trade only: Syrup 10 mg/5 mL, Supps 25, 100 mg.] ▶LK ♀C ▬ $$$

FLUPHENAZINE (*Prolixin, ✦Modecate, Modeten*)   1.25 to 10 mg/day IM divided q 6 to 8 h. Start 0.5 to 10 mg/day PO divided q 6 to 8 h. Usual effective dose 1 to 20 mg/d. Depot (fluphenazine decanoate/enanthate): 12.5 to 25 mg IM/SC q 3 weeks is equivalent to 10 to 20 mg/day PO fluphenazine. [Generic/Trade: Tabs 1, 2.5, 5, 10 mg. Elixir 2.5 mg/5 mL. Oral concentrate 5 mg/mL.] ▶LK ♀C ▶? $$$

HALOPERIDOL (*Haldol*)   2 to 5 mg IM. Start 0.5 to 5 mg PO bid to tid, usual effective dose 6 to 20 mg/day. Therapeutic range 2 to 15 ng/mL. Depot haloperidol (haloperidol decanoate): 100 to 200 mg IM q 4 weeks is equivalent to 10 mg/day oral haloperidol. [Generic only: Tabs 0.5, 1, 2, 5, 10, 20 mg. Oral concentrate 2 mg/mL.] ▶LK ♀C ▬ $$

PERPHENAZINE   Start 4 to 8 mg PO tid or 8 to 16 mg PO bid to qid (hospitalized patients), maximum 64 mg/day PO. Can give 5 to 10 mg IM q 6 h, maximum 30 mg/day IM. [Generic only: Tabs 2, 4, 8, 16 mg. Oral concentrate 16 mg/5 mL.] ▶LK ♀C ▶? $$$

PIMOZIDE (*Orap*)   <u>Tourette's:</u> Start 1 to 2 mg/day PO in divided doses, increase q 2 days to usual effective dose of 1 to 10 mg/day. [Trade only: Tabs 1, 2 mg.] ▶L ♀C ▬ $$$

THIORIDAZINE (*Mellaril, ✦Rideril*)   Start 50 to 100 mg PO tid, usual dose 200 to 800 mg/day. Not first line therapy. Causes QTc prolongation, torsades de pointes, and sudden death. Contraindicated with SSRIs, propranolol, pindolol. Monitor baseline ECG and potassium. Pigmentary retinopathy with doses >800 mg/day. [Generic only: Tabs 10, 15, 25, 50, 100, 150, 200 mg. Oral concentrate 30, 100 mg/mL.] ▶LK ♀C ▶? $$

THIOTHIXENE (*Navane*) Start 2 mg PO tid. Usual effective dose is 20 to 30 mg/day, maximum 60 mg/day PO. [Generic/Trade: Caps 1, 2, 5, 10. Oral concentrate 5 mg/mL. Trade only: Caps 20 mg.] ▶LK ♀C ▶? $$$

TRIFLUOPERAZINE (*Stelazine*) Start 2 to 5 mg PO bid. Usual effective dose is 15 to 20 mg/day. [Generic/Trade: Tabs 1, 2, 5, 10 mg. Trade only: Oral concentrate 10 mg/mL.] ▶LK ♀C ▶– $$$

Antipsychotics—2nd Generation (Atypical)

ARIPIPRAZOLE (*Abilify, Abilify Discmelt*) Schizophrenia: Start 10 to 15 mg PO daily. Max 30 mg daily. Bipolar disorder: Start 15 mg PO daily. Max 30 mg/day. Agitation associated with schizophrenia or Bipolar disorder: 9.75 mg IM recommended. May consider 5.25 to 15 mg if indicated. May repeat in 2 h up to max 30 mg/day. Depression, adjunctive therapy: Start 2 to 5 mg PO daily. Max 15 mg/day. [Trade only: Tabs 2, 5, 10, 15, 20, 30 mg. Oral soln 1 mg/mL (150 mL). Orally disintegrating tabs (Discmelt) 10, 15, 20, 30 mg.] ▶L ♀C ▶? $$$$$

ASENAPINE (*Saphris*) Schizophrenia: Initial and maintenance 5 mg SL bid. Max 10 mg/d. Bipolar disorder: Initial and maintenance, 10 mg SL bid. May reduce to 5 mg SL bid if needed. Max 20 mg/d. [Trade: Sublingual tabs 5, 10 mg] ▶L - Glucuronidation ♀C ▶–

CLOZAPINE (*Clozaril, FazaClo ODT*) Start 12.5 mg PO daily or bid. Usual effective dose is 300 to 450 mg/day divided bid, max 900 mg/day. Agranulocytosis 1 to 2%; check WBC and ANC weekly for 6 months, then q 2 weeks. Seizures, myocarditis, cardiopulmonary arrest. [Generic/Trade: Tabs 25, 100 mg. Generic only: Tabs 12.5, 50, 200 mg. Trade only: Orally disintegrating tab (Fazaclo ODT) 12.5, 25, 100 mg (scored).] ▶L ♀B ▶– $$$$$

ILOPERIDONE (*Fanapt*) Start 1 mg PO bid. Increase to 2 mg PO bid on day 2, then by 2 mg per dose each day to usual effective range of 6 to 12 mg PO bid. Max 24 mg/day. [Trade: Tabs 1, 2, 4, 6, 8, 10, 12 mg.] ▶L ♀C ▶–?

OLANZAPINE (*Zyprexa, Zyprexa Zydis, Zyprexa Relprevv*) Agitation in acute bipolar mania or schizophrenia: Start 10 mg IM (2.5 to 5 mg in elderly or debilitated patients); may repeat in 2 h to max 30 mg/day. Schizophrenia, oral therapy: Start 5 to 10 mg PO daily; usual effective dose is 10 to 15 mg/day. Schizophrenia, long-acting injection: dose based on prior oral dose and ranges from 150 mg to 300 mg deep IM (gluteal) q 2 weeks or 300 mg to 405 mg q 4 weeks. See package insert. Bipolar disorder, maintenance treatment or monotherapy for acute manic or mixed episodes: Start 10 to 15 mg PO daily. Increase by 5 mg/day at intervals after 24 h to usual effective dose of 5 to 20 mg/day, max 20 mg/day. Bipolar disorder, adjunctive for acute manic or mixed episodes: Start 10 mg PO daily; usual effective dose is 5 to 20 mg/day, max 20 mg/day. Bipolar depression, olanzapine + fluoxetine: Start 5 mg olanzapine + 20 mg fluoxetine daily in the evening. Increase to usual range of 5 to 12.5 mg olanzapine plus 20 to 50 mg fluoxetine as tolerated. Treatment-resistant depression, olanzapine + fluoxetine: Start 5 mg olanzapine + 20 mg fluoxetine daily in the evening. Increase to usual range of 5 to 20 mg olanzapine plus 20 to 50 mg fluoxetine as tolerated. [Trade only: Tabs 2.5, 5, 7.5, 10, 15, 20 mg. Tabs orally-disintegrating (Zyprexa Zydis) 5, 10, 15, 20 mg. Long-acting injection (Zyprexa Relprevv) 210, 300, 405 mg/vial.] ▶L ♀C ▶– $$$$$

ANTIPSYCHOTIC RELATIVE ADVERSE EFFECTS[a]

Generation	Antipsychotic	Anticholinergic	Sedation	Hypotension	EPS	Weight Gain	Diabetes/Hyperglycemia	Dyslipidemia
1st	chlorpromazine	+++	+++	++	++	++	?	?
1st	fluphenazine	++	+	+	++++	++	?	?
1st	haloperidol	+	+	+	++++	++	0	?
1st	loxapine	++	+	+	++	+	?	?
1st	molindone	++	++	+	++	+	?	?
1st	perphenazine	++	++	+	++	+	+/?	?
1st	pimozide	+	+	+	+++	?	?	?
1st	thioridazine	++++	+++	+++	+	+++	+/?	?
1st	thiothixene	+	++	++	+++	++	?	?
1st	trifluoperazine	++	+	+	+++	++	?	?
2nd	aripiprazole	++	+	0	0	0/+	0	0
2nd	clozapine	++++	+++	+++	0	+++	+	+
2nd	olanzapine	+++	++	+	0b	+++	+	+
2nd	risperidone	+	++	+	+b	++	+	?
2nd	quetiapine	+	+++	++	0	++	?	?
2nd	ziprasidone	+	+	0	0	0/+	0	0

[a]Risk of specific adverse effects is graded from 0 (absent) to ++++ (high). ? = Limited or inconsistent comparative data. [b]EPS (EPS) are dose-related and are more likely for risperidone >6-8 mg/day / olanzapine >20 mg/day. Akathisia risk remains unclear and may not be reflected in these ratings. There are limited comparative data for aripiprazole relative to other second generation antipsychotics.
References: Goodman & Gilman 11e p461-500, Applied Therapeutics 8e p78, APA schizophrenia practice guideline, Psychiatry Q 2002; 73:297, Diabetes Care 2004; 27:596.

PALIPERIDONE (*Invega, Invega Sustenna*) <u>Schizophrenia and schizoaffective disorder (adjunctive and monotherapy):</u> Start 6 mg PO every morning. 3 mg/day may be sufficient in some. Max 12 mg/day. Extended-release injection: Start 234 mg IM (deltoid) and then 156 mg IM one week later. Recommended monthly dose 117 mg IM (deltoid or gluteal) or within range of 36 to 234 mg, based on response. [Trade only: Extended-release tabs 1.5, 3, 6, 9 mg.] ▶KL ♀C ▶– $$$$$
QUETIAPINE (*Seroquel, Seroquel XR*) <u>Schizophrenia:</u> Start 25 mg PO bid (regular tabs); increase by 25 to 50 mg bid to tid on day 2 and 3, and then to target dose of 300 to 400 mg/day divided bid to tid on day 4. Usual effective dose is 150 to 750 mg/day, max 800 mg/day. <u>Schizophrenia, extended-release tabs:</u> Start 300 mg PO daily in evening, increase by up to 300 mg/day at intervals of more than 1 day to usual effective range of 400 to 800 mg/day. <u>Acute bipolar mania, monotherapy, or adjunctive:</u> Start 50 mg PO bid on day 1,

(cont.)

then increase to no higher than 100 mg bid on day 2, 150 mg bid on day 3, and 200 mg bid on day 4. May increase prn to 300 mg bid on days 5 and 400 mg bid thereafter. Usual effective dose is 400 to 800 mg/day. <u>Acute bipolar mania, monotherapy or adjunctive, extended release:</u> Start 300 mg PO on evening day 1, 600 mg day 2, and 400 to 800 mg/day thereafter. <u>Bipolar depression, regular and extended release:</u> 50 mg PO hs on day 1, 100 mg hs day 2, 200 mg hs day 3, and 300 mg hs day 4. May increase prn to 400 mg hs on day 5 and 600 mg hs on day 8. <u>Bipolar maintenance:</u> Continue dose required to maintain remission. <u>Major depressive disorder, adjunctive to antidepressants, extended release:</u> Start 50 mg evening of day 1, may increase to 150 mg on day 3. Max 300 mg/day. Eye exam for cataracts recommended q 6 months. [Trade only: Tabs 25, 50, 100, 200, 300, 400 mg. Extended-release tabs 50, 150, 200, 300, 400 mg.] ▶LK ♀C ▶– $$$$$

RISPERIDONE (*Risperdal, Risperdal Consta*) <u>Schizophrenia</u> (adults): Start 2 mg/day PO given once daily or divided bid (0.5 mg bid in the elderly, debilitated, or with hypotension, severe renal or hepatic disease); increase by 1 to 2 mg/day (no more than 0.5 mg bid in elderly and debilitated) at intervals of 24 h or more to usual effective dose of 4 to 8 mg/day given once daily or divided bid, max 16 mg/day. Long-acting injection (Consta): <u>Schizophrenia, Bipolar type I</u> maintenance: start 25 mg IM q 2 weeks while continuing oral dose for 3 weeks. May increase at 4 week intervals to max 50 mg q 2 weeks. <u>Schizophrenia</u> (13 to 17 yo): Start 0.5 mg PO daily; increase by 0.5 to 1 mg/day at intervals of 24 h or more to target dose of 3 mg/day. Max 6 mg/day. <u>Bipolar mania</u> (adults): Start 2 to 3 mg PO daily; may increase by 1 mg/day at 24 h intervals to max 6 mg/day. <u>Bipolar mania</u> (10 to 17 yo): Start 0.5 mg PO daily; increase by 0.5 to 1 mg/day at intervals of 24 h to recommended dose of 2.5 mg/day. Max 6 mg/day. <u>Autistic disorder irritability</u> (age 5 to 16 yo): Start 0.25 mg (for wt less than 20 kg) or 0.5 mg (wt 20 kg or greater) PO daily. May increase after 4 days to 0.5 mg/day (for wt less than 20 kg) or 1.0 mg/day (wt 20 kg or greater). Maintain at least 14 days. May then increase at 14 days intervals or more by increments of 0.25 mg/day (for wt less than 20 kg) or 0.5 mg/day (wt 20 kg or greater) to max 1.0 mg/day (for wt less than 20 kg), 2.5 mg/day (20 to 44 kg) or 3.0 mg/day (wt more than 45 kg). [Generic/Trade: Tabs 0.25, 0.5, 1, 2, 3, 4 mg. Oral soln 1 mg/mL (30 mL). Orally disintegrating tabs 0.5, 1, 2, 3, 4 mg. Generic only: Orally disintegrating tabs 0.25 mg.] ▶LK ♀C ▶– $$$$$

ZIPRASIDONE (*Geodon*) <u>Schizophrenia:</u> Start 20 mg PO bid with food; may adjust at more than 2 day intervals to max 80 mg PO bid. <u>Acute agitation:</u> 10 to 20 mg IM, max 40 mg/day. <u>Bipolar mania:</u> Start 40 mg PO bid; may increase to 60 to 80 mg bid on day 2. Usual effective dose is 40 to 80 mg bid. [Trade only: Caps 20, 40, 60, 80 mg, Susp 10 mg/mL.] ▶L ♀C ▶– $$$$$

Anxiolytics/Hypnotics—Benzodiazepines—Long Half-Life (25-100 h)

BROMAZEPAM (*✦Lectopam*) Canada only. 6 to 18 mg/day PO in divided doses. [Generic/Trade: Tabs 1.5, 3, 6 mg.] ▶L ♀D ▶– $

CHLORDIAZEPOXIDE (*Librium*) Anxiety: 5 to 25 mg PO or 25 to 50 mg IM/IV tid to qid. Acute alcohol withdrawal: 50 to 100 mg PO/IM/IV, repeat q 3 to 4 h prn up to 300 mg/day. Half-life 5 to 30 h. [Generic/Trade: Caps 5, 10, 25 mg.] ▶LK ♀D ▶– ©IV $$

CLONAZEPAM (*Klonopin, Klonopin Wafer, ✦Rivotril, Clonapam*) Panic disorder: Start 0.25 to 0.5 mg PO bid to tid, max 4 mg/day. Half-life 18 to 50 h. Epilepsy: Start 0.5 mg PO tid. Max 20 mg/day. [Generic/Trade: Tabs 0.5, 1, 2 mg. Orally disintegrating tabs (approved for panic disorder only) 0.125, 0.25, 0.5, 1, 2 mg.] ▶LK ♀D ▶– ©IV $

CLORAZEPATE (*Tranxene, Tranxene SD*) Start 7.5 to 15 mg PO at bedtime or bid to tid, usual effective dose is 15 to 60 mg/day. Acute alcohol withdrawal: 60 to 90 mg/day on first day divided bid to tid, reduce dose to 7.5 to 15 mg/day over 5 days. [Generic/Trade: Tabs 3.75, 7.5, 15 mg. Trade only (Tranxene SD): Tabs extended-release 11.25, 22.5 mg.] ▶LK ♀D ▶– ©IV $

DIAZEPAM (*Valium, Diastat, Diastat AcuDial, ✦Vivol, E Pam, Diazemuls*) Active seizures: 5 to 10 mg IV q 10 to 15 min to max 30 mg, or 0.2 to 0.5 mg/kg rectal gel PR. Skeletal muscle spasm, spasticity related to cerebral palsy, paraplegia, athetosis, stiff man syndrome: 2 to 10 mg PO/PR tid to qid. Anxiety: 2 to 10 mg PO bid to qid. Half-life 20 to 80 h. Alcohol withdrawal: 10 mg PO tid to qid for 24 h then 5 mg PO tid to qid prn. [Generic/Trade: Tabs 2, 5, 10 mg. Generic only: Oral soln 5 mg/5 mL. Oral concentrate (Intensol) 5 mg/mL. Trade only: Rectal gel (Diastat) 2.5, 5, 10, 15, 20 mg. Rectal gel (Diastat AcuDial) 10, 20 mg.] ▶LK ♀D ▶– ©IV $

FLURAZEPAM (*Dalmane*) 15 to 30 mg PO at bedtime. Half-life 70 to 90 h. [Generic/Trade: Caps 15, 30 mg.] ▶LK ♀X ▶– ©IV $

Anxiolytics/Hypnotics—Benzodiazepines—Medium Half-Life (10 to 15 h)

ESTAZOLAM (*ProSom*) 1 to 2 mg PO at bedtime. [Generic/Trade: Tabs 1, 2 mg.] ▶LK ♀X ▶– ©IV $$

LORAZEPAM (*Ativan*) Anxiety: 0.5 to 2 mg IV/IM/PO q 6 to 8 h, max 10 mg/day. Half-life 10 to 20 h. Status epilepticus: Adult: 4 mg IV over 2 min; may repeat in 10 to 15 min. Status epilepticus: Peds: 0.05 to 0.1 mg/kg (max 4 mg) IV over 2 to 5 min; may repeat 0.05 mg/kg once in 10 to 15 min. [Generic/Trade: Tabs 0.5, 1, 2 mg. Generic only: Oral concentrate 2 mg/mL.] ▶LK ♀D ▶– ©IV $

TEMAZEPAM (*Restoril*) 7.5 to 30 mg PO at bedtime. Half-life 8 to 25 h. [Generic/Trade: Caps 7.5, 15, 22.5, 30 mg.] ▶LK ♀X ▶– ©IV $

Anxiolytics/Hypnotics—Benzodiazepines—Short Half-Life (< 12 h)

NOTE *To avoid withdrawal, gradually taper when discontinuing after prolonged use. Sedative-hypnotics have been associated with severe allergic reactions and complex sleep behaviors including sleep driving. Use caution and discuss with patients.*

ALPRAZOLAM (*Xanax, Xanax XR, Niravam*) 0.25 to 0.5 mg PO bid to tid. Half-life 12 h. Multiple drug interactions. [Generic/Trade: Tabs 0.25, 0.5, 1, 2 mg. Tabs

(cont.)

extended-release 0.5, 1, 2, 3 mg. Orally disintegrating tab (Niravam) 0.25, 0.5, 1, 2 mg. Generic only: Oral concentrate (Intensol) 1 mg/mL.] ▶LK ♀D ▶– ©IV $

OXAZEPAM (***Serax***) 10 to 30 mg PO tid to qid. Half-life 8 h. [Generic/Trade: Caps 10, 15, 30 mg. Trade only: Tabs 15 mg.] ▶LK ♀D ▶– ©IV $$$

TRIAZOLAM (***Halcion***) 0.125 to 0.5 mg PO at bedtime. 0.125 mg/day in elderly. Half-life 2 to 3 h. [Generic/Trade: Tabs 0.125, 0.25 mg.] ▶LK ♀X ▶– ©IV $

Anxiolytics/Hypnotics—Other

BUSPIRONE (***BuSpar, Vanspar***) Anxiety: Start 15 mg "dividose" daily (7.5 mg PO bid), usual effective dose 30 mg/day. Max 60 mg/day. [Generic/Trade: Tabs 5, 10, Dividose Tabs 15, 30 mg (scored to be easily bisected or trisected). Generic only: Tabs 7.5 mg.] ▶L ♀B ▶– $$$

CHLORAL HYDRATE (***Aquachloral Supprettes, Somnote***) 25 to 50 mg/kg/day up to 1000 mg PO/PR. Many physicians use higher than recommended doses in children (eg, 75 mg/kg). [Generic only: Syrup 500 mg/5 mL, rectal supps 500 mg. Trade only: Caps 500 mg. Rectal supps: 325, 650 mg.] ▶LK ♀C ▶+ ©IV $

ESZOPICLONE (***Lunesta***) 2 mg PO at bedtime prn. Max 3 mg. Elderly: 1 mg PO at bedtime prn, max 2 mg. [Trade only: Tabs 1, 2, 3 mg.] ▶L ♀C ▶? ©IV $$$$

RAMELTEON (***Rozerem***) Insomnia: 8 mg PO at bedtime. [Trade only: Tabs 8 mg.] ▶L ♀C ▶? $$$$

ZALEPLON (***Sonata, ✦Starnoc***) 5 to 10 mg PO at bedtime prn, max 20 mg. Do not use for benzodiazepine or alcohol withdrawal. [Generic/Trade: Caps 5, 10 mg.] ▶L ♀C ▶– ©IV $$$$

ZOLPIDEM (***Ambien, Ambien CR, Zolpimist, Edluar***) Adult: Insomnia: Standard tabs: 10 mg PO at bedtime. For age older than 65 yo or debilitated: 5 mg PO at bedtime. Oral spray: 10 mg PO at bedtime. For age older than 65 yo or debilitated: 5 mg PO at bedtime. Control-release tabs: 12.5 mg PO at bedtime. For age older than 65 yo or debilitated: give 6.25 mg PO at bedtime. Do not use for benzodiazepine or alcohol withdrawal. [Generic/Trade: Tabs 5, 10 mg. Trade only: Controlled-release tabs 6.25, 12.5 mg. Oral spray 5 mg/actuation (Zolpimist), sublingual tab 5, 10 mg (Edluar).] ▶L ♀B ▶+ ©IV $$$$

ZOPICLONE (***✦Imovane***) Canada only. Adults: 5 to 7.5 mg PO at bedtime. Reduce dose in elderly. [Generic/Trade: Tabs 5, 7.5 mg. Generic only: Tabs 3.75 mg.] ▶L ♀D ▶– $

Combination Drugs

SYMBYAX (olanzapine + fluoxetine) Bipolar type 1 with depression and treatment-resistant depression: Start 6/25 mg PO at bedtime. Max 18/75 mg/day. [Trade only: Caps (olanzapine/fluoxetine) 3/25, 6/25, 6/50, 12/25, 12/50 mg.] ▶LK ♀C ▶– $$$$$

Drug Dependence Therapy

ACAMPROSATE (***Campral***) Maintenance of abstinence from alcohol: 666 mg (2 tabs) PO tid. Start after alcohol withdrawal and when patient is abstinent. [Trade only: Tabs delayed-release 333 mg.] ▶K ♀C ▶? $$$$

DISULFIRAM (*Antabuse*) <u>Sobriety:</u> 125 to 500 mg PO daily. Patient must abstain from any alcohol for ≥ 12 h before using. Metronidazole and alcohol in any form (cough syrups, tonics, etc.) contraindicated. [Trade only: Tabs 250, 500 mg.] ▶L ♀C ▶? $$$

NALTREXONE (*ReVia, Depade, Vivitrol*) <u>Alcohol/opioid dependence:</u> 25 to 50 mg PO daily. Avoid if recent ingestion of opioids (past 7 to 10 days). Hepatotoxicity with higher than approved doses. [Generic/Trade: Tabs 50 mg. Trade only (Vivitrol): Extended-release injectable susp kits 380 mg.] ▶LK ♀C ▶? $$$$

NICOTINE GUM (*Nicorette, Nicorette DS*) <u>Smoking cessation:</u> Gradually taper: 1 piece q 1 to 2 h for 6 weeks, 1 piece q 2 to 4 h for 3 weeks, then 1 piece q 4 to 8 h for 3 weeks, max 30 pieces/day of 2 mg or 24 pieces/day of 4 mg. Use Nicorette DS 4 mg/piece in high cigarette use (more than 24 cigarettes/day). [OTC/Generic/Trade: Gum 2, 4 mg.] ▶LK ♀D ▶- $$$

NICOTINE INHALATION SYSTEM (*Nicotrol Inhaler, ✦Nicorette inhaler*) 6 to 16 cartridges/day for 12 weeks. [Trade only: Oral inhaler 10 mg/cartridge (4 mg nicotine delivered), 42 cartridges/box.] ▶LK ♀D ▶- $$$$$

NICOTINE LOZENGE (*Commit, Nicorette*) <u>Smoking cessation:</u> In those who smoke within 30 min of waking use 4 mg lozenge; others use 2 mg. Take 1 to 2 lozenges q 1 to 2 h for 6 weeks, then q 2 to 4 h in weeks 7 to 9, then q 4 to 8 h in weeks 10 to 12. Length of therapy 12 weeks. [OTC Generic/Trade: Lozenge 2, 4 mg in 48, 72, 168 count packages.] ▶LK ♀D ▶- $$$$$

NICOTINE NASAL SPRAY (*Nicotrol NS*) <u>Smoking cessation:</u> 1 to 2 doses q 1 h, each dose is 2 sprays, 1 in each nostril (1 spray contains 0.5 mg nicotine). Minimum recommended: 8 doses/day, max 40 doses/day. [Trade only: Nasal soln 10 mg/mL (0.5 mg/inhalation); 10 mL bottles.] ▶LK ♀D ▶- $$$$$

NICOTINE PATCHES (*Habitrol, NicoDerm CQ, Nicotrol, ✦Prostep*) <u>Smoking cessation:</u> Start 1 patch (14 to 22 mg) daily, taper after 6 weeks. Ensure patient has stopped smoking. [OTC/Rx/Generic/Trade: Patches 11, 22 mg/24 h. 7, 14, 21 mg/24 h (Habitrol and NicoDerm). OTC/Trade: Patches 15 mg/16 h (Nicotrol).] ▶LK ♀D ▶- $$$$

SUBOXONE (buprenorphine + naloxone) Treatment of <u>opioid dependence:</u> Maintenance: 16 mg SL daily. Can individualize to range of 4 to 24 mg SL daily. [Trade only: SL tabs 2/0.5 mg and 8/2 mg buprenorphine/naloxone.] ▶L ♀C ▶- ⊙III $$$$$

VARENICLINE (*Chantix*) <u>Smoking cessation:</u> Start 0.5 mg PO daily for day 1 to 3, then 0.5 mg bid days 4 to 7, then 1 mg bid thereafter. Take after meals with full glass of water. Start 1 week prior to cessation and continue for 12 weeks. [Trade only: Tabs 0.5, 1 mg.] ▶K ♀C ▶? $$$$

Stimulants/ADHD/Anorexiants

ADDERALL (dextroamphetamine + amphetamine) (*Adderall XR*) <u>ADHD, standard-release tabs:</u> Start 2.5 mg (3 to 5 yo) or 5 mg (age 6 yo or older) PO daily to bid, increase by 2.5 to 5 mg q week, max 40 mg/day. <u>ADHD, extended-release caps</u> (Adderall XR): If age 6 to 12 yo, then start 5 to 10 mg PO daily

(cont.)

to a max of 30 mg/day. If 13 to 17 yo, then start 10 mg PO daily to a max of 20 mg/day. If adult, then 20 mg PO daily. Narcolepsy, standard-release: Start 5 to 10 mg PO every morning, increase to 5 to 10 mg q week, max 60 mg/day. Avoid evening doses. Monitor growth and use drug holidays when appropriate. [Generic/Trade: Tabs 5, 7.5, 10, 12.5, 15, 20, 30 mg. Trade only: Caps extended-release (Adderall XR) 5, 10, 15, 20, 25, 30 mg.] ▶L ♀C ▶- ©II $$$$

ARMODAFINIL (*Nuvigil*) Obstructive sleep apnea/hypopnea syndrome and narcolepsy: 150 to 250 mg PO every morning. Inconsistent evidence for improved efficacy of 250 mg/day dose. Shift work sleep disorder: 150 mg PO 1 h prior to start of shift. [Trade only: Tabs 50, 100, 150, 200, 250 mg.] ▶L ♀C ▶? ©IV $$$$$

ATOMOXETINE (*Strattera*) ADHD: All ages wt greater than 70 kg: Start 40 mg PO daily, then increase after more than 3 days to target of 80 mg/day divided daily to bid. Max 100 mg/day. [Trade only: Caps 10, 18, 25, 40, 60, 80, 100 mg.] ▶K ♀C ▶? $$$$$

CAFFEINE (*NoDoz, Vivarin, Caffedrine, Stay Awake, Quick-Pep, Cafcit*) 100 to 200 mg PO q 3 to 4 h prn. [OTC Generic/Trade: Tabs/Caps 200 mg. Oral soln caffeine citrate (Cafcit) 20 mg/mL. OTC Trade only: Tabs extended-release 200 mg. Lozenges 75 mg.] ▶L ♀B/C ▶? $

DEXMETHYLPHENIDATE (*Focalin, Focalin XR*) ADHD, extended-release, not already on stimulants: Start 5 mg (children) or 10 mg (adults) PO every morning. Max 30 mg/day (children) or 40 mg/day (Adults). Immediate-release, not already on stimulants: 2.5 mg PO bid. Max 20 mg/day. If taking racemic methylphenidate, use conversion of 2.5 mg for each 5 mg of methylphenidate. [Generic/Trade: Tabs immediate-release 2.5, 5, 10 mg. Trade only: Caps extended-release (Focalin XR) 5, 10, 15, 20, 30 mg] ▶L ♀C ▶? ©II $$$

DEXTROAMPHETAMINE (*Dexedrine, Dextrostat*) Narcolepsy: Age 6 to 12 yo: Start 5 mg PO every morning, increase by 5 mg/day q week. Age older than 12 yo: Start 10 mg PO every morning, increase by 10 mg/day q week. Usual dose range 5 to 60 mg/day in divided doses (tabs) or daily (extended-release). ADHD: 2.5 to 5 mg PO every morning, usual max 40 mg/day. Avoid evening doses. Monitor growth and use drug holidays when appropriate. [Generic/Trade: Caps extended-release 5, 10, 15 mg. Generic only: Tabs 5, 10 mg. Oral soln 5 mg/5 mL.] ▶L ♀C ▶- ©II $$$$

BODY MASS INDEX*		Heights are in feet and inches; weights are in pounds					
BMI	*Class.*	*4' 10"*	*5' 0"*	*5' 4"*	*5' 8"*	*6' 0"*	*6' 4"*
<19	Underweight	<91	<97	<110	<125	<140	<156
19–24	Healthy Weight	91–119	97–127	110–144	125–163	140–183	156–204
25–29	Overweight	120–143	128–152	145–173	164–196	184–220	205–245
30–40	Obese	144–191	153–204	174–233	197–262	221–293	246–328
>40	Very Obese	>191	>204	>233	>262	>293	>328

*BMI = kg/m² = (wt in pounds)(703)/(height in inches)². Anorectants appropriate if BMI ≥30 (with comorbidities ≥27); surgery an option if BMI >40 (with comorbidities 35–40). www.nhlbi.nih.gov

GUANFACINE (*Intuniv*)   Start 1 mg PO q AM. Increase by 1 mg/week to max 4 mg/day. [Trade only: Tabs 1, 2, 3, 4 mg.]   ▶LK – ♀B ▶?

LISDEXAMFETAMINE (*Vyvanse*)   <u>ADHD</u> adults and children ages 6 to 12 yo: Start 30 mg PO every morning. May increase weekly by 10 to 20 mg/day to max 70 mg/day. Avoid evening doses. Monitor growth and use drug holidays when appropriate. [Trade: Caps 20, 30, 40, 50, 60, 70 mg.]   ▶L ♀C ▶ –©II $$$$

METHYLPHENIDATE (*Ritalin, Ritalin LA, Ritalin SR, Methylin, Methylin ER, Metadate ER, Metadate CD, Concerta, Daytrana, ✦Biphentin*)   <u>ADHD/ Narcolepsy:</u> 5 to 10 mg PO bid to tid or 20 mg PO every morning (sustained and extended-release), max 60 mg/day. Or 18 to 36 mg PO every morning (Concerta), max 72 mg/day. Avoid evening doses. Monitor growth and use drug holidays when appropriate. [Trade only: Tabs 5, 10, 20 mg (Ritalin, Methylin, Metadate). Tabs extended-release 10, 20 mg (Methylin ER, Metadate ER). Tabs extended-release 18, 27, 36, 54 mg (Concerta). Caps extended-release 10, 20, 30, 40, 50, 60 mg (Metadate CD) May be sprinkled on food. Tabs sustained-release 20 mg (Ritalin SR). Caps extended-release 10, 20, 30, 40 mg (Ritalin LA). Tabs chewable 2.5, 5, 10 mg (Methylin). Oral soln 5 mg/5 mL, 10 mg/5 mL (Methylin). Transdermal patch (Daytrana) 10 mg/9 h, 15 mg/9 h, 20 mg/9 h, 30 mg/9 h. Generic only: Tabs 5, 10, 20 mg, tabs extended-release 10, 20 mg, tabs sustained-release 20 mg.]   ▶LK ♀C ▶? ©II $$

MODAFINIL (*Provigil, ✦Alertec*)   <u>Narcolepsy and sleep apnea/hypopnea:</u> 200 mg PO every morning. <u>Shift work sleep disorder:</u> 200 mg PO 1 h before shift. [Trade only: Tabs 100, 200 mg.]   ▶L ♀C ▶? ©IV $$$$$

PHENTERMINE (*Adipex-P, Ionamin, Pro-Fast*)   8 mg PO tid or 15 to 37.5 mg/day every morning or 10 to 14 h before retiring. For short-term use. [Generic/Trade: Caps 15, 30, 37.5 mg. Tabs 37.5 mg. Trade only: Caps extended-release 15, 30 mg (Ionamin). Generic only (Pro-Fast): Caps 18.75 mg, Tabs 8 mg.]   ▶LK ♀C ▶ –©IV $$

SIBUTRAMINE (*Meridia*)   Start 10 mg PO every morning, max 15 mg/day. Monitor pulse and BP. [Trade only: Caps 5, 10, 15 mg.]   ▶KL ♀C ▶ –©IV $$$$

PULMONARY

Beta Agonists—Short-Acting

ALBUTEROL (*AccuNeb, Ventolin HFA, Proventil HFA, ProAir HFA, VoSpire ER, ✦Airomir, Asmavent, salbutamol*)   MDI: 2 puffs q 4 to 6 h prn. Soln: 0.5 mL of 0.5% soln (2.5 mg) nebulized tid to qid. One 3 mL unit dose (0.083%) nebulized tid to qid. Caps for inhalation: 200 to 400 mcg q 4 to 6 h. Tabs: 2 to 4 mg PO tid to qid or extended-release 4 to 8 mg PO q 12 h up to 16 mg PO q 12 h. Peds: 0.1 to 0.2 mg/kg/dose PO tid up to 4 mg tid for age 2 to 5 yo, 2 to 4 mg or extended-release 4 mg PO q 12 h for age 6 to 12 yo. <u>Prevention of exercise-induced bronchospasm:</u> MDI: 2 puffs 15 to 30 min before exercise. [Trade only: MDI 90 mcg/actuation, 200 metered doses/canister. "HFA"

(cont.)

inhalers use hydrofluoroalkane propellant instead of CFCs but are otherwise equivalent. Generic/Trade: Soln for inhalation 0.021% (AccuNeb), 0.042% (AccuNeb), and 0.083% in 3 mL vials, 0.5% (5 mg/mL) in 20 mL with dropper. Tabs extended-release 4, 8 mg (VoSpire ER). Tabs only: Syrup 2 mg/5 mL. Tabs immediate-release 2, 4 mg.] ▶L ♀C ▶? $$

FENOTEROL (✦*Berotec*) Canada only. 1 to 2 puffs prn tid to qid. Nebulizer: Up to 2.5 mg q 6 h. [Soln for inhalation: 20 mL bottles of 1 mg/mL (with preservatives that may cause bronchoconstriction in those with hyperreactive airways).] ▶L ♀C ▶? $

LEVALBUTEROL (*Xopenex, Xopenex HFA*) MDI 2 puffs q 4 to 6 h prn. Nebulizer 0.63 to 1.25 mg q 6 to 8 h. Peds: 0.31 mg nebulized tid for age 6 to 11 yo. [Generic/Trade: Soln for inhalation 0.31, 0.63, 1.25 mg in 3 mL and 1.25 mg in 0.5 mL unit-dose vials. Trade only: HFA MDI 45 mcg/actuation, 15 g 200/canister. "HFA" inhalers use hydrofluoroalkane propellant.] ▶L ♀C ▶? $$$

METAPROTERENOL (*Alupent, ✦orciprenaline*) MDI: 2 to 3 puffs q 3 to 4 h. Soln: 0.2 to 0.3 mL 5% soln nebulized q 4 h. Peds: Tabs: 20 mg PO tid to qid age older than 9 yo, 10 mg PO tid to qid if age 6 to 9 yo, 1.3 to 2.6 mg/kg/day divided tid to qid if age 2 to 5 yo. [Trade only: MDI 0.65 mg/actuation, 14 g 200/canister. Generic/Trade: Soln for inhalation 0.4%, 0.6% in 2.5 mL unit-dose vials. Generic only: Syrup 10 mg/5 mL, Tabs 10, 20 mg.] ▶L ♀C ▶? $$

PIRBUTEROL (*Maxair Autohaler*) MDI: 1 to 2 puffs q 4 to 6 h. [Trade only: MDI 200 mcg/actuation, 14 g 400/canister.] ▶L ♀C ▶? $$$$

Beta Agonists—Long-Acting

ARFORMOTEROL (*Brovana*) COPD: 15 mcg nebulized bid. [Trade only: Soln for inhalation 15 mcg in 2 mL vial.] ▶L ♀C ▶? $$$$$

FORMOTEROL (*Foradil, Perforomist, ✦Oxeze Turbuhaler*) 1 puff bid. Nebulized: 20 mcg q 12 h. Not for acute bronchospasm. Use only in combination with corticosteroids. [Trade only: DPI 12 mcg, 12, 60 blisters/pack (Foradil). Soln for inhalation: 20 mcg in 2 mL vial (Perforomist). Canada only (Oxeze): DPI 6, 12 mcg 60 blisters/pack.] ▶L ♀C ▶? $$$

SALMETEROL (*Serevent Diskus*) 1 puff bid. Not for acute bronchospasm. Use only in combination with corticosteroids. [Trade only: DPI (Diskus): 50 mcg, 60 blisters.] ▶L ♀C ▶? $$$$

Combinations

ADVAIR (fluticasone - inhaled + salmeterol) (*Advair HFA*) Asthma: DPI: 1 puff bid (all strengths). MDI: 2 puffs bid (all strengths). COPD: DPI: 1 puff bid (250/50 only). [Trade only: DPI: 100/50, 250/50, 500/50 mcg fluticasone/ salmeterol per actuation; 60 doses/DPI. Trade only (Advair HFA): MDI 45/21, 115/21, 230/21 mcg fluticasone/salmeterol per actuation; 120 doses/ canister.] ▶L ♀C ▶? $$$$$

COMBIVENT (albuterol + ipratropium) 2 puffs qid, max 12 puffs/day. Contraindicated with soy or peanut allergy. [Trade only: MDI: 90 mcg albuterol/18 mcg ipratropium per actuation, 200/canister.] ▶L ♀C ▶? $$$$

DUONEB (albuterol + ipratropium) (←**Combivent inhalation soln**) 1 unit dose qid. [Generic/Trade: Unit dose: 2.5 mg albuterol/0.5 mg ipratropium per 3 mL vial, premixed; 30, 60 vials/carton.] ▶L ♀C ▶? $$$$$

SYMBICORT (budesonide + formoterol) Asthma: 2 puffs bid (both strengths). COPD: 2 puffs bid (160/4.5). [Trade only: MDI: 80/4.5, 160/4.5 mcg budesonide/formoterol per actuation; 120 doses/canister.] ▶L ♀C ▶? $$$$

Inhaled Steroids

NOTE *See Endocrine-Corticosteroids when oral steroids necessary.*

BECLOMETHASONE—INHALED (*QVAR*) 1 to 4 puffs bid (40 mcg). 1 to 2 puffs bid (80 mcg). [Trade only: HFA MDI: 40, 80 mcg/actuation, 7.3 g 100 actuations/canister.] ▶L ♀C ▶? $$$

BUDESONIDE—INHALED (*Pulmicort Respules, Pulmicort Flexhaler*) 1 to 2 puffs daily up to 4 puffs bid. Respules: 0.5 to 1 mg daily or divided bid. [Trade only: DPI (Flexhaler) 90, 180 mcg powder/actuation 60, 120 doses, respectively/canister, Respules 1 mg/2 mL unit dose. Generic/Trade: Respules 0.25, 0.5 mg/2 mL unit dose.] ▶L ♀B ▶? $$$$

CICLESONIDE—INHALED (*Alvesco*) 80 mcg/puff: 1 to 4 puffs bid. 160 mcg/puff: 1 to 2 puffs bid. [Trade only: 80 mcg/actuation, 60 per canister. 160 mcg/actuation, 60, 120 per canister.] ▶L ♀C ▶? $$$$

FLUNISOLIDE—INHALED (*AeroBid, AeroBid-M, Aerospan*) 2 to 4 puffs bid. [Trade only: MDI: 250 mcg/actuation, 100 metered doses/canister. AeroBid-M (AeroBid + menthol flavor). Aerospan HFA MDI: 80 mcg/actuation, 60, 120 metered doses/canister.] ▶L ♀C ▶? $$$

FLUTICASONE—INHALED (*Flovent HFA, Flovent Diskus*) 2 to 4 puffs bid. [Trade only: HFA MDI: 44, 110, 220 mcg/actuation 120/canister. DPI (Diskus): 50, 100, 250 mcg/actuation delivering 44, 88, 220 mcg, respectively.] ▶L ♀C ▶? $$$$

MOMETASONE—INHALED (*Asmanex Twisthaler*) 1 to 2 puffs in the evening or 1 puff bid. If prior oral corticosteroid therapy: 2 puffs bid. [Trade only: DPI: 110 mcg/actuation with #30 dosage units, 220 mcg/actuation with #30, 60, 120 dosage units.] ▶L ♀C ▶? $$$$

PREDICTED PEAK EXPIRATORY FLOW (liters/min)   *Am Rev Resp Dis* 1963; 88:644

Age (yr)	Women (height in inches)					Men (height in inches)					Child (height in inches)	
	55″	60″	65″	70″	75″	60″	65″	70″	75″	80″		
20 yr	390	423	460	496	529	554	602	649	693	740	44″	160
30 yr	380	413	448	483	516	532	577	622	664	710	46″	187
40 yr	370	402	436	470	502	509	552	596	636	680	48″	214
50 yr	360	391	424	457	488	486	527	569	607	649	50″	240
60 yr	350	380	412	445	475	463	502	542	578	618	52″	267
70 yr	340	369	400	432	461	440	477	515	550	587	54″	293

INHALED STEROIDS: ESTIMATED COMPARATIVE DAILY DOSES*

Drug	Form	≥12 yo & ADULTS Low Dose	Medium Dose	High Dose	CHILDREN (5–11 yo) Low Dose	Medium Dose	High Dose
beclomethasone HFA MDI	40 mcg/puff 80 mcg/puff	2–6 1–3	6–12 3–6	>12 >6	2–4 1–2	4–8 2–4	>8 >4
budesonide DPI	90 mcg/dose 180 mcg/dose	2–6 1–3	6–13 3–7	>13 >7	2–4 1–2	4–9 2–4	>9 >4
budesonide	soln for nebs	—	—	—	0.5 mg 0.25–0.5 mg (0–4 yo)	1 mg >0.5–1 mg (0–4 yo)	2 mg >1 mg (0–4 yo)
flunisolide MDI	250 mcg/puff	2–4	4–8	>8	2–3	4–5	>5
flunisolide HFA MDI	80 mcg/puff	4	5–8	>8	2	4	≥8
fluticasone HFA MDI	44 mcg/puff 110 mcg/puff 220 mcg/puff	2–6 1–2 1	6–10 2–4 1–2	>10 >4 >2	2–4 (0–11 yo) 1–2 (0–11 yo) n/a	4–8 (0–11 yo) 2–3 (0–11 yo) 1–2 (0–11 yo)	>8 (0–11 yo) >4 (0–11 yo) >2 (0–11 yo)
fluticasone DPI	50 mcg/dose 100 mcg/dose 250 mcg/dose	2–6 1–3	6–10 3–5 2	>10 >5 >2	2–4 1–2 n/a	4–8 2–4 1	>8 >4 >1
mometasone DPI	220 mcg/dose	1	2	>2	n/a	n/a	n/a
triamcinolone MDI	75 mcg/puff	4–10	10–20	>20	4–8	8–12	>12

*HFA = Hydrofluoroalkane (propellant). MDI = metered dose inhaler. DPI = dry powder inhaler. All doses in puffs (MDI) or inhalations (DPI) Reference: http://www.nhlbi.nih.gov/guidelines/asthma/asthsumm.pdf

INHALER COLORS (Body then cap—Generics may differ)

Advair:	purple	Atrovent HFA:	clear/green	Proventil HFA:	yellow/orange	
Advair HFA:	purple/light purple	Azmacort:	white/white	Pulmicort:	white/brown	
Aerobid:	grey/purple	Combivent:	clear/orange	QVAR 40 mcg:	beige/grey	
Aerobid-M:	grey/green			QVAR 80 mcg:	mauve/grey	
Aerospan:	purple/grey	Flovent HFA:	orange/peach			
Alupent:	clear/blue			Serevent		
Alvesco 80 mcg:	brown/red	Foradil:	grey/beige	Diskus:	green	
		Intal:	white/blue	Spiriva:	grey	
Alvesco 160 mcg:	red/red	Maxair:	white/white	Ventolin HFA:	light blue/navy	
Asmanex:	white/pink	Maxair Autohaler:	white/white	Xopenex HFA:	blue/red	
		ProAir HFA:	red/white			

TRIAMCINOLONE—INHALED (Azmacort) 2 puffs tid to qid or 4 puffs bid; max dose 16 puffs/day. [Trade only: MDI: 75 mcg/actuation, 240/canister. Built-in spacer.] ▶L ♀C ▶? $$$$

Leukotriene Inhibitors

MONTELUKAST (Singulair) Adults: 10 mg PO daily. Chronic Asthma, Allergic rhinitis: give 5 mg PO daily for age 6 to 14 yo, give 4 mg (chew tab or oral granules) PO daily for age 2 to 5 yo. Asthma age 12 to 23 mo: 4 mg (oral granules) PO daily. Allergic rhinitis age 6 to 23 mo: 4 mg (oral granules) PO daily. Prevention of exercise-induced bronchoconstriction: 10 mg PO 2 h before exercise. [Trade only: Tabs 10 mg. Oral granules 4 mg packet, 30/box. Chewable tabs (cherry flavored) 4, 5 mg.] ▶L ♀B ▶? $$$$

ZAFIRLUKAST (Accolate) 20 mg PO bid. Peds age 5 to 11 yo, 10 mg PO bid. Take 1 h before or 2 h after meals. Potentiates warfarin and theophylline. [Trade only: Tabs 10, 20 mg.] ▶L ♀B ▶— $$$$

ZILEUTON (Zyflo CR) 1200 mg PO bid. Hepatotoxicity, potentiates warfarin, theophylline, and propranolol. [Trade only: Tabs extended-release 600 mg.] ▶L ♀C ▶? $$$$$

Other Pulmonary Medications

ACETYLCYSTEINE—INHALED (Mucomyst) Mucolytic: 3 to 5 mL of 20% or 6 to 10 mL of 10% soln nebulized tid to qid. [Generic/Trade: Soln for inhalation 10, 20% in 4, 10, 30 mL vials.] ▶L ♀B ▶? $

AMINOPHYLLINE (✦Phyllocontin) Acute asthma: Loading dose: 6 mg/kg IV over 20 to 30 min. Maintenance 0.5 to 0.7 mg/kg/h IV. [Generic only: Tabs 100, 200 mg. Oral liquid 105 mg/5 mL. Canada Trade only: Tabs controlled-release (12 h) scored 225, 350 mg.] ▶L ♀C ▶? $

CROMOLYN—INHALED (Intal, Gastrocrom, ✦Nalcrom) Asthma: 2 to 4 puffs qid or 20 mg nebs qid. Prevention of exercise-induced bronchospasm: 2 puffs 10 to 15 min prior to exercise. Mastocytosis: Oral concentrate 200 mg PO qid for adults, 100 mg qid in children 2 to 12 yo. [Trade only: MDI 800 mcg/actuation, 112, 200/canister. Oral concentrate 100 mg/5 mL in 8 amps/foil pouch (Gastrocrom). Generic/Trade: Soln for nebs: 20 mg/2 mL.] ▶LK ♀B ▶? $$$

DORNASE ALFA (*Pulmozyme*) <u>Cystic fibrosis:</u> 2.5 mg nebulized daily to bid. [Trade only: Soln for inhalation: 1 mg/mL in 2.5 mL vials.] ▶L ♀B ▶? $$$$$

EPINEPHRINE RACEMIC (*S-2*, ✦*Vaponefrin*) <u>Severe croup:</u> 0.05 mL/kg/dose diluted to 3 mL w/NS. Max dose 0.5 mL. [Trade only: Soln for inhalation: 2.25% epinephrine in 15, 30 mL.] ▶Plasma ♀C ▶– $

IPRATROPIUM—INHALED (*Atrovent, Atrovent HFA*) 2 puffs qid, or one 500 mcg vial neb tid to qid. Contraindicated with soy or peanut allergy (Atrovent MDI only). [Trade only: Atrovent HFA MDI: 17 mcg/actuation, 200/canister. Generic/Trade: Soln for nebulization: 0.02% (500 mcg/vial) in unit dose vials.] ▶Lung ♀B ▶? $$$$

KETOTIFEN (✦*Zaditen*) Canada only. For age 6 mo to 3 yo: give 0.05 mg/kg PO bid. Age older than 3 yo: give 1 mg PO bid. [Generic/Trade: Tabs 1 mg. Syrup 1 mg/5 mL.] ▶L ♀C ▶– $$

THEOPHYLLINE (*Elixophyllin, Uniphyl, Theo-24, T-Phyl*, ✦*Theo-Dur, Theolair*) 5 to 13 mg/kg/day PO in divided doses. Max dose 900 mg/day. Peds dosing variable. [Generic/Trade: Elixir 80 mg/15 mL. Trade only: Caps: Theo-24: 100, 200, 300, 400 mg. T-Phyl: 12 Hr SR tabs 200 mg. Theolair: Tabs 125, 250 mg. Generic only: 12 Hr tabs 100, 200, 300, 450 mg, 12 Hr caps 125, 200, 300 mg.] ▶L ♀C ▶+ $

TIOTROPIUM (*Spiriva*) <u>COPD:</u> Handihaler: 18 mcg inhaled daily. [Trade only: Caps for oral inhalation 18 mcg. To be used with "Handihaler" device only. Packages of 5, 30, 90 caps with Handihaler device.] ▶K ♀C ▶– $$$$

TOXICOLOGY

ACETYLCYSTEINE (*N-acetylcysteine, Mucomyst, Acetadote*, ✦*Parvolex*) <u>Contrast nephropathy prophylaxis:</u> 600 mg PO bid on the day before and on the day of contrast. <u>Acetaminophen toxicity:</u> Mucomyst: Loading dose 140 mg/kg PO or NG, then 70 mg/kg q 4 h for 17 doses. May be mixed in water or soft drink diluted to a 5% soln. Acetadote (IV): Loading dose 150 mg/kg in 200 mL of D5W infused over 60 min; maintenance dose 50 mg/kg in 500 mL of D5W infused over 4 h followed by 100 mg/kg in 1000 mL of D5W infused over 16 h. [Generic/Trade: Soln 10%, 20%. Trade only: IV (Acetadote).] ▶L ♀B ▶? $$$$

CHARCOAL (*activated charcoal, Actidose-Aqua, CharcoAid, EZ-Char*, ✦*Charcodate*) 25 to 100 g (1 to 2 g/kg) PO or NG as soon as possible. May repeat q 1 to 4 h prn at doses equivalent to 12.5 g/h. When sorbitol is coadministered, use only with the first dose if repeated doses are to be given. [OTC/Generic/Trade: Powder 15, 30, 40, 120, 240 g. Soln 12.5 g/60 mL, 15 g/75 mL, 15 g/120 mL, 25 g/120 mL, 30 g/120 mL, 50 g/240 mL. Susp 15 g/120 mL, 25 g/120 mL, 30 g/150 mL, 50 g/240 mL. Granules 15 g/120 mL.] ▶Not absorbed ♀+ ▶+ $

DEFEROXAMINE (*Desferal*) <u>Chronic iron overload:</u> 500 to 1000 mg IM daily and 2 g IV infusion (no faster than 15 mg/kg/h) with each unit of blood or 1 to 2 g SC daily (20 to 40 mg/kg/day) over 8 to 24 h via continuous infusion pump. <u>Acute iron toxicity:</u> IV infusion up to 15 mg/kg/h (consult poison center). ▶K ♀C ▶? $$$$$

ANTIDOTES

Toxin	Antidote/Treatment	Toxin	Antidote/Treatment
acetaminophen	N-acetylcysteine	digoxin	dig immune Fab
TCAs	sodium bicarbonate	ethylene glycol	fomepizole
		heparin	protamine
arsenic, mercury	dimercaprol (BAL)	iron	deferoxamine
benzodiazepine	flumazenil	lead	BAL, EDTA, succimer
beta blockers	glucagon	methanol	fomepizole
calcium channel blockers	calcium chloride, glucagon	methemoglobin	methylene blue
		opioids/opiates	naloxone
cyanide	cyanide antidote kit, Cyanokit (hydroxo-cobalamin)	organophosphates	atropine+pralidoxime
		warfarin	vitamin K, FFP

FLUMAZENIL (*Romazicon*) <u>Benzodiazepine sedation reversal:</u> 0.2 mg IV over 15 sec, then 0.2 mg q 1 min prn up to 1 mg total dose. <u>Overdose reversal:</u> 0.2 mg IV over 30 sec, then 0.3 to 0.5 mg q 30 sec prn up to 3 mg total dose. Contraindicated in mixed drug OD or chronic benzodiazepine use. ▶LK ♀C ▶? $$$$

HYDROXOCOBALAMIN (*Cyanokit*) <u>Cyanide poisoning:</u> 5 g IV over 15 min; may repeat prn. ▶K ♀C ▶? $$$$$

IPECAC SYRUP 30 mL PO for adults, 15 mL age 1 to 12 yo. [OTC Generic only: Syrup 30 mL.] ▶Gut ♀C ▶? $

METHYLENE BLUE (*Urolene blue*) <u>Methemoglobinemia:</u> 1 to 2 mg/kg IV over 5 min. <u>Dysuria:</u> 65 to 130 mg PO tid after meals with liberal water. May turn urine/contact lenses blue. [Trade only: Tabs 65 mg.] ▶K ♀C ▶? $

PRALIDOXIME (*Protopam, 2-PAM*) <u>Organophosphate poisoning:</u> consult poison center: 1 to 2 g IV infusion over 15 to 30 min or slow IV injection over 5 min or longer (max rate 200 mg/min). May repeat dose after 1 h if muscle weakness persists. High dose regimen (unapproved): 2 g over 30 min, followed by 1 g/h for 48 h, then 1 g/h every 4 h until improved. Peds: 20 to 50 mg/kg/dose IV over 15 to 30 min. ▶K ♀C ▶? $$$$

SUCCIMER (*Chemet*) <u>Lead toxicity in children 1 yo or older:</u> Start 10 mg/kg PO or 350 mg/m2 q 8 h for 5 days, then reduce the frequency to q 12 h for 2 wks. [Trade only: Caps 100 mg.] ▶K ♀C ▶? $$$$$

UROLOGY

Benign Prostatic Hyperplasia

ALFUZOSIN (*UroXatral, ✦Xatral*) 10 mg PO daily after a meal. [Trade only: Tab extended-release 10 mg.] ▶KL ♀B ▶– $$$

DUTASTERIDE (*Avodart*) 0.5 mg PO daily. [Trade only: Caps 0.5 mg.] ▶L ♀X ▶– $$$$

FINASTERIDE (*Proscar, Propecia*) Proscar: 5 mg PO daily alone or in combination with doxazosin to reduce the risk of symptomatic progression of BPH. <u>Androgenetic alopecia in men:</u> Propecia: 1 mg PO daily. [Generic/Trade: Tabs 1 mg (Propecia), 5 mg (Proscar).] ▶L ♀X ▶– $$$

TAMSULOSIN (*Flomax*) 0.4 mg PO daily, 30 min after a meal. Maximum 0.8 mg/day. [Generic/Trade: Caps 0.4 mg.] ▶LK ♀B ▶– $$$$

Bladder Agents—Anticholinergics & Combinations

DARIFENACIN (*Enablex*) <u>Overactive bladder with symptoms of urinary urgency, frequency, and urge incontinence:</u> 7.5 mg PO daily. May increase to max dose 15 mg PO daily in 2 weeks. Max dose 7.5 mg PO daily with moderate liver impairment or when coadministered with potent CYP3A4 inhibitors (ketoconazole, itraconazole, ritonavir, nelfinavir, clarithromycin, and nefazodone). [Trade only: Tabs extended-release 7.5, 15 mg.] ▶LK ♀C ▶– $$$$

FESOTERODINE (*Toviaz*) <u>Overactive bladder:</u> 4 to 8 mg PO daily. [Trade only: Tabs extended-release 4, 8 mg.] ▶plasma ♀C ▶– $$$$

OXYBUTYNIN (*Ditropan, Ditropan XL, Gelnique, Oxytrol, ✦Oxybutyn, Uromax*) <u>Bladder instability:</u> 2.5 to 5 mg PO bid to tid, max 5 mg PO qid. Extended-release tabs: 5 to 10 mg PO daily, increase 5 mg/day q week to 30 mg/day. Oxytrol: 1 patch twice a week on abdomen, hips, or buttocks. Gelnique: Apply gel once daily to abdomen, upper arms/shoulders, or thighs. [Generic/Trade: Syrup 5 mg/5 mL. Tabs extended-release 5, 10, 15 mg. Trade only: Transdermal patch (Oxytrol) 3.9 mg/day. Gelnique 10% gel, 1 g unit dose.] ▶LK ♀B ▶? $

PROSED/DS (methenamine + phenyl salicylate + methylene blue + benzoic acid + hyoscyamine) <u>Bladder spasm:</u> 1 tab PO qid with liberal fluids. May turn urine/contact lenses blue. [Trade only: Tabs (methenamine 81.6 mg/phenyl salicylate 36.2 mg/methylene blue 10.8 mg/benzoic acid 9.0 mg/hyoscyamine sulfate 0.12 mg).] ▶KL ♀C ▶? $$

SOLIFENACIN (*VESIcare*) <u>Overactive bladder with symptoms of urinary urgency, frequency, or urge incontinence:</u> 5 mg PO daily. Max dose: 10 mg daily (5 mg daily if CrCl < 30 mL/min, moderate hepatic impairment, or concurrent ketoconazole or other potent CYP3A4 inhibitors). [Trade only: Tabs 5, 10 mg.] ▶LK ♀C ▶– $$$$

TOLTERODINE (*Detrol, Detrol LA, ✦Unidet*) <u>Overactive bladder:</u> 1 to 2 mg PO bid (Detrol) or 2 to 4 mg PO daily (Detrol LA). [Trade only: Tabs 1, 2 mg. Caps extended-release 2, 4 mg.] ▶L ♀C ▶– $$$$

TROSPIUM (*Sanctura, Sanctura XR, ✦Trosec*) <u>Overactive bladder with urge incontinence:</u> 20 mg PO bid; give 20 mg qhs if CrCl < 30 mL/min. If age 75 yo or older may taper down to 20 mg daily. Extended-release: 60 mg PO qam, 1 h before food. [Trade only: Tabs 20 mg, Caps extended-release 60 mg.] ▶LK ♀C ▶? $$$$

URISED (methenamine + phenyl salicylate + atropine + hyoscyamine + benzoic acid + methylene blue) <u>Dysuria:</u> 2 tabs PO qid. May turn urine/contact lenses blue. Don't use with sulfa. [Trade only: Tabs (methenamine 40.8 mg/phenyl salicylate 18.1 mg/atropine 0.03 mg/hyoscyamine 0.03 mg/4.5 mg benzoic acid/5.4 mg methylene blue).] ▶K ♀C ▶? $

UTA (methenamine + sodium phosphate + phenyl salicylate + methylene blue + hyoscyamine) <u>Bladder spasm:</u> 1 cap PO qid with liberal fluids. [Trade only: Caps (methenamine 120 mg/sodium phosphate 40.8 mg/phenyl salicylate 36 mg/methylene blue 10 mg/hyoscyamine 0.12 mg).] ▶KL ♀C ▶? $

UTIRA-C (methenamine + sodium phosphate + phenyl salicylate + methylene blue + hyoscyamine) Bladder spasm: 1 cap PO qid with liberal fluids. [Trade only: Tabs (methenamine 81.6 mg/sodium phosphate 40.8 mg/phenyl salicylate 36.2 mg/methylene blue 10.8 mg/hyoscyamine 0.12 mg).] ▶KL ♀C ▶? $$

Bladder Agents—Other

BETHANECHOL (*Urecholine, Duvoid, ✦Myotonachol*) Urinary retention: 10 to 50 mg PO tid-qid. [Generic/Trade: Tabs 5, 10, 25, 50 mg.] ▶L ♀C ▶? $$$$

PHENAZOPYRIDINE (*Pyridium, Azo-Standard, Urogesic, Prodium, Pyridiate, Urodol, Baridium, UTI Relief, ✦Phenazo*) Dysuria: 200 mg PO tid for 2 days. May turn urine/contact lenses orange. [OTC Generic/Trade: Tabs 95, 97.2 mg. Rx Generic/Trade: Tabs 100, 200 mg.] ▶K ♀B ▶? $

Erectile Dysfunction

ALPROSTADIL (*Muse, Caverject, Caverject Impulse, Edex, Prostin VR Pediatric, prostaglandin E1, ✦Prostin VR*) 1 intraurethral pellet (Muse) or intracavernosal injection (Caverject, Edex) at lowest dose that will produce erection. Onset of effect is 5 to 20 min. [Trade only: Syringe system (Edex) 10, 20, 40 mcg. (Caverject) 5, 10, 20, 40 mcg. (Caverject Impulse) 10, 20 mcg. Pellet (Muse) 125, 250, 500, 1000 mcg. Intracorporeal injection of locally compounded combination agents (many variations): "Bi-mix" can be 30 mg/mL papaverine + 0.5 to 1 mg/mL phentolamine, or 30 mg/mL papaverine + 20 mcg/mL alprostadil in 10 mL vials. "Tri-mix" can be 30 mg/mL papaverine + 1 mg/mL phentolamine + 10 mcg/mL alprostadil in 5, 10, or 20 mL vials.] ▶L ♀- ▶- $$$$

SILDENAFIL (*Viagra*) Start 50 mg PO 0.5 to 4 h prior to intercourse. Max 1 dose/day. Usual effective range 25 to 100 mg. Start at 25 mg if for age 65 yo or older or liver/renal impairment. Contraindicated with nitrates. [Trade only (Viagra): Tabs 25, 50, 100 mg. Unscored tab but can be cut in half.] ▶LK ♀B ▶- $$$$

TADALAFIL (*Cialis*) 2.5 to 5 mg PO daily without regard to timing of sexual activity. As needed dosing: Start 10 mg PO at least 30 to 45 min prn prior to sexual activity. May increase to 20 mg or decrease to 5 mg prn. Max 1 dose/day. Start 5 mg (max 1 dose/day) if CrCl 31 to 50 mL/min. Max 5 mg/d if CrCl < 30 mL/min on dialysis. Max 10 mg/day if mild to moderate hepatic impairment; avoid in severe hepatic impairment. Max 10 mg once in 72 h if concurrent potent CYP3A4 inhibitors. Contraindicated with nitrates and alpha-blockers (except tamsulosin 0.4 mg daily). Not FDA approved for women. [Trade only (Cialis): Tabs 2.5, 5, 10, 20 mg.] ▶L ♀B ▶- $$$$

VARDENAFIL (*Levitra*) Start 10 mg PO 1 h before sexual activity. Usual effective dose range 5 to 20 mg. Max 1 dose/day. Use lower dose (5 mg) if age 65 yo or older or moderate hepatic impairment (max 10 mg). Contraindicated with nitrates and alpha-blockers. Not FDA approved in women. [Trade only: Tabs 2.5, 5, 10, 20 mg.] ▶LK ♀B ▶- $$$$

YOHIMBINE (*Yocon, Yohimex*)   5.4 mg PO tid. Not FDA approved. [Generic/Trade: Tabs 5.4 mg.]   ▶L ♀– ▶– $

Nephrolithiasis

CITRATE (*Polycitra-K, Urocit-K, Bicitra, Oracit, Polycitra, Polycitra-LC*) <u>Urinary alkalinization:</u> 1 packet in water/juice PO tid to qid. [Generic/Trade: Polycitra-K packet 3300 mg potassium citrate/ea, Polycitra-K oral soln (1100 mg potassium citrate/5 mL, 480 mL). Oracit oral soln (490 mg sodium citrate/5 mL, 15, 30, 480 mL). Bicitra oral soln (500 mg sodium citrate/5 mL, 480 mL). Urocit-K wax (potassium citrate) Tabs 5, 10 mEq. Polycitra-LC oral soln (550 mg potassium citrate/500 mg sodium citrate per 5 mL, 480 mL). Polycitra oral syrup (550 mg potassium citrate/500 mg sodium citrate per 5 mL, 480 mL.]   ▶K ♀C ▶? $$$

INDEX

To facilitate speed of use, index entries are shown with page number and approximate position on the page ("t" is top; "m" is middle; "b" is bottom). Although the PDA edition of the *Tarascon Pocket Pharmacopoeia* contains more than 5000 drug names, it is physically impossible to include all in pocket-sized manuals. Therefore, rarely used or specialized drugs appear in the PDA only (noted as "PDA" in the index) or in both the PDA and Deluxe edition (noted as "D" in the index).

165
Index

t = top of page
m = middle of page
b = bottom of page
D,PDA = see page 163

166
Index

t = top of page
m = middle of page
b = bottom of page
D,PDA = see page 163

167
Index

t = top of page
m = middle of page
b = bottom of page
D,PDA = see page 163

169
Index
t = top of page
m = middle of page
b = bottom of page
D,PDA = see page 163

170
Index

t = top of page
m = middle of page
b = bottom of page
D,PDA = see page 163

171
Index
t = top of page
m = middle of page
b = bottom of page
D,PDA = see page 163

176
Index
t = top of page
m = middle of page
b = bottom of page
D,PDA = see page 163

179
Index
t = top of page
m = middle of page
b = bottom of page
D,PDA = see page 163

180
Index

t = top of page
m = middle of page
b = bottom of page
D,PDA = see page 163

184
Index

t = top of page
m = middle of page
b = bottom of page
D,PDA = see page 163

185
Index

t = top of page
m = middle of page
b = bottom of page
D,PDA = see page 163

186
Index

t = top of page
m = middle of page
b = bottom of page
D,PDA = see page 163

187
Index

t = top of page
m = middle of page
b = bottom of page
D,PDA = see page 163

189
Index

t = top of page
m = middle of page
b = bottom of page
D,PDA = see page 163

APPENDIX

ADULT EMERGENCY DRUGS (selected)

ALLERGY	diphenhydramine (*Benadryl*): 50 mg IV/IM. epinephrine: 0.1–0.5 mg IM (1:1000 solution), may repeat after 20 minutes. methylprednisolone (*Solu-Medrol*): 125 mg IV/IM.
HYPERTENSION	esmolol (*Brevibloc*): 500 mcg/kg IV over 1 minute, then titrate 50–200 mcg/kg/min. fenoldopam (*Corlopam*): Start 0.1 mcg/kg/min, titrate up to 1.6 mcg/kg/min. labetalol (*Normodyne*): Start 20 mg slow IV, then 40–80 mg IV q10 min prn up to 300 mg total cumulative dose. nitroglycerin (*Tridil*): Start 10–20 mcg/min IV infusion, then titrate prn up to 100 mcg/min. nitroprusside (*Nipride*): Start 0.3 mcg/kg/min IV infusion, then titrate prn up to 10 mcg/kg/min.
DYSRHYTHMIAS / ARREST	adenosine (*Adenocard*): PSVT (not A-fib): 6 mg rapid IV & flush, preferably through a central line or proximal IV. If no response after 1–2 minutes, then 12 mg. A third dose of 12 mg may be given prn. amiodarone (*Cordarone, Pacerone*): V-fib or pulseless V-tach: 300 mg IV/IO; may repeat 150 mg just once. Life-threatening ventricular arrhythmia: Load 150 mg IV over 10 min, then 1 mg/min × 6 h, then 0.5 mg/min × 18 h. atropine: 0.5 mg IV, repeat prn to maximum of 3 mg. diltiazem (*Cardizem*): Rapid A-fib: bolus 0.25 mg/kg or 20 mg IV over 2 min. May repeat 0.35 mg/kg or 25 mg 15 min after 1st dose. Infusion 5–15 mg/h. epinephrine: 1 mg IV/IO q 3–5 minutes for cardiac arrest. [1:10,000 solution]. lidocaine (*Xylocaine*): Load 1 mg/kg IV, then 0.5 mg/kg q 8–10 min prn to max 3 mg/kg. Maintenance 2 g in 250 mL D5W (8 mg/mL) at 1–4 mg/min drip (7–30 mL/h).
PRESSORS	dobutamine (*Dobutrex*): 2–20 mcg/kg/min. 70 kg: 5 mcg/kg/min with 1 mg/mL concentration (eg, 250 mg in 250 mL D5W) = 21 mL/h. dopamine (*Intropin*): Pressor: Start at 5 mcg/kg/min, increase prn by 5–10 mcg/kg/min increments at 10 min intervals, max 50 mcg/kg/min. 70 kg: 5 mcg/kg/min with 1600 mcg/mL concentration (eg, 400 mg in 250 mL D5W) = 13 mL/h. Doses in mcg/kg/min: 2–4 = (traditional renal dose, apparently ineffective) dopaminergic receptors; 5–10 = (cardiac dose) dopaminergic and beta1 receptors; >10 = dopaminergic, beta1, and alpha1 receptors. norepinephrine (*Levophed*): 4 mg in 500 mL D5W (8 mg/mL) at 2–4 mcg/min. 22.5 mL/h = 3 mcg/min. phenylephrine (*Neo-Synephrine*): Infusion for hypotension: 20 mg in 250 mL D5W (80 mcg/mL) at 40–180 mcg/min (35–160 mL/h).
INTUBATION	etomidate (*Amidate*): 0.3 mg/kg IV. methohexital (*Brevital*): 1–1.5 mg/kg IV. propofol (*Diprivan*): 2.0–2.5 mg/kg IV. rocuronium (*Zemuron*): 0.6–1.2 mg/kg IV. succinylcholine (*Anectine*): 1 mg/kg IV. Peds (<5 yo): 2 mg/kg IV. thiopental (*Pentothal*): 3–5 mg/kg IV.
SEIZURES	diazepam (*Valium*): 5–10 mg IV, or 0.2–0.5 mg/kg rectal gel up to 20 mg PR. fosphenytoin (*Cerebyx*): Load 15–20 "phenytoin equivalents" per kg either IM, or IV no faster than 100–150 mg/min. lorazepam (*Ativan*): 0.05–0.15 mg/kg up to 3–4 mg IV/IM. phenobarbital: 200–600 mg IV at rate ≤60 mg/min; titrate prn up to 20 mg/kg. phenytoin (*Dilantin*): 15–20 mg/kg up to 1000 mg IV no faster than 50 mg/min.

CARDIAC DYSRHYTHMIA PROTOCOLS (for adults and adolescents)

Chest compressions ~100/min. Ventilations 8–10/min if intubated; otherwise 30:2 compression/ventilation ratio. Drugs that can be administered down ET tube (use 2–2.5 × usual dose): epinephrine, atropine, lidocaine, naloxone, vasopressin*.

V-Fib, Pulseless V-Tach
Airway, oxygen, CPR until defibrillator ready
Defibrillate 360 J (old monophasic), 120–200 J (biphasic), or with AED
Resume CPR × 2 minutes (5 cycles)
Repeat defibrillation if no response
Vasopressor during CPR:
- Epinephrine 1 mg IV/IO q 3–5 minutes, or
- Vasopressin* 40 units IV to replace 1st or 2nd dose of epinephrine
Rhythm/pulse check every ~2 minutes
Consider antiarrhythmic during CPR:
- Amiodarone 300 mg IV/IO; may repeat 150 mg just once
- Lidocaine 1.0–1.5 mg/kg IV/IO, then repeat 0.5–0.75 mg/kg to max 3 doses or 3 mg/kg
- Magnesium sulfate 1–2 g IV/IO if suspect torsades de pointes

Asystole or Pulseless Electrical Activity (PEA)
Airway, oxygen, CPR
Vasopressor (when IV/IO access):
- Epinephrine 1 mg IV/IO q3–5 minutes, or
- Vasopressin* 40 units IV/IO to replace 1st or 2nd dose of epinephrine
Consider atropine 1 mg IV/IO for asystole or slow PEA. Repeat q 3–5 min up to 3 doses.
Rhythm/pulse check every ~2 minutes
Consider 6 H's: hypovolemia, hypoxia, H+ acidosis, hyper / hypokalemia, hypoglycemia, hypothermia
Consider 5 T's: Toxins, tamponade-cardiac, tension pneumothorax, thrombosis (coronary or pulmonary), trauma

Bradycardia, <60 bpm and Inadequate Perfusion
Airway, oxygen, IV
Prepare for transcutaneous pacing; don't delay if advanced heart block
Consider atropine 0.5 mg IV; may repeat q 3–5 min to max 3 mg
Consider epinephrine (2–10 mcg/min) or dopamine (2–10 mcg/kg/min)
Prepare for transvenous pacing

Tachycardia with Pulses
Airway, oxygen, IV
If unstable and heart rate >150 bpm, then synchronized cardioversion
If stable narrow-QRS (<120 ms):
- Regular: Attempt vagal maneuvers. If no success, adenosine 6 mg IV, then 12 mg prn (may repeat × 1)
- Irregular: Control rate with diltiazem or beta blocker (caution in CHF or severe obstructive pulmonary disease).
If stable wide-QRS (>120 ms):
- Regular and suspect V-tach: Amiodarone 150 mg IV over 10 min; repeat prn to max 2.2 g/24 h. Prepare for elective synchronized cardioversion.
- Regular and suspect SVT with aberrancy: adenosine as per narrow-QRS above.
- Irregular and A-fib: Control rate with diltiazem or beta blocker (caution in CHF/ severe obstructive pulmonary disease).
- Irregular and A-fib with pre-excitation (WPW): Avoid AV nodal blocking agents; consider amiodarone 150 mg IV over 10 minutes.
- Irregular and torsades de pointes: magnesium 1–2 g IV load over 5–60 minutes, then infusion.

bpm=beats per minute; CPR=cardiopulmonary resuscitation; ET=endotracheal; IO=intraosseous; J=Joules; ms=milliseconds; WPW=Wolff-Parkinson-White. Sources: *Circulation* 2005; 112, suppl IV; *NEJM* 2008;359:21-30 (demonstrated no benefit over epinephrine and worse long-term neurological outcomes).

ANTIVIRAL DRUGS FOR INFLUENZA A	Treatment* (Duration of 5 days)	Prevention (Duration of 10 days post-exposure)
OSELTAMIVIR (*Tamiflu*)		
Adults and adolescents age 13 years and older		
	75 mg PO bid	75 mg PO once daily
Children, 1 year of age and older†		
Body weight ≤15 kg	30 mg PO bid	30 mg PO once daily
Body weight >15 to 23 kg	45 mg PO bid	45 mg PO once daily
Body weight >23 to 40 kg	60 mg PO bid	60 mg PO once daily
Body weight >40 kg	75 mg PO bid	75 mg PO once daily
Infants, newborn to 11 months of age†, ‡		
Age 3 to 11 months old	3 mg/kg/dose PO bid	3 mg/kg/dose PO once daily
Age younger than 3 months old¶	3 mg/kg/dose PO bid	Not for routine prophylaxis in infants <3 mo
ZANAMIVIR (*Relenza*)§		
Adults and children (age 7 years and older for treatment, age 5 years and older for prophylaxis)		
	10 mg (two 5-mg inhalations) bid	10 mg (two 5-mg inhalations) once daily

Adapted from http://www.cdc.gov/h1n1flu/recommendations.htm

*Start treatment as soon as possible; benefit is greatest when started within 2 days of symptom onset. Hospitalized patients with severe infection might require treatment for longer than 5 days.

†A dosing syringe with graduations of 30, 45, and 60 mg is provided with *Tamiflu* oral suspension. The 75 mg dose can be measured by combining 30 mg and 45 mg. For infants less than 1 year old, a different oral syringe must be used to measure the dose. The concentration of oseltamivir differs between commercial *Tamiflu* suspension (12 mg/mL) and pharmacist-compounded suspension (15 mg/mL). Capsules can be opened and mixed with sweetened fluids to mask bitter taste. Make sure units of measure on dosing instructions match dosing device provided.

‡Oseltamivir is not FDA-approved for use in infants less than 1 year old. An Emergency Use Authorization for use in infants expired in June 2010.

¶This dose is not intended for premature infants. Immature renal function may lead to slow clearance and high concentrations of oseltamivir in this age group.

§Zanamivir should not be used by patients with underlying pulmonary disease. Do not attempt to use *Relenza* in a nebulizer or ventilator; lactose in the formulation may cause the device to malfunction.